D1557822

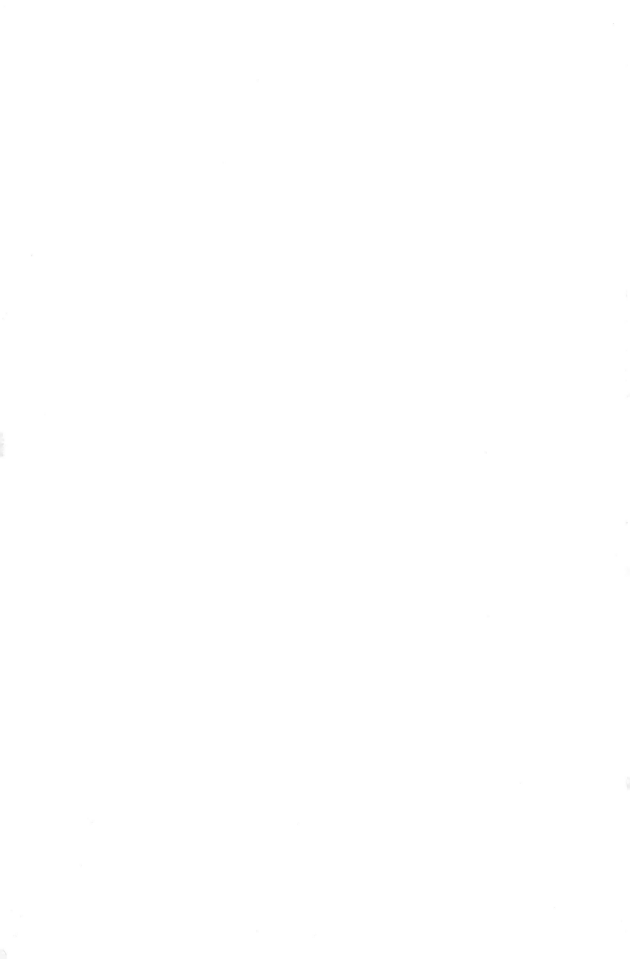

Contemporary Endoscopic Spine Surgery

(Volume 2)

Lumbar Spine

Edited by

Kai-Uwe Lewandrowski
Center For Advanced Spine Care
Tucson
Arizona
USA

Jorge Felipe Ramírez León
Fundación Universitaria Sanitas
Clínica Reina Sofía – Clínica Colsanitas
Centro de Columna – Cirugía Mínima Invasiva
Bogotá, D.C.
Colombia

Anthony Yeung
University of New Mexico
School of Medicine
Albuquerque
New Mexico

Hyeun-Sung Kim
Department of Neurosurgery
Nanoori Gangnam Hospital
Seoul
Republic of Korea

Xifeng Zhang
Department of Orthopedics
First Medical Center
PLA General Hospital
Beijing 100853
China

Gun Choi
Neurosurgeon and Minimally Invasive Spine Surgeon
President Pohang Wooridul Hospital
South Korea

Stefan Hellinger
Department of Orthopedic Surgery
Arabellaklinik
Munich
Germany

Álvaro Dowling
Endoscopic Spine Clinic
Santiago
Chile

Contemporary Endoscopic Spine Surgery

(Volume 2)

Lumbar Spine

Editors: Kai-Uwe Lewandrowski, Jorge Felipe Ramírez León, Anthony Yeung,

Hyeun-Sung Kim, Xifeng Zhang, Gun Choi, Stefan Hellinger and Álvaro Dowling

ISBN (Online): 978-981-5051-51-3

ISBN (Print): 978-981-5051-52-0

ISBN (Paperback): 978-981-5051-53-7

©2022, Bentham Books imprint.

Published by Bentham Science Publishers Pte. Ltd. Singapore. All Rights Reserved.

need for a court order if at any point you breach any terms of this License Agreement. In no event will any delay or failure by Bentham Science Publishers in enforcing your compliance with this License Agreement constitute a waiver of any of its rights.

3. You acknowledge that you have read this License Agreement, and agree to be bound by its terms and conditions. To the extent that any other terms and conditions presented on any website of Bentham Science Publishers conflict with, or are inconsistent with, the terms and conditions set out in this License Agreement, you acknowledge that the terms and conditions set out in this License Agreement shall prevail.

Bentham Science Publishers Pte. Ltd.
80 Robinson Road #02-00
Singapore 068898
Singapore
Email: subscriptions@benthamscience.net

BENTHAM SCIENCE

ENDORSEMENTS

ISASS

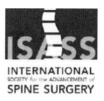

The International Society for the Advancement of Spine Surgery (ISASS; formerly The Spine Arthroplasty Society) has its roots in motion preservation as an alternative to fusion. Since then, it has worked to achieve its mission of acting as a global, scientific and educational society with a surgeon-centered focus. ISASS was organized to provide an independent venue to discuss and address the issues involved with all aspects of basic and clinical science of motion preservation, stabilization, innovative technologies, MIS procedures, biologics, and other fundamental topics to restore and improve motion and function of the spine. ISASS has a robust international membership of orthopedic and neurosurgery spine surgeons and scientists. ISASS is dedicated to advancing evolutionary and innovative spinal techniques and procedures such as endoscopic spine surgery. Every editor of Contemporary Endoscopic Spine Surgery represents ISASS as a member, author, reviewer, or editor of its quarterly circulation – The International Journal of Spine Surgery (IJSS). The contributors of *Contemporary Endoscopic Spinal Surgery* have succeeded in compiling an exhaustive and up-to-date reference text. It is an example of our society's mission pursuit of surgeon education and scientific study. It is my pleasure to endorse this comprehensive text on behalf of ISASS.

Domagoj Coric
President
International Society for the Advancement of Spine Surgery (ISASS)
Illinois
USA

SBC

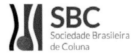

Founded on October 12, 1994, the Brazilian Spine Society (Sociedade Brasileira de Coluna - SBC) is a scientific, non-profit organization whose primary objective is the advancement of spine surgery through basic research and clinical study in orthopedics and neurosurgery. SBC is actively engaged in the accreditation and continued education of spine surgeons in Brazil. It prides itself on bringing the latest high-grade scientific evidence on novel technological advances and therapies to its professional members. SBC pursues this mission with its quarterly circulation Coluna/ Columna and its online courses, including Introduction to Endoscopy. The authors and editors of Contemporary Endoscopic Spine Surgery have put forward a comprehensive reference text essential to SBC's core curriculum of teaching spinal endoscopy to the next generation of surgeons. The presented clinical protocols for the endoscopic treatment of cervical and lumbar spine conditions are vetted and validated by peer-reviewed articles published by its contributors. It is my pleasure to endorse Contemporary Endoscopic Spine Surgery on behalf of the Brazilian Spine Society.

Cristiano Magalhães Menezes
President of the Brazilian Spine Society (Sociedade Brasileira de Coluna - SBC)
São Paulo
Brazil

MISS OF COA

The Minimally Invasive Spine Surgery (MISS) of Chinese Orthopaedic Association (COA) was founded in 2003, which is one of the most special subsidiary societies of Chinese Medical Association, aiming to promote and develop minimally invasive orthopedics especially spine surgeries in China.

The MISS society organizes global discussions and encourages our members to participate international efforts and cooperation to improve surgeon education. With this mission in mind, it is my pleasure to endorse Contemporary Endoscopic Spine Surgery on behalf of the MISS of COA. Many international editors and contributors are from China, who have made great efforts, contributions and dedications to this book. They share with and update readers all over the world about the latest endoscopic spinal surgery techniques. I am confident that *Contemporary Endoscopic Spinal Surgery* can be a textbook for spine surgeons. It should be used as medical school advanced lessons materials for continuing education courses. In sum, it is my pleasure and honor to support it on behalf of the MISS of COA.

Huilin Yang
Chairman of MISS of COA
Professor & Chairman of Orthopedic Department
The First Affiliated Hospital of Soochow University
Suzhou
China

SICCMI

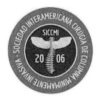

SICCMI (Sociedad Interamericana De Cirugia De Columna Minimamente Invasive) was founded in 2006 with similar objectives pursued by the editors of Contemporary Endoscopic Spine Surgery: the advancement and mainstreaming of minimally invasive spine surgery (MIS). SICMII members joined to implement MIS in all countries of South America, the Caribbean, Central America, and North America. Endoscopic surgery is performed by many of its key opinion leaders at the highest level, some of which have contributed to this multi-volume text. Four of the editors are active SICCMI members in leadership positions. The book contents are exhaustive and comprehensive, encompassing topics of the cervical and lumbar spine and advanced technology applications. Contemporary Endoscopic Spine Surgery will serve as SICCMI's core curriculum and course material for endoscopic surgery of the spine. It is my pleasure to endorse it on behalf of SICCMI.

President of SICCMI
Manuel Rodriguez
President-Elect of SICCMI, Department of Neurosurgery
ABC Medical Center
Ciudad de México, Mexico

SBMT

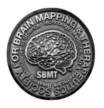

As a nonprofit organization, the Society for Brain Mapping and Therapeutics (SBMT) focuses on improving patient care by translating new technologies into life-saving diagnostic and therapeutic procedures. Contemporary Endoscopic Spine Surgery is a prime example of achieving excellence in education and scientific discovery. Authors and editors from around the globe came together to present the reader with the most up-to-date endoscopic spine surgery protocols and their supporting clinical evidence. SBMT has an active spine section led by productive innovator surgeons – some of which have demonstrated their leadership with their editorial contributions to *Contemporary Endoscopic Spinal Surgery*. The editors have embraced multidisciplinary collaborations across many cultural and geographic barriers. Their effort represents one of the core principles of SBMT's mission: to identify and bridge gaps in modern patient care with technological advances. It is my pleasure to endorse *Contemporary Endoscopic Spinal Surgery* on behalf of SBMT.

Babak Kateb
Founding Chairman of the Board of Directors
CEO and Scientific Director of SBMT
Californias
USA

SILACO

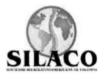

SILICO (Sociedad Ibero Latinoamericana de Columna) had its beginnings in the meetings of the Scoliosis Research Society with the first Hispano-American Congress held in 1991 in Buenos Aires Argentina. Since then, it has morphed into an organization that promotes the study of treatments and prevention of spinal conditions by bringing together spine care professionals from all subspecialties. The scientific activities of our biannual Ibero-Latin American Congress are focused on the promotion of surgeon education to the highest academic standards via international relationships between members from the Americas, Spain and Portugal.

Contemporary Endoscopic Spine Surgery resembles such a collaborative effort where authors worldwide have come together to update the reader on the latest endoscopic spinal surgery techniques.

SILACO has incorporated Contemporary Endoscopic Spine Surgery into its core curriculum and plans on using it as course material for its continuing education courses. It is my pleasure to endorse it on behalf of SILACO.

Jaime Moyano
President of SILACO
Editor Revista De Sociedad Ecuatoriana De Ortopedia y Traumatología
de la Sociedad Ecuatoriana De Ortopedia Y Traumatología
Quito, Ecuador

SOMEEC

SOMEEC- Sociedad Mexicana de Endoscopia de Columna- is Mexico's prime organization uniting spine surgeons with a diverse training background having a fundamental interest in endoscopic surgery. SOMEEC organizes annual meetings where member surgeons and international faculty update each other on their latest clinical research to promote spine care *via* endoscopic spinal surgery technique. Two of the senior lead editors of *Contemporary Endoscopic Spinal Surgery* have been active international supporters of SOMEEC. I am pleased to endorse their latest three-volume reference text, which will become an integral centerpiece of SOMEEC's continuing medical educational programs.

Cecilio Quinones
Past President of the Sociedad Mexicana de Endoscopia de Columnas

KOSESS

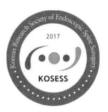

The Korean Research Society of Endoscopic Spine Surgery (KOSESS) was established in 2017. KOSESS was founded to bring endoscopic spine surgeons in the Republic of Korea together to advance the subspecialty of endoscopic spine surgery with high-quality clinical research. It is reflected in *Contemporary Endoscopic Spine Surgery* by the numerous contributions of Korean authors. It is *Contemporary Endoscopic Spine Surgery*. It is my pleasure to endorse it on behalf of KOSESS.

Hyeun-Sung Kim (Harrison Kim)
President of the Korean Research Society of the Endoscopic Spine Society
(KOSESS)
Seoul

Republic of Korea

KOMISS

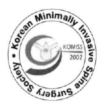

Since its establishment in 2002, the *Korean Minimally Invasive Spinal Surgery Society* (KOMISS) has had a leading role in developing new clinically applicable technologies to advance patient care with less invasive yet more effective therapies. The superiority of minimally invasive spine surgery in Korea is demonstrated by its competitiveness on the world stage at the highest academic level. It is reflected in *Contemporary Endoscopic Spine Surgery* by the numerous Korean authors who have contributed to this timely reference text with their groundbreaking clinical research on endoscopic spine surgery. I am proud of their accomplishments and want to congratulate them on acting as KOMISS ambassadors by carrying the message of Korean excellence in minimally invasive spinal surgery the world over within *Contemporary Endoscopic Spine Surgery*. It is my pleasure to endorse it on behalf of KOMISS.

Dae Hyun Kim
President of KOMISS
Seoul
Republic of Korea

NATIONAL ACADEMY OF MEDICINE OF COLOMBIA

After reviewing the table of content and some representative chapters, I am happy to inform you that the Board of Directors of the National Academy of Medicine of Colombia grants academic endorsement of your book series entitled Contemporary Endoscopy Spine Surgery. Kai-Uwe Lewandrowski, Jorge Felipe Ramírez, and Anthony Yeung produced a text of great interest and scientific impact.

On behalf of the National Academy of Medicine, I would like to express my admiration and respect for your dedication to scientific research that led to this great work's culmination. It meets the high standards required by our National Academy to support such a production spearheaded by one of our most esteemed members - Dr. Jorge Felipe Ramírez.

Gustavo Landazabal Bernal
General Secretary
National Academy of Medicine of Colombia
Bogota, Colombia

IITS

International Intradiscal Therapy Society

The International Intradiscal Therapy Society (IITS) was founded in 1987, initially headquartered in Belgium, Wisconsin, and led by Dr. Eugene Nordby, the first Executive Director of IITS. Members were primarily orthopaedic surgeons, anesthesiologists, radiologists, and rheumatologists dedicated to the treatment, research, and education involving The FDA-approved and validated level I studies that supported intradiscal spinal therapies.

From 2013-2017, the society began operating under International Intradiscal and Transforaminal Therapy Society (IITTSS) to reflect the advancements in endoscopic spine surgery augmenting Intradiscal therapy. The organization wanted to include and reflect the state-of-the-art evolution in intradiscal therapy with advances by intradiscal visualization of pain generators through the endoscope. However, the society reverted to IITS.

IITS now sponsors workshops on intradiscal therapy in conjunction with other International societies when it lost its original pharma support. IITS disseminates a newsletter to provide its membership, other healthcare professionals, and the general public information on the safest and cost-effective techniques to treat conditions such as herniated nucleus pulposus and other intradiscal spinal disorders.

IITS is a 501C3 non-profit organization whose focus is on intradiscal therapy aided by the endoscope as the least invasive, visually-guided treatment for discogenic pain, including extra-discal and complex foraminal decompression and stabilization procedures. The disc has been validated as the primary initial source of common back pain.

Two of the senior lead editors of Contemporary Endoscopic Spinal Surgery have been in active leadership roles in International Spine Organizations as consultants, full and associate professors, and directors. I am pleased to endorse their latest three-volume reference text, which will become integral to IITS' ongoing course programs.

Anthony Yeung
Executive Director of IITS
Desert Institute for Spine Care
Phoenix, Arizona
USA

SLAOT

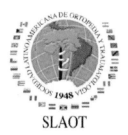

SLAOT

The Sociedad Latinoamericana de Ortopedia y Traumatologia (SLAOT)/ Latin American Society of Orthopaedics and Traumatology is a non-profit, autonomous, scientific organization of orthopaedic surgeons and orthopaedic care professionals. SLAOT has an organization structure that brings together professionals with a diverse scientific interest. It promotes continuous professional development and education at the highest level. *Contemporary Endoscopic Spine Surgery* is of interest to SLAOT because of its illustrative use of cutting-edge technology and discussion of validated clinical endoscopic spinal surgery protocols. It is my pleasure to endorse *Contemporary Endoscopic Spine Surgery* on behalf of SLAOT.

Horacio Caviglia
President of SLAOT FEDERACION
USA

CONTENTS

PREFACE

Nowadays, lumbar spinal endoscopy is well accepted. Not too long ago, its critics scrutinized it for lack of sufficient high-grade clinical evidence to endorse the implementation of endoscopic spinal surgery protocols to treat the common painful conditions of the lumbar spine. Traditionally trained spine surgeons still heavily rely on image-based medical necessity criteria for surgical intervention. These include stenosis, deformity, and instability. In essence, endoscopic spinal surgery replaces these established open lumbar spinal surgery protocols with more targeted miniaturized surgeries that largely ignore these traditional image-based criteria when establishing the indication for surgery. Instead, it focuses on treating validated pain generators, many of which escape detection by conventional advanced imaging studies such as the magnetic resonance image (MRI) scan. It is undeniable even to the untrained bystander that this amounts to a culture clash.

Contemporary Endoscopic Spine Surgery: Lumbar Spine's editors are internationally renowned key opinion leaders with decades of experience in endoscopic spinal surgery. They have come together to develop a multi-authored and clinically focused medical monograph to give the reader a most up-to-date review of modern lumbar spinal endoscopic surgeries. Moreover, they intended to disperse the myth of endoscopic lumbar spine surgery being experimental - a procedure that can only be consistently be mastered by the talented few. Therefore, the editors asked the contributing authors to illustrate their results with the endoscopic lumbar surgery in the context of the peer-reviewed literature by thoroughly discussing the available high-grade clinical evidence. The editors have authored many of these landmark articles that pushed the envelope of clinical research far beyond the initial level of personal opinion and case series reports. They went on to validate them with sophisticated statistical analysis of multi-arm clinical studies.

The publication is intended for Orthopedic Spine & Neurosurgeons interested in treating common painful conditions including herniated disc, stenosis, tumor, and infection with minimally invasive endoscopic techniques. The selection of chapters was based on contemporary trends in lumbar endoscopic spinal surgery. For this purpose, a wide array of highly timely and clinically relevant topics have been assembled based on historical and anatomical considerations. They range from the review of modern transforaminal and interlaminar decompression methods, their hybridized versions, the mobile outside-in approach for far-migrated disc herniations, the over-the-top and contralateral decompression techniques, endoscopic treatment of facet cysts, visualized rhizotomy procedures of painful facet disease, and other denervation techniques of the sinuvertebral- and basivertebral nerve, the application of endoscopic procedures in the elderly, to the illustrative discussion of challenging endoscopic indications and endoscopic and endoscopically assisted fusions. The editors identified these less costly yet safe endoscopic treatments for the lumbar spine's common painful degenerative conditions in response to patients' demand for less burdensome and less risky therapies with a shorter time to recovery and return to work. Contemporary Endoscopic Spine Surgery: Lumbar Spine was written with these goals in mind. The editors hope that the readers will find it an informative knowledge resource they will continue to revert to when implementing a lumbar endoscopic spinal surgery program in their practice setting.

Kai-Uwe Lewandrowski
Center For Advanced Spine Care
Tucson
Arizona
USA

Jorge Felipe Ramírez León
Fundación Universitaria Sanitas
Clínica Reina Sofía – Clínica Colsanitas
Centro de Columna – Cirugía Mínima Invasiva
Bogotá, D.C.
Colombia

Anthony Yeung
University of New Mexico
School of Medicine
Albuquerque
New Mexico

Hyeun-Sung Kim
Department of Neurosurgery
Nanoori Gangnam Hospital
Seoul
Republic of Korea

Xifeng Zhang
Department of Orthopedics
First Medical Center
PLA General Hospital
Beijing 100853
China

Gun Choi
Neurosurgeon and Minimally Invasive Spine Surgeon
President Pohang Wooridul Hospital
South Korea

Stefan Hellinger
Department of Orthopedic Surgery
Arabellaklinik
Munich
Germany

Álvaro Dowling
Endoscopic Spine Clinic
Chile

List of Contributors

Anthony Yeung	University of New Mexico School of Medicine, Albuquerque, New Mexico Desert Institute for Spine Care, Phoenix, AZ, USA
An Sixing	Department of orthopedics, First Medical Center, PLA General Hospital, Beijing, 100853, China
Álvaro Dowling	Endoscopic Spine Clinic, Santiago, Chile Department of Orthopaedic Surgery, USP, Ribeirão Preto, Brazil
Bu Rongqiang	Department of Orthopedics, First Medical Center, PLA General Hospital, Beijing 100853, China
Carolina Ramírez Martínez	Minimally Invasive Spine Center for Latinamerican Endoscopic Spine Surgeons, LESS Invasiva Academy, Bogotá, D.C. Colombia, USA
Cong Qiang	Department of Orthopedics Shenyang, Department of orthopedics, Shenyang 242 Hospital, Shenyang 110034, China
Friedrich Tieber	Am Webereck 6 1/2 - 86157 Augsburg, Germany
Gabriel Oswaldo Alonso Cuéllar	Minimally Invasive Spine Center for Latinamerican Endoscopic Spine Surgeons, LESS Invasiva Academy, Bogotá, D.C. Colombia, USA
Harshavardhan Dilip Raorane	Department of Neurosurgery, Nanoori Hospital, Gangnam, South Korea
Hyeun Sung Kim	Department of Neurosurgery, Nanoori Gangnam Hospital, Seoul, South Korea
Il-Tae Jang	Department of Neurosurgery, Nanoori Gangnam Hospital, Seoul, Republic of Korea, Beijing 100048, China
Jin-Sung Kim	Spine Center, Department of Neurosurgery, Seoul St. Mary's Hospital, College of Medicine, The Catholic University of Korea, 222 Banpo Daero, Seocho-gu, Seoul, 137-701, Korea
Ji-Yeon Kim	Department of Neurosurgery, Nanoori Hospital, Seoul City, South Korea
Jiyeon Kim	Department of Neurosurgery, Nanoori Hospital, Gangnam, South Korea
José Gabriel Rugeles Ortíz	Minimally Invasive Spine Center for Latinamerican Endoscopic Spine Surgeons, LESS Invasiva Academy, Bogotá, D.C. Colombia, USA
Jorge Felipe Ramírez León	Minimally Invasive Spine Center for Latinamerican Endoscopic Spine Surgeons, Bogotá, D.C. Colombia, USA Universidad El Bosque, Bogotá, D.C. Colombia, USA
Kai-Uwe Lewandrowski	Center for Advanced Spine Care of Southern Arizona and Surgical Institute of Tucson, Tucson, AZ, USA Department of Orthopaedic Surgery, UNIRIO, Rio de Janeiro, Brazil Department of Orthoapedic Surgery, Fundación Universitaria Sanitas, Bogotá, D.C., Colombia, USA
Nicolás Prada Ramírez	Minimally Invasive Spine Center for Latinamerican Endoscopic Spine Surgeons, LESS Invasiva Academy, Bogotá, D.C. Colombia, USA Colombia Clínica Foscal, Bucaramanga, Colombia, USA
Nimar Salari	Desert Institute for Spine Care, Phoenix, AZ, USA

Nitin Maruti Adsul Department of Neurosurgery, Nanoori Gangnam Hospital, Seoul, South Korea
Ortho-Spine Surgery, Sir Ganga Ram Hospital, New Delhi, India

Pang Hung Wu Department of Neurosurgery, Nanoori Gangnam Hospital, Seoul, South Korea
Departments of Orthopaedic Surgery, National University Health System, Jurong Health Campus, Singapore

Ramon Torres Orthopedic Surgeon/ Spine surgery fellowship Universidad de Chile Instituto Traumatologico Santiago, Chile, USA

Ravindra Singh Department of Neurosurgery, Halifax Infirmary Hospital, Dalhousie University, Canada

Ralf Rothoerl Department of Neurosurgery, Isar Clinic, Munich, Germany

Rômulo Pedroza Pinheiro Orthopeadic Spine Surgery Department of Orthopedics and Anestesiology, Ribeirão Preto Medical School, University of São Paulo, Ribeirão Preto - SP, Brazil

Said G Osman Department of Orthopedic and Spine Surgery, Arabellaklinik, Munich, Germany

Stefan Hellinger Sky Spine Endoscopy Institute 1003 W 7th St, Frederick, MD 21701, USA

Tae Jang IL Department of Neurosurgery, Nanoori Hospital, Gangnam, South Korea

Wu Shang Department of orthopedics, Affiliated Hospital of Yangzhou University, Yangzhou, 225001, China

Yan Yu-qiu Department of orthopedics, Beijing Yuho Rehabilitation Hospital, Beijing 100853, China

Yuan Huafeng Department of orthopedics Shenyang, Department of Orthopedics, Shenyang 242 Hospital, Shenyang 110034, China

Zhang Xi-feng Department of Orthopedics, First Medical Center, PLA General Hospital, Beijing 100853, China

CHAPTER 1

Lumbar Endoscopy: Historical Perspectives, Present & Future

Kai-Uwe Lewandrowski[1,2,3,*], **Jin-Sung Kim**[4], **Friedrich Tieber**[6] and **Anthony Yeung**

[1] *Center for Advanced Spine Care of Southern Arizona and Surgical Institute of Tucson, Tucson AZ, USA*

[2] *Associate Professor of Orthopaedic Surgery, Universidad Colsanitas, Bogota, Colombia, USA*

[3] *Visiting Professor, Department Orthopaedic Surgery, UNIRIO, Rio de Janeiro, Brazil*

[4] *Professor, Spine Center, Department of Neurosurgery, Seoul St. Mary's Hospital, College of Medicine, The Catholic University of Korea 222 Banpo Daero, Seocho-gu, Seoul, 137-701, Korea*

[5] *Clinical Professor, University of New Mexico School of Medicine, Albuquerque, New Mexico Desert Institute for Spine Care, Phoenix, AZ, USA*

[6] *Am Webereck 6 1/2 - 86157 Augsburg, Germany*

Abstract: Endoscopy of the lumbar spine has traditionally found much broader adoption than those endoscopic procedures of other areas of the spine. Initially, a herniated disc was the target of endoscopic spine surgery techniques. Stenosis indications were later identified as technological advancements permitted. Many endoscopic spinal surgeries commenced in the domain of interventional pain management. Lasers and radiofrequency were applied to some of the procedures that nowadays are aided by direct videoendosocopic visualization of the painful pathology. In this chapter, the authors briefly reviewed the history of spinal endoscopy and its key opinion leaders. Giving credit to the most prominent pioneers of this fast-moving field sets the stage for what the reader is about to discover in this most-up-to-date publication: Contemporary Spinal Endoscopy: Lumbar Spine.

Keywords: Lumbar spine, disc herniation, stenosis, impingement, degeneration, decompression, open, minimally invasive, endoscopic, historical considerations, lasers, radiofrequency.

---

* **Corresponding author Kai-Uwe Lewandrowski:** Center for Advanced Spine Care of Southern Arizona and Surgical Institute of Tucson, Tucson, AZ, USA, Department of Orthopaedic Surgery, UNIRIO, Rio de Janeiro, Brazil and Department of Orthoapedic Surgery, Fundación Universitaria Sanitas, Bogotá, D.C., Colombia, USA; Tel: +1 520 204-1495; Fax: +1 623 218-1215; E-mail: business@tucsonspine.com

INTRODUCTION

Many historical perspectives have been revisited by repurposing existing technologies in new surgical approaches within the last ten years, during which spinal endoscopy has gained significant traction among spine surgeons. Likewise, have we witnessed the resurgence of previously employed surgical techniques that have been applied in the early years of spinal endoscopy. As in the fashion industry, where specific trends reappear in a modernized form by fusing different design elements or materials to create new products and marketing strategies, spine surgeons are similarly susceptible to embracing modern trends in spinal endoscopy in their quest to overcome shortcomings of existing treatment protocols for common degenerative conditions of the spine. Industry recycles existing medical know-how and often modernizes them by technology transfer from other commercial areas, such as the aerospace or the automotive industry, by innovation mechanisms of adoption, miniaturizations, automation, and system integration to develop advanced surgical instruments-, and equipment of improved performance, reliability, and durability. Innovations widely adopted in other industries are making their way into medical applications. Examples include high-definition (HD) video technology with touch-screen displays, high-speed HD recording equipment, robotics- and navigation tools, 3D heads-up display goggles for surgeons to be worn during surgery to improve eye-hand coordination, and many others. Rapid endoscopic spine surgery product development with a myriad of instruments being pushed by an army of sales associates is another area of rapid change that has been playing itself out in the operating room — endoscopes with larger inner working channels, sturdy enough to withstand the abuse of more frequent short sterilization cycles to respond to the rising caseload, motorized shavers, drills, and large Ø rongeurs employed during rapid decompression. Endoscopes previously rated for 200 to 250 simple discectomy surgeries are now used in more complex and demanding advanced endoscopic spine procedures. These include intradiscal therapies with heat-generating lasers or radiofrequency devices for the early stages of the disease and the late stages where aggressive decompression and reconstructive procedures may be needed for spinal stenosis instability-related neural element encroachment. Endoscopic placement of spinal implants, such as interbody fusion cages and posterior supplemental fixation with pedicle screw-rod constructs, are other examples of contemporary advancements in endoscopic spinal surgery. This increasing quality and durability demand on spinal endoscopes to work in a large variety of surgical indication scenarios has widened the field of industry competitors, with some front-runners pushing clinical product portfolios, reimbursement, and coding agendas. Traditional German endoscopic equipment makers are being displaced in China, Korea, and Japan by domestic Asian manufacturers whose technological know-how has now risen to a competitive level at lower acquisition costs. In some cases, Asian spinal endoscopy, radiofrequency, and motorized decompression equipment have even advanced beyond what European competitors can put forward, mainly because of progressive clinical agendas with broader indications for endoscopic spinal surgery.

Whether all of these innovations are genuinely impactful and leaps forward that ultimately improve patient outcomes and are not just vogue trends at an increased cost to patients and the health care system, on the whole, is not always obvious and often requires vetting them in the operating room with investigational clinical studies - all of which requires clinical testing, resources, and most of all, time. Spine surgeons have little of the latter and, by their very nature, may be innovation enthusiasts in their quest to overcome shortcomings of existing clinical protocols.

The authors of this chapter attempted to put some of these new trends in perspective within the historical context of spinal endoscopy by reviewing the contributions of some of the early key players in an attempt to help the aspiring endoscopic spine surgeon to position her-, or himself in the increasingly complex field of surgical procedures. With spinal endoscopy becoming more mainstream, many North American and European national and international spine surgeons' organizations are struggling with its adoption. They have just begun to embrace it by spelling out clinical treatment guidelines and figuring out how to establish an accredited core curriculum with validated training programs. On the contrary, if endoscopic spinal surgery training had made it into the mainstream core curriculum many years ago, informal education sources would be less and less relevant. For the time being, many novice endoscopic spine surgeons in many parts of the world – particularly in North America and Europe - have to rely on an industry-sponsored weekend cadaver- and other short instructional courses. While some of them are lucky enough to be mentored by veteran key opinion leaders (KOLs), the vast majority - by default - are autodidacts and primarily self-taught, having to go through an endoscopic learning curve that many find out is steeper than with other procedures they are routinely performing.

THE TRANSFORMATION

The final goal of spinal surgery is to decompress neural elements and stabilize unstable spinal motion segments. Traditionally, this required extensive exposure and stripping of soft tissues, which in turn may devitalize and degenerate the very structures whose integrity is paramount to maintaining a healthy spinal motion segment. Problems such as post-laminectomy instability and epidural fibrosis have long been recognized as some of the potential follow-up problems that could arise from traditional open spinal surgery [1 - 3]. Other well-recognized problems include disruption of vascular supply and denervation of paraspinal muscles with resultantly decreased trunk strength and chronic pain syndromes that at least in part arise from extensive spinal exposures [4]. At ten years, the cumulative rate of development of adjacent level disease in the cervical and lumbar spine in previously healthy spinal motion segments adjacent to fusions has been reported to be as high as 25%. This is not a small number, and recognition of this problem has prompted surgeons to look for alternative ways to accomplish the two fundamental goals of each spinal surgical procedure: Neural element decompression and stabilization of unstable motion segments [5 - 8].

From the patient's point of view, reducing blood loss and surgical time, with rapid recovery and return to work, are clear advantages that are now being openly discussed. With the overall online availability of educational information, patients have become more educated, curious, at times critical, and hopeful that their specific problem can be solved with less aggressive procedures. To many patients, spinal endoscopy intuitively presents itself as such a solution. From a surgeon's point of view, these advantages are no less critical as they lessen the burden to patients and drive patient satisfaction: lower blood loss, complications, infection rates, faster return to work, and social reintegration. Less time to narcotic independence are clinical upsides of spinal endoscopy that can easily be communicated to patients, families, and in due to time to hospitals, health insurance companies, and third-party payers, who still frequently deem spinal endoscopy as an experimental procedure. Since the first edition of Spinal Endoscopy, several high-grade clinical evidence studies have been published. A large body of literature on spinal endoscopy has emerged out of Asia and China in particular. In North America and Europe, however, spinal endoscopy is still yet to be included in treatment and coverage guidelines despite a substantial increase of peer-reviewed journal articles on the safety, efficacy, and equivalency of endoscopic decompression to other minimally invasive (MIS) and open spinal surgeries. Regional variations of the degree of acceptance and utilization of endoscopic spine surgery and changes from the previously dominating transforaminal to the now more popular interlaminar and full endoscopic approach have been discovered. The differences in the surgeon's endoscopic approach preference reflect a shift to more complex decompression and reconstructive procedures. Historically a method developed for simple discectomies, spinal endoscopy is now the most commonly employed minimally invasive spinal surgery technique the world over which has found use in a much more comprehensive range of surgical application.

HISTORY PERSPECTIVES OF ENDOSCOPIC SPINAL SURGERY

Mixter and Barr, in 1934, performed the first microdiscectomy procedures for radicular pain due to a herniated disc. They reported on 19 patients who underwent laminectomy [9]. The concept of a less aggressive decompression was first introduced by Hult, who performed nucleotomy through an extraperitoneal approach in 1951 [10]. In the 1960s, the concept of chemonucleolysis evolved after Lyman and Smith discovered that percutaneous injection of Chymopapain could hydrolyze a herniated nucleus pulposus in a patient with sciatica due to the herniated disc [11].

In 1973, Parvis Kambin introduced a transforaminal approach using percutaneously placed Craig's cannula through which he performed microdiscectomy in a non-visualized fashion [12]. Hijikata reported on the non-visualized posterolateral percutaneous nucleotomy in 1975 [13]. William Friedman introduced the direct lateral approach for percutaneous nucleotomy in 1983. A higher rate of bowel injury was noted, though [14]. The introduction of a specially modified arthroscope into the intervertebral disc, and, thus, the first visualized microdiscectomy, was first reported by Forst and Hausman in 1983 [15]. Coaxial endoscopes with a central working channel soon emerged as an alternative to traditional arthroscopic systems, often using a separate tubular working channel for instruments. They were developed because they offered the option to visualize and remove the painful pathology with a wide range of surgical instruments or thermal therapy equipment. Onik described the addition of a motorized shaver in 1985, which led to the coining of the term "Automated Percutaneous Nucleotomy" [16].

Kambin published his first "discoscopic views" from within the disc in 1988 and later emphasized the importance of epidural visualization [17]. One year later, Schreiber described the injection of indigo carmine dye into the disc to stain abnormal nucleus pulposus and annular fissures [18]. Kambin also first described the "safe" or "working" zone in 1990 as the triangle bordered by the exiting nerve root, the inferior endplate and the superior articular process of the inferior vertebra, and medially by the traversing nerve root (Fig. **1**) [19]. Ultimately, a larger diameter working cannula allowed for more sophisticated instruments and endoscopes to be used (Fig. **2**) [20].

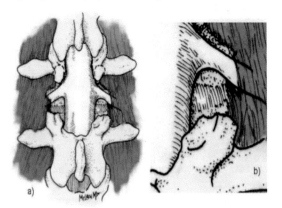

Fig. (1). Surgical anatomy of the "safe zone": The safe zone is formed by the lateral border of the exiting nerve root above, medially by the border of the traversing root or thecal sack, inferiorly by the endplate and dorsally by the superior articular process of the inferior vertebral body. Safe zone is located within the axilla between the exiting and traversing nerve roots (with permission from R.F. McLain).

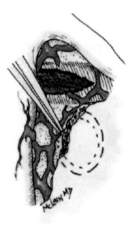

Fig. (2). The "safe zone" is entered by removing parts of the superior articular process of the inferior vertebral body thus performing a foraminoplasty (with permission from R.F. McLain).

Schreiber and Leu (Zurich) contributed to the development of multichannel endoscopes [18] in cooperation with Karl Storz Endoskopie, Tuttlingen (Fig. **3**), and by Hal Matthews in partnership with Danek Inc., Memphis [21 - 23]. Since the endoscope was directed *via* the posterolateral approach into the lumbar neuroforamen, the surgical technique was called "Foraminoscopy".

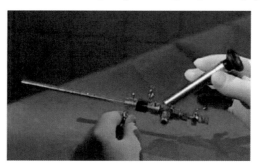

Fig. (3). First Storz™ working channel endoscope developed by Leu.

These authors recognized that it was necessary to direct the foraminoscope in different trajectories to reach all types of a herniated disc in the various foraminal zones and the possible cranial to caudal locations (Fig. **4**).

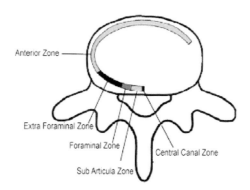

Fig. (4). Zone classification to describe the location of a herniated lumbar disc proposed by Schreiber & Leu in 1993.

Citation Medical Corp., Reno NV, produced the Danek endoscope. Hal Matthews introduced it at the Laser Conference in 1991 in San Francisco [21]. Its 0°-viewing angle is dictated by the glass fiber bundles used for image transmission. This endoscope allowed the introduction of instruments of up to 3.5 mm. The single-use Danek design failed because of cost and poor image quality. Moreover, it did not fit into the lumbar foramen, and the 0° optic was impractical for visualized treatment of central herniation. It was taken off the market in 1994.

The Leu foraminoscope was designed for the treatment of foraminal and extraforaminal herniations. Karl Storz produced it, and its clinical use was demonstrated by Dr. Leu in 1991 (Fig. **5**) [24]. The Storz-built endoscope used a Hopkins rod lens system with a 6° viewing angle acceptable for the chosen indications.

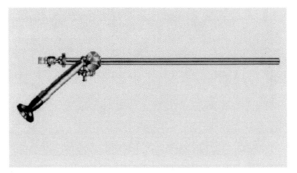

Fig. (5). The Leu foraminoscope produced by Karl Storz, Tuttlingen, Germany in 1991. It had a Hopkins rod lens system with a 6° viewing, a working length of 145 mm and the inner working channel large enough to accommodate instruments of up to 3.0 mm in Ø.

Karl Storz offered the foraminoscope designed by Hans-Jörg Leu until 2012 when more current products replaced it after a 21-year run. Popular design features included a working length of 145 mm, and an inner working channel Ø of 3.0 mm (Fig. **4**). It had several advantages with a brilliant image and the great tools required to do endoscopic discectomy surgery. It could be sterilized and therefore was suitable for multi-use. Moreover, large capital purchases for proprietary videoendoscopic tower equipment were unnecessary since the Leu-designed and Storz-produced foraminoscope easily connected to existing Video Towers. Storz also provided the first interlaminar endoscopic nucleotomy set, popularized by Vogl (Fig. **6**).

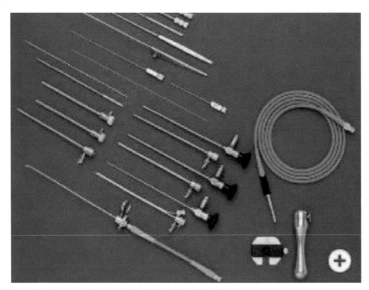

Fig. (6). Storz™ interlaminar nucleotomy developed by Vogl.

In 1992, Dr. Thomas Hoogland recognized the need to innovate endoscopic spine surgery beyond the scope of what the Danek foraminoscope was able to do. Shortcomings in the treatment of intracanal, foraminal, extraforaminal herniations with free fragments were the basis for innovations that followed. He first reported the utility of a foraminoplasty to deal with these types of herniations in 1994. His technique deployed reamers and drills over a guidewire introduced over the „Tom Shidi" guide cannula - one of the critical elements of his outside-in technique [25]. A comparison of the specifications of the early foraminoscopes produced between 1992 – 1997 is shown in Table **1**.

Table 1. Comparison of specifications of the early foraminoscopes 1992 – 1997.

Geometric Data & Specs	Karl Storz 1992 (Leu)	Danek Inc. 1992 (Hoodland)	Richard Wolf YESS 1997 (Yeung)
Working Length	145 mm	210 mm	207 mm
Outer Ø	6.0 mm	6.3 mm	Oval
Working Channel Ø	3.1 mm for 3.5 mm Ø Instruments	3.6 mm for 3.5 mm Ø Instruments	2.7 mm for 2.5 mm Ø Instruments
Optic	Rod-Lens System	Fiber Optic Cable	Rod-Lens System
Two Irrigation Channels	YES	YES	YES
Connector For Video Camera	YES	YES	YES

In 1993, Schreiber started working with large working channel endoscopes allowing direct visualization of annular tears [18]. Kambin and Zhou demonstrated using a 30-degree endoscope, recognizing that lateral recess stenosis can hamper the procedure's effectiveness. In 1996, they established foraminoplasty *via* endoscopic removal of facet overhang, osteophytes, and annulectomy using specialized forceps and trephines [20, 26]. Foley, Mathews, and Ditsworth published their transforaminal series in 1998 and 1999 [27 - 29]. In 1998, Yeung introduced The Yeung Endoscopic Spine System (YESS) using a rod-lense multichannel, wide-angled endoscope with integrated suction irrigation channels produced by Richard Wolf [30]. The oval-shaped device had a 207 mm working channel of 2.7 mm Ø suitable for 2.5 mm surgical instruments. The YESS system was designed for the inside-out technique employing foraminoplasty with trephines, lasers, and radiofrequency (Fig. **7**) [66].

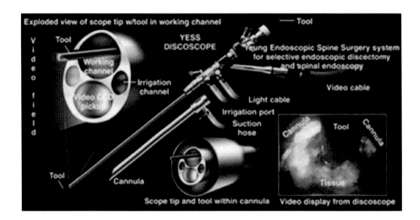

Fig. (7). The Yeung Endoscopic Spine System (YESS) produced by Richard Wolf consisted of an oval-shaped multichannel, wide-angled endoscope with a 207 mm working channel of 2.7 mm in Ø for use of 2.5 mm surgical instruments, an irrigation channel, and a rod lens system. It was designed for intradiscal decompression for protrusions, for foraminal and extraforaminal herniations and for foraminoplasty with lasers and radiofrequency.

In 1998, Dr. Hoogland pioneered a multichannel 1.9 mm Ø rod-lens endoscope with a length of 180 mm, and capable of accomodating Ø 3.5 mm instruments. The system had excellent image quality and an irrigation channel and was based on a fiberglass illumination system that came with a 0° and a 30° optic (Fig. **8**). To date, this OEM offers still the broadest range of coaxial endoscopes with a working channel in many different lengths, diameters of the inlet, and outer diameter.

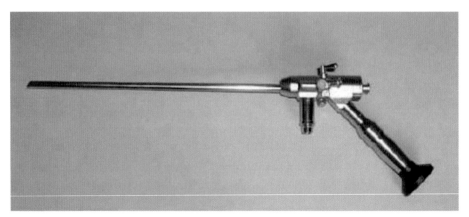

Fig. (8). Hoogland's multichannel endoscope produced by a German OEM manufacturer in 1998 with the following specifications: length 180 mm, working channel Ø of 3.6 mm for instruments up to Ø 3.5 mm, irrigation channel, 0° and 30° optic fiber glass illumination system, outer Ø 6.3 mm, and 1.9 mm Ø rod-lens system delivering excellent image quality.

In 2001, Knight *et al.* published on endoscopic foraminoplasty employing a side-firing Ho: YAG laser [31]. The advent of lasers also stimulated electrothermal annuloplasty for low back pain, which Tsou and Yeung described in 2002 [32]. Soon after that, more modern systems were introduced by the senior author of this chapter (Anthony Yeung) in 1998-2002, with the launch of the new Yeung Endoscopic Spine System (YESS), followed by additional decompression instruments and cannula modifications which were designed around the transforaminal endoscopic approach for intradiscal and epiduroscopic procedures [33]. Yeung *et al.* describe the utility of provocative intraoperative discography, thermal discoplasty, and annuloplasty, annular resection for creating an annular window to perform foraminoplasty using endoscopic Kerrison, abrasive drills, burrs, and lasers. Bipolar electro-frequency probes were introduced by Tsou and Yeung, who performed a thermal electro-annuloplasty for chronic discogenic low back pain. This technique was done on the direct visualization targeting disc nucleus and annular fissures [34]. A variety of intradiscal conditions, including delamination and fissuring and entrapment of herniated disc material into annular fissures, have been described by the senior author of this chapter (Anthony Yeung), who has employed the inside-out technique to diagnose and treat these intradiscal entities.

Another leap forward was achieved by Ruetten *et al.*, who dealt with poor visualization of the epidural space with the popularization of the direct lateral approach with the uniportal use of a foraminoscope [35]. Ruetten and his group also validated the indications of the interlaminar and full endoscopic techniques [36 - 46]. Hoogland and Schubert dealt with the problem alternatively by describing foraminoplasty with transforaminal reamers in 2005 [47]. This technique made it easier to access sequestered disc fragments that migrated in locations far from the interspace. Lee further analyzed this problem in 2006 and found that patients with severe canal and lateral recess stenosis had less favorable clinical outcomes due to a higher risk for remnant disc fragments responsible for persistent clinical symptoms [48].

Lee *et al.* also pioneered the definition and application of a classification system for the location of a herniated disc by dividing them into near-migrated (zone two and zone three), and upward (zone one), or downward (zone four) far-migrated disc fragments [49]. The first author's own clinical experience underlines the importance of using radiographic classification systems for both herniated disc and spinal stenosis. Another chapter of this text demonstrates the utility of a radiographic classification system for foraminal and lateral recess stenosis. The division of the neuroforamen into entry-, mid-, and exit zone is helpful when stratifying patients and selecting appropriate surgical candidates [50].

THE NITZE-LEITER MUSEUM FOR ENDOSCOPY

The International Nitze-Leiter Research Society for Endoscopy houses many historical instruments, writings, and construction drawings. The highlight is the original light conductor by the Frankfurt doctor Philipp Bozzini from 1806. It is recognized in the professional world as the first endoscope, with all the properties still the basis for modern endoscopes today. The collection includes the significant achievements in endoscopy through to the developments of the 20th century. In its entirety, the Endoscopy Museum houses items from the first endoscopic aids to modern endoscopic technologies of the computer age. More than 3000 exhibits show the viewer the milestone development over more than two centuries and many individual pieces (Figs. **9** and **10**). Each in itself represents a piece of medical history and shows doctors' will to develop ever-better medical devices to improve the treatment of patients.

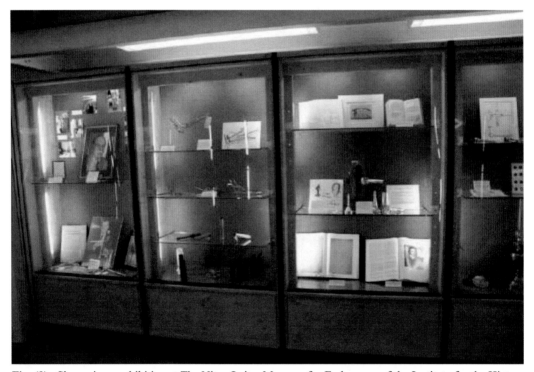

Fig. (9). Shown is an exhibition at The Nitze-Leiter Museum for Endoscopy of the Institute for the History of Medicine at the University of Vienna. The chair has existed since 1848. The museum was opened in 1996.

Particular emphasis is placed in the urology department with urethroscopes, cystoscopes, blind and optical lithotriptors, resectoscopes in various development phases, and gastroenterology esophagoscopes gastro-, recto-colonoscopes, and laparoscopes of all development stages.

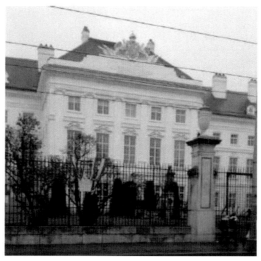

Fig. (10). The Endoscopy Museum has been housed for a long time in the Josefinum since 1920. The building was created in 1785 by Emperor Josef II near the Center of Vienna, Austria.

Donations to the International Nitze-Leiter Research Society for Endoscopy, consisting of instruments, equipment, catalogs, image and video material from closed ordinations, hospital departments, or international instrument manufacturers, as well as numerous bequests, form the holdings of the Nitze-Leiter collection. The collection also contains treasures from the history of bronchoscopy, ophthalmology, gynecology, and ENT. Instruments from international manufacturers provide information about the individual development steps in lighting, optics, and mechanics and show therapeutic applications' progress. With a steady influx of objects, aspects of the more recent endoscopy history are also on display.

THE EVOLUTION OF LASERS IN SPINAL ENDOSCOPY

Lasers have always been appealing for surgeons when applied in minimally invasive procedures. Peter Ascher demonstrated it by employing neodymium:yttrium-aluminum-garnet (Nd: YAG) laser through an 18 gauge needle introduced fluoroscopically into the intervertebral disc [51]. His technique ablated and vaporized intradiscal tissue in short bursts without heat damage to adjacent tissues. This procedure was ideally suitable for an outpatient setting as the patient was discharged off the needle is withdrawn in the puncture wound was covered with a small Band-Aid.

The Ho: YAG laser was compared to the Nd: YAG laser in a clinical trial conducted by Quigley *et al*. in 1991 [52]. He noted that the Ho: YAG laser was the best to compromise between the efficacy of absorption and the convenience of fiber-optic delivery at that time. In 1990, Davis *et al*. reported clinical success in 85% of his 40 patients who underwent laser discectomy with the potassium-titanyl-phosphate (KTP 532-nm) laser [53]. Only six of the 40 patients required revision with open discectomy procedures because of clinical failures. In 1995, Casper *et al*. described using the side-firing Ho: YAG laser [54], which was also employed later by Yeung *et al*. [55]. At a one-year follow-up, Casper *et al*. reported an 84% success rate [55]. Siebert *et al*. published a 78% success rate on 100 patients with a mean follow-up of 17 months treated with the Nd: YAG laser [56].

Mayer *et al*. were the first to suggest the combined use of an endoscope with laser ablation through an endoscopically introduced fiber. Extensive clinical trials followed and were very supportive of the clinical use of lasers to remove the herniated disc [57]. Hellinger reported in 1999 on more than 2500 patients he treated with the help of the Ascher technique with an 80% success rate over 13 years [58]. Yeung *et al*. noted an 84% success rate on more than 500 patients he treated with the KTP laser [59].

The current state-of-the-art has been summarized by Ahn *et al*. in a recent article [60]. Open microscopic laser surgery, percutaneous endoscopic laser surgery, and laser-tissue modulation for spinal pain comprise the three ways lasers are currently applied in interventional and minimally invasive spinal surgery. Ahn et a. encouraged further study of the select clinical indications demonstrating efficacy to substantiate the lack of evidence with randomized clinical trials [60]. A multicenter randomized prospective trial by Brouwer *et al*. failed to show a difference in clinical outcomes between 57 conventional microdiscectomy patients to another 55 percutaneous laser disc decompression patients [61, 62]. The needle-based (18G) percutaneous laser procedure placed a 600-micron glass fiber into the center of the disc employing a diode laser (Biolitec, 980 nm, 7 W, 0.6 s pulses, interval 1 s) to total energy delivered of 1500 J. Nonetheless, the reoperation rate was higher in the laser group (52%) than in the microdiscectomy (21%) group [63, 64]. The cost-effectiveness of laser- over standard microdiscectomy has been demonstrated for a simple herniated disc. However, it remains to be seen when integrated with an endoscopic platform and applied in more complex clinical scenarios such as foraminal and lateral recess stenosis [65]. At a minimum, the concern for nerve root injury with laser application in the spine remains [66, 67].

RADIOFREQUENCY ABLATION

High-frequency radiofrequency ablation has found several applications in neurosurgery, endoscopic spine, orthopedic and pain management. High (RF) radio frequency with low temperatures has been employed for tissue dissection (monopolar) and coagulating mode (mono and bipolar). Five years ago, when the first edition of Spinal Endoscopy was published, only one radiofrequency product was dominating the market. Nowadays, nearly every vendor selling spinal endoscopes also has a radiofrequency probe in the portfolio produced in-house or by a third party. Typically, radiofrequency probes are compatible with the working channel of the spinal endoscope are used for hemostasis, shrinkage, or ablative effects in the soft tissue to dissect them of a herniated disc.

Radiofrequency ablation of tissues is well accepted in other areas such as plastic surgery, oral maxillofacial surgery, and dental procedures. These devices have found their way into spinal surgery for thermal ablation of disc tissue. With further miniaturization and reduced acquisition costs, they nowadays present an attractive alternative to lasers. While the acquisition cost of lasers nowadays may be comparable to the expense of capital equipment purchase of a complete radiofrequency system, radiofrequency is found in most operating rooms. In a routine clinical application in high-turn-over operating rooms, radiofrequency with disposable probes is perceived more practical by most and less cumbersome. Besides, lasers may impose additional safety issues for patients, surgeons, and supporting staff that does not exist with the radiofrequency application.

The utility of High (RF) radio frequency with low temperatures tissue ablation has been investigated in at least one study. In 2004, Tsou *et al.* reviewed 113 consecutive patients with a minimum postoperative follow-up of 2 years. Patients were treated for discogenic low back pain [34]. Their clinical analysis showed excellent results in 15%, good in 28.3%, fair in 30.1%, and poor results in 26.5% of patients, respectively. The authors concluded that the treatment interrupted the purported annular defect pain sensitization process [34].

In 2016, Pan *et al.* demonstrated the benefit of using radiofrequency treatment of annular tears and adhesions to the dural sac due to inflammatory granulomas in 63 consecutive patients with discogenic low back pain [68]. The authors claimed that concordant pain could be triggered by stimulating the inflammatory granulation tissue within the annular tears or between the posterior longitudinal ligament and the dural sac with a bipolar radiofrequency probe. The authors concluded that the debridement of the granuloma with the radiofrequency probe was essential in achieving favorable clinical outcomes. Others have corroborated the observations. In 2013, Wang used radiofrequency to alleviate refractory pain of spinal metastasis patients with ablation during transforaminal endoscopy [69], and Sairyo employed it to treat low back pain in professional athletes [70]. Similar radiofrequency applications were demonstrated in 2016 by Pereira *et al.* and Bellini *et al.* They both reported improved clinical outcomes in patients with postoperative epidural fibrosis following epiduroscopic rather than endoscopic visualization [71, 72]. Nowadays, high radio frequency with low temperatures tissue ablation is useful in spinal endoscopy when controlling bleeding and shrinking tissue to facilitate visualization. The need for a modernized radiofrequency application may arise from advances in endoscopic spinal decompression and reconstructive procedures.

NEW LANDMARK CLINICAL OUTCOME STUDIES

Until recently, randomized prospective trials comparing the traditional open *versus* the endoscopically performed lumbar microdiscectomy procedure were unavailable. Earlier studies, however, suggested that successful outcomes can be achieved. In 2006 and 2007, Choi *et al.* reported a 92% success rate with their extraforaminal fragmentectomy technique [73, 74]. In his 2007 study, he wrote on 41 patients in whom soft extraforaminal disc herniations were treated in such a way with a more medialized trajectory [74]. In the same year, Lee *et al.* demonstrated high clinical success rates with downward migrated disc fragments (91.8%), in upward migrated disc fragments (88.9%), in near-migrated disc fragments (97%), and slightly less favorable clinical results with far-migrated disc fragments (78.9%) [49]. The authors concluded that this type of herniation is the hardest to reach and demands proficient surgical skills. In 2009, Ruetten *et al.* popularized his lateral recess endoscopic stenosis decompression with the interlaminar approach and compared it to the conventional microsurgical technique [43]. This prospective randomized controlled trial on 161 patients proved that full endoscopic decompression was just as effective as the established technique with similar recurrence rates of 6.2%. Another study on 78 patients corroborated these findings by reporting complete relief of leg pain in 82% of the patients at two-year follow-up [44]. Ruetten's studies proved equal patient VAS and ODI patient satisfaction data at two-year follow-up [41, 44].

In 2013, Birkenmeier *et al.* published a metanalysis of comparative controlled clinical trials on endoscopic and microsurgical standard procedures [39]. Based on four randomized controlled trials (RCTs) and one controlled study (CS), he concluded that the endoscopic technique resulted in more favorable numbers of operating time, blood loss, complication- and revision rates, surgical pain, postoperative rehabilitation, hospital stay, and return to work than with the microsurgical techniques. These five studies demonstrated similar clinical outcomes regardless of whether the endoscopic or the microsurgical was used.

In 2018, Kong *et al.* prospectively randomized patients with lumbar disc herniation and lateral recess stenosis to either endoscopic lumbar discectomy (PELD) or microsurgical laminotomy (ML) technique [75]. At the Third

Affiliated Hospital of Sun Yat-sen University of Medical Sciences in Guangzhou, China, Limin Rong's team conducted an open-label randomized single-center study comparing percutaneous transforaminal endoscopic discectomy (PTSD) to mid-line microendoscopic discectomy (MED) [76]. One-year follow-up data were available in 89.5% of the 153 patients. The authors did not find any statistically significant differences in the primary clinical and secondary perioperative outcome measures (length of surgery and hospital stay, time to mobilization, cost of surgery and total hospital cost, complications-, and reoperations rates). However, the authors reported less favorable clinical outcomes with medially located disc herniations at one year (p = 0.028). Far lateral disc herniation treated with MED hod lower ODI reductions at 3 months (p = 0.008), 6 months (p = 0.028), and 1 year (p = 0.028) postoperatively. The complication rates were similar, with 13.75% in the PTSD group and 16.44% in the MED group (p = 0.642) [78].

THE ASIAN LEADERSHIP ROLE

Over the past five years, endoscopic spinal surgery has gained popularity in Asian countries. The development of endoscopic spine surgery in Asia is mainly concentrated in East Asia and India. A review of the publication activities shows that the authors in five countries in Asia publish the most significant number of articles in endoscopic spine surgery each year. There are many academic activities in Asian countries with formalized training programs during congresses, national and international meetings, and workshops. In Table **2**, the timeline of the implementation of contemporary endoscopic and MIS techniques for the top 5 major Asian countries – China, South Korea, India, Japan, and Taiwan. They are now undisputed leaders in the field of endoscopic spine surgery.

Table 2. Year of the first MIS and endoscopic surgery in top 5 major Asia.

-	MED	FESS Or PELD	Endoscopic Laminotomy For Spinal Stenosis
China	1998	2005	2012
India	2000s	2000	2017
Japan	1998	2003	2009
South Korea	1990s	1992	2014
Taiwan	2001	1997	2010
MED, microendoscopic discectomy; FESS, full-endoscopic spinal surgery; PELD, percutaneous endoscopic lumbar discectomy			

There is no doubt that the strong support of MIS associations and societies in these top 5 Asian countries played an important role. In 2002 and earlier than in most western countries, CK Park established the MIS association South Korea to promote and develop the MIS field. It was named KOMISS – The Korean Minimally Invasive Spine Surgery Society. In 2003, the COA-CMISS and CSSA-CMISS were founded in China. Subsequently, JASMISS (Japanese Society of Minimally Invasive Spine Surgery), TSMISS (Taiwan Society of Minimally Invasive Spine Surgery), and MISSION (Minimally Invasive Spine Surgeons of India) also established their respective MIS associations. These associations have made significant contributions to the development of endoscopic spine surgery in Asian countries. Of the major countries in Asia, the role of the surgeons at the Wooridul Spine Hospitals in Korea has been most prominent. These surgeons continue to improve the expertise and surgical techniques of MIS of the spine by actively encouraging the surgeons to perform endoscopic spine surgery in other regions of Asia, thereby setting new clinical standards with high acceptance amongst their peers [48, 76 - 80]. Today, endoscopic spinal surgery in Asia has become mainstream for the treatment of herniated discs and spinal stenosis. There are now Korean and Chinese manufacturers able to produce endoscopic spine systems of good quality and durability competitive enough to have established a foothold in these Asian markets, where it is easier for them to compete because of lower production cost, and familiarity, and in some cases preferential treatment they receive, with the regulatory process involved trying to get their products to the market. The proximity of Asian manufacturers to the local market and their ability to interact with their surgeons closely has broadened the scope of endoscopic spine surgery even further, which now even includes endoscopically assisted lumbar interbody fusion procedures [81 - 84].

Additional advances have been pioneered by Korean KOLs, including the unilateral bi-portal endoscopic (UBE) technique that is gaining some traction among Korean spine surgeons. The method is not a full-endoscopic spine surgery but an endoscopy-assisted surgical procedure designed as a stepping stone for spine surgeons with limited endoscopic surgery experience. Dr. Daniel Julio De Antoni reported the original concept of UBE from Argentina in the 1980ies, who published it in the Revista Argentina De Artroscopia Vol 1, No.1 pp 81-85, in 1981 and later again in 1996 [85]. In this context, the Destandeau endoscopic spine system should not be forgotten [86]. Storz developed it after problems arose with its early UBE system. The Destandeau System employs interlaminar biportal endoscopy with a fixed optical system and a nerve hook (Fig. **11**).

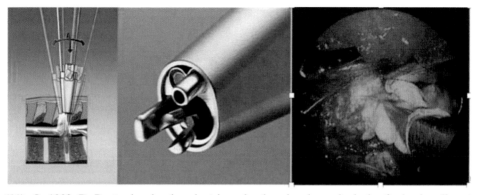

Fig. (11). In 1992, Dr Destandau developed a triangular dorsal endoscopic device for lumbar discectomy, which was deployed through a 20 mm incision. It is equipped with an endoscope, a suction cannula an integrated separator to push the dura away from instrument and an 8 mm working channel.

Consequently, the modern UBE surgery is a combination of familiar mini-open and other retractor-based MIS exposure with the endoscope to aid in the visualization of areas that are not directly accessible or cannot be visualized as part of the surgical exposure [87 - 89]. Whether it is because of cultural differences, high acceptance of modern technologies amongst Asian patients and surgeons alike, or the drive to perfect a surgical technique beyond its original design limitations is academic from the point of view of this chapter's authors. The fact remains that Asia spine surgeons have not only embraced MIS and endoscopic spine surgery but have excelled at it by combining elegant tactical improvements in surgical techniques with those of advanced instruments and other ancillary technologies. Nowadays, the expectations are high, and it became apparent that much larger spinal surgical procedures could be performed with modern MIS techniques using the endoscopic platform that had previously been unimaginable.

CONCLUSION

This historical review of endoscopic spinal surgery demonstrated that many treatment concepts have been around and recycled several times. Time-proven solutions have been repurposed and reinvented in the quest of expanding the indications for spinal endoscopy. In the authors' opinion, reviewing the historical context is not just a matter of crediting the KOL's of the past and present for their contributions. Still, it is also a necessity to position procedural innovations proposed for current clinical practice appropriately. The authors hope that the reader of Contemporary Spinal Endoscopy: Lumbar Spine has gained interest in further studying the diagnostic and therapeutic concepts behind modern spinal endoscopy procedures as they have developed and from where they have evolved.

CONSENT FOR PUBLICATION

Not applicable.

CONFLICT OF INTEREST

The authors declare no conflict of interest, financial or otherwise.

ACKNOWLEDGEMENT

Declared none.

REFERENCES

[1]   Papagelopoulos PJ, Peterson HA, Ebersold MJ, Emmanuel PR, Choudhury SN, Quast LM. Spinal column deformity and instability after lumbar or thoracolumbar laminectomy for intraspinal tumors in children and young adults. Spine 1997; 22(4): 442-51.
[http://dx.doi.org/10.1097/00007632-199702150-00019] [PMID: 9055374]

[2]   Mullin BB, Rea GL, Irsik R, Catton M, Miner ME. The effect of postlaminectomy spinal instability on the outcome of lumbar spinal stenosis patients. J Spinal Disord 1996; 9(2): 107-16.
[http://dx.doi.org/10.1097/00002517-199604000-00004] [PMID: 8793776]

[3]   Alkalay RN, Kim DH, Urry DW, Xu J, Parker TM, Glazer PA. Prevention of postlaminectomy epidural fibrosis using bioelastic materials. Spine 2003; 28(15): 1659-65.
[http://dx.doi.org/10.1097/01.BRS.0000083161.67605.40] [PMID: 12897488]

[4]   Keller A, Brox JI, Reikerås O. Predictors of change in trunk muscle strength for patients with chronic low back pain randomized to lumbar fusion or cognitive intervention and exercises. Pain Med 2008; 9(6): 680-7.
[http://dx.doi.org/10.1111/j.1526-4637.2007.00333.x] [PMID: 18828199]

[5]   Harrop JS, Youssef JA, Maltenfort M, et al. Lumbar adjacent segment degeneration and disease after arthrodesis and total disc arthroplasty. Spine 2008; 33(15): 1701-7.
[http://dx.doi.org/10.1097/BRS.0b013e31817bb956] [PMID: 18594464]

[6]   Hilibrand AS, Carlson GD, Palumbo MA, Jones PK, Bohlman HH. Radiculopathy and myelopathy at segments adjacent to the site of a previous anterior cervical arthrodesis. J Bone Joint Surg Am 1999; 81(4): 519-28.
[http://dx.doi.org/10.2106/00004623-199904000-00009] [PMID: 10225797]

[7]   Rihn JA, Lawrence J, Gates C, Harris E, Hilibrand AS. Adjacent segment disease after cervical spine fusion. Instr Course Lect 2009; 58: 747-56.
[PMID: 19385583]

[8]   Kepler CK, Hilibrand AS. Management of adjacent segment disease after cervical spinal fusion. Orthop Clin North Am 2012; 43(1): 53-62.
[http://dx.doi.org/10.1016/j.ocl.2011.08.003]

[9]   Mixter WJ, Barr J. Rupture of the intervertebral disc with involvement of the spinal canal. N Engl J Med 1934; 211(5): 210-5.
[http://dx.doi.org/10.1056/NEJM193408022110506]

[10]   Hult L. Retroperitoneal disc fenestration in low-back pain and sciatica; a preliminary report. Acta Orthop Scand 1951; 20(4): 342-8.
[http://dx.doi.org/10.3109/17453675108991181] [PMID: 14894204]

[11]   Smith L. Enzyme dissolution of the nucleus pulposus in humans. JAMA 1964; 187(2): 137-40.
[http://dx.doi.org/10.1001/jama.1964.03060150061016] [PMID: 14066733]

[12]   Kambin P, Ed. Arthroscopic Microdiscectomy: Minimal Intervention Spinal Surgery. Baltimore, MD: Urban & Schwarenburg 1990.

[13]   Hijikata S, Yamagishi M, Nakayma T. Percutaneous discectomy. J Todenhosp 1975; 5: 5-13.

[14]   Friedman WA. Percutaneous discectomy: an alternative to chemonucleolysis? Neurosurgery 1983; 13(5): 542-7.
[http://dx.doi.org/10.1227/00006123-198311000-00010] [PMID: 6227832]

[15]   Hausmann B. Nucleoscopy- a new examination technique. Arch Orthop Trauma Surg 1983; 13: 542-7.

[16]   Onik G, Helms CA, Ginsberg L, Hoaglund FT, Morris J. Percutaneous lumbar diskectomy using a new aspiration probe: porcine and cadaver model. Radiology 1985; 155(1): 251-2.
[http://dx.doi.org/10.1148/radiology.155.1.3975407] [PMID: 3975407]

[17]   Kambin P, Nixon JE, Chait A, Schaffer JL. Annular protrusion: pathophysiology and roentgenographic appearance. Spine 1988; 13(6): 671-5.
[http://dx.doi.org/10.1097/00007632-198813060-00013] [PMID: 2972071]

[18]   Schreiber A, Suezawa Y, Leu H. Does percutaneous nucleotomy with discoscopy replace conventional discectomy? Eight years of experience and results in treatment of herniated lumbar disc. Clin Orthop Relat Res 1989; 238: 35-42.
[http://dx.doi.org/10.1097/00003086-198901000-00005] [PMID: 2910617]

[19]   Kambin P, Zhou L. History and current status of percutaneous arthroscopic disc surgery. Spine 1996; 21(24) (Suppl.): 57S-61S.
[http://dx.doi.org/10.1097/00007632-199612151-00006] [PMID: 9112325]

[20]   Kambin P, Schaffer JL. Percutaneous lumbar discectomy. Review of 100 patients and current practice. Clin Orthop Relat Res 1989; 238: 24-34.
[http://dx.doi.org/10.1097/00003086-198901000-00004] [PMID: 2910608]

[21]   Mathews HH. First International Symposium on Laser in Orthopaedics. San Francisco. 1991.

[22]   Mathews HH, Kyles MK, Lang BH, Fiore SM, Gordon CL. Spinal endoscopy: Indications, approaches and applications. Orthop Trans 1995; 19: 219.

[23]   Mathews HH. Transforaminal endoscopic microdiscectomy. Neurosurg Clin N Am 1996; 7(1): 59-63.
[http://dx.doi.org/10.1016/S1042-3680(18)30405-4] [PMID: 8835146]

[24]   Leu Hj, Hauser R. Die perkutan posterolaterale Foraminoskopie: Prinzip, Technik und Erfahrungen seit 1991. Arthroskopie 1996; 9: 26-31.

[25]   Hoogland T. Transforaminal endoscopic discectomy with foraminoplasty for lumbar disc herniation Surgical Techniques in Orthopaedics and Traumatology 2003. 55-120-C-40, p6

[26]   Kambin P, O'Brien E, Zhou L, Schaffer JL. Arthroscopic microdiscectomy and selective fragmentectomy. Clin Orthop Relat Res 1998; (347): 150-67.
[PMID: 9520885]

[27]   Foley KT, Smith MM, Rampersaud YR. Microendoscopic approach to far-lateral lumbar disc herniation. Neurosurg Focus 1999; 7(5): e5.
[http://dx.doi.org/10.3171/foc.1999.7.5.8] [PMID: 16918212]

[28]   Mathews HH. Transforaminal endoscopic microdiscectomy. Neurosurg Clin N Am 1996; 7(1): 59-63.
[http://dx.doi.org/10.1016/S1042-3680(18)30405-4] [PMID: 8835146]

[29]   Ditsworth DA. Endoscopic transforaminal lumbar discectomy and reconfiguration: a postero-lateral approach into the spinal canal. Surg Neurol 1998; 49(6): 588-97.
[http://dx.doi.org/10.1016/S0090-3019(98)00004-4] [PMID: 9637618]

[30]   Yeung AT. Minimally Invasive Disc Surgery with the Yeung Endoscopic Spine System (YESS). Surg Technol Int 1999; 8: 267-77.
[PMID: 12451541]

[31]   Knight MT, Ellison DR, Goswami A, Hillier VF. Review of safety in endoscopic laser foraminoplasty for the management of back pain. J Clin Laser Med Surg 2001; 19(3): 147-57.
[http://dx.doi.org/10.1089/104454701152927982] [PMID: 11469307]

[32]   Yeung AT, Tsou PM. Posterolateral endoscopic excision for lumbar disc herniation: Surgical technique, outcome, and complications in 307 consecutive cases. Spine 2002; 27(7): 722-31.
[http://dx.doi.org/10.1097/00007632-200204010-00009] [PMID: 11923665]

[33]   Yeung AT, Yeung CA. Advances in endoscopic disc and spine surgery: foraminal approach. Surg Technol Int 2003; 11: 255-63. [Review].
[PMID: 12931309]

[34]   Tsou PM, Alan Yeung C, Yeung AT. Posterolateral transforaminal selective endoscopic discectomy and thermal annuloplasty for chronic lumbar discogenic pain: a minimal access visualized intradiscal surgical procedure. Spine J 2004; 4(5): 564-73.
[http://dx.doi.org/10.1016/j.spinee.2004.01.014] [PMID: 15363430]

[35]   Ruetten S, Komp M, Godolias G. An extreme lateral access for the surgery of lumbar disc herniations inside the spinal canal using the full-endoscopic uniportal transforaminal approach-technique and prospective results of 463 patients. Spine 2005; 30(22): 2570-8.
[http://dx.doi.org/10.1097/01.brs.0000186327.21435.cc] [PMID: 16284597]

[36]   Ruetten S, Hahn P, Oezdemir S, *et al.* Full-endoscopic uniportal decompression in disc herniations and stenosis of the thoracic spine using the interlaminar, extraforaminal, or transthoracic retropleural approach. J Neurosurg Spine 2018; 29(2): 157-68.
[http://dx.doi.org/10.3171/2017.12.SPINE171096] [PMID: 29856303]

[37]   Ruetten S, Hahn P, Oezdemir S, Baraliakos X, Godolias G, Komp M. Operation of Soft or Calcified Thoracic Disc Herniations in the Full-Endoscopic Uniportal Extraforaminal Technique. Pain Physician 2018; 21(4): E331-40.
[http://dx.doi.org/10.36076/ppj.2018.4.E331] [PMID: 30045599]

[38]   Komp M, Hahn P, Oezdemir S, *et al.* Bilateral spinal decompression of lumbar central stenosis with the full-endoscopic interlaminar *versus* microsurgical laminotomy technique: a prospective, randomized, controlled study. Pain Physician 2015; 18(1): 61-70.
[http://dx.doi.org/10.36076/ppj/2015.18.61] [PMID: 25675060]

[39]   Birkenmaier C, Komp M, Leu HF, Wegener B, Ruetten S. The current state of endoscopic disc surgery: review of controlled studies comparing full-endoscopic procedures for disc herniations to standard procedures. Pain Physician 2013; 16(4): 335-44.
[http://dx.doi.org/10.36076/ppj.2013/16/335] [PMID: 23877449]

[40]   Ruetten S, Komp M, Hahn P, Oezdemir S. [Decompression of lumbar lateral spinal stenosis: full-endoscopic, interlaminar technique]. Oper Orthop Traumatol 2013; 25(1): 31-46.
[http://dx.doi.org/10.1007/s00064-012-0195-2] [PMID: 23371002]

[41]   Ruetten S. Full-endoscopic Operations of the Spine in Disk Herniations and Spinal Stenosis. Surg Technol Int 2011; 21: 284-98.
[PMID: 22505003]

[42]   Komp M, Hahn P, Merk H, Godolias G, Ruetten S. Bilateral operation of lumbar degenerative central spinal stenosis in full-endoscopic interlaminar technique with unilateral approach: prospective 2-year results of 74 patients. J Spinal Disord Tech 2011; 24(5): 281-7.
[http://dx.doi.org/10.1097/BSD.0b013e3181f9f55e] [PMID: 20975592]

[43]   Ruetten S, Komp M, Merk H, Godolias G. Surgical treatment for lumbar lateral recess stenosis with the full-endoscopic interlaminar approach *versus* conventional microsurgical technique: a prospective, randomized, controlled study. J Neurosurg Spine 2009; 10(5): 476-85.
[http://dx.doi.org/10.3171/2008.7.17634] [PMID: 19442011]

[44]   Ruetten S, Komp M, Merk H, Godolias G. Full-endoscopic interlaminar and transforaminal lumbar

discectomy *versus* conventional microsurgical technique: a prospective, randomized, controlled study. Spine 2008; 33(9): 931-9.
[http://dx.doi.org/10.1097/BRS.0b013e31816c8af7] [PMID: 18427312]

[45] Ruetten S, Komp M, Merk H, Godolias G. Use of newly developed instruments and endoscopes: full-endoscopic resection of lumbar disc herniations *via* the interlaminar and lateral transforaminal approach. J Neurosurg Spine 2007; 6(6): 521-30.
[http://dx.doi.org/10.3171/spi.2007.6.6.2] [PMID: 17561740]

[46] Ruetten S, Komp M, Godolias G. A New full-endoscopic technique for the interlaminar operation of lumbar disc herniations using 6-mm endoscopes: prospective 2-year results of 331 patients. Minim Invasive Neurosurg 2006; 49(2): 80-7.
[http://dx.doi.org/10.1055/s-2006-932172] [PMID: 16708336]

[47] Schubert M, Hoogland T. Endoscopic transforaminal nucleotomy with foraminoplasty for lumbar disk herniation. Oper Orthop Traumatol 2005; 17(6): 641-61.
[http://dx.doi.org/10.1007/s00064-005-1156-9] [PMID: 16369758]

[48] Lee SH, Kang BU, Ahn Y, *et al.* Operative failure of percutaneous endoscopic lumbar discectomy: a radiologic analysis of 55 cases. Spine 2006; 31(10): E285-90.
[http://dx.doi.org/10.1097/01. brs.0000216446.13205.7a] [PMID: 16648734]

[49] Lee S, Kim SK, Lee SH, *et al.* Percutaneous endoscopic lumbar discectomy for migrated disc herniation: classification of disc migration and surgical approaches. Eur Spine J 2007; 16(3): 431-7.
[http://dx.doi.org/10.1007/s00586-006-0219-4] [PMID: 16972067]

[50] Lewandrowski KU. "Outside-in" technique, clinical results, and indications with transforaminal lumbar endoscopic surgery: a retrospective study on 220 patients on applied radiographic classification of foraminal spinal stenosis. Int J Spine Surg 2014; 8: 8.
[http://dx.doi.org/10.14444/1026] [PMID: 25694915]

[51] Ascher PW. Status quo and new horizons of laser therapy in neurosurgery. Lasers Surg Med 1985; 5(5): 499-506.
[http://dx.doi.org/10.1002/lsm.1900050509] [PMID: 4068883]

[52] Quigley MR, Maroon JC, Shih T, Elrifai A, Lesiecki ML. Laser discectomy. Comparison of systems. Spine 1994; 19(3): 319-22.
[http://dx.doi.org/10.1097/00007632-199402000-00011] [PMID: 8171364]

[53] Davis JK. Percutaneous discectomy improved with KTP laser. Clin Laser Mon 1990; 8(7): 105-6.
[PMID: 10149820]

[54] Casper GD, Hartman VL, Mullins LL. Percutaneous laser disc decompression with the holmium: YAG laser. J Clin Laser Med Surg 1995; 13(3): 195-203.
[http://dx.doi.org/10.1089/clm.1995.13.195] [PMID: 10150646]

[55] Yeung AT. The evolution of percutaneous spinal endoscopy and discectomy: state of the art. Mt Sinai J Med 2000; 67(4): 327-32.
[PMID: 11021785]

[56] Siebert WE. Percutaneous laser discectomy, state of the art reviews. Spine 1993; 7: 129-30.

[57] Mayer HM, Brock M, Berlien HP, Weber B. Percutaneous endoscopic laser discectomy (PELD). A new surgical technique for non-sequestrated lumbar discs. Acta Neurochir Suppl (Wien) 1992; 54: 53-8.
[http://dx.doi.org/10.1007/978-3-7091-6687-1_7] [PMID: 1595409]

[58] Hellinger J. Technical aspects of the percutaneous cervical and lumbar laser-disc-decompression and -nucleotomy. Neurol Res 1999; 21(1): 99-102.
[http://dx.doi.org/10.1080/01616412.1999.11740902] [PMID: 10048065]

[59] Yeung AT. The Evolution and Advancement of Endoscopic Foraminal Surgery: One Surgeon's Experience Incorporating Adjunctive Techologies. SAS J 2007; 1(3): 108-17.

[http://dx.doi.org/10.1016/S1935-9810(07)70055-5] [PMID: 25802587]

[60]   Ahn Y, Lee U. Expert Rev Med Devices. Use of lasers in minimally invasive spine surgery 2018; 15(6): 423-33.

[61]   Brouwer PA, Peul WC, Brand R, *et al.* Effectiveness of percutaneous laser disc decompression *versus* conventional open discectomy in the treatment of lumbar disc herniation; design of a prospective randomized controlled trial. BMC Musculoskelet Disord 2009; 10(1): 49.
[http://dx.doi.org/10.1186/1471-2474-10-49] [PMID: 19439098]

[62]   Brouwer PA, Brand R, van den Akker-van Marle ME, *et al.* Percutaneous laser disc decompression *versus* conventional microdiscectomy in sciatica: a randomized controlled trial. Spine J 2015; 15(5): 857-65.
[http://dx.doi.org/10.1016/j.spinee.2015.01.020] [PMID: 25614151]

[63]   Brouwer PA, Brand R, van den Akker-van Marle ME, *et al.* Percutaneous laser disc decompression *versus* conventional microdiscectomy for patients with sciatica: Two-year results of a randomised controlled trial. Interv Neuroradiol 2017; 23(3): 313-24.
[http://dx.doi.org/10.1177/1591019917699981] [PMID: 28454511]

[64]   Cselik Z, Aradi M, von Jako RA, *et al.* Impact of infrared laser light-induced ablation at different wavelengths on bovine intervertebral disc ex vivo: evaluation with magnetic resonance imaging and histology. Lasers Surg Med 2012; 44(5): 406-12.
[http://dx.doi.org/10.1002/lsm.22034] [PMID: 22532099]

[65]   van den Akker-van Marle ME, Brouwer PA, Brand R, *et al.* Percutaneous laser disc decompression *versus* microdiscectomy for sciatica: Cost utility analysis alongside a randomized controlled trial. Interv Neuroradiol 2017; 23(5): 538-45.
[http://dx.doi.org/10.1177/1591019917710297] [PMID: 28679342]

[66]   Chang MC. Sacral root injury during trans-sacral epiduroscopic laser decompression: A case report. Medicine (Baltimore) 2017; 96(42): e8326.
[http://dx.doi.org/10.1097/MD.0000000000008326] [PMID: 29049245]

[67]   Kobayashi S, Uchida K, Takeno K, *et al.* A case of nerve root heat injury induced by percutaneous laser disc decompression performed at an outside institution: technical case report. Neurosurgery 2007; 60(2 Suppl 1): ONSE171-2.
[http://dx.doi.org/10.1227/01.NEU.0000249228.82365.D2]

[68]   Pan F, Shen B, Chy SK, *et al.* Transforaminal endoscopic system technique for discogenic low back pain: A prospective Cohort study. Int J Surg 2016; 35: 134-8.
[http://dx.doi.org/10.1016/j.ijsu.2016.09.091] [PMID: 27693825]

[69]   Wang D, Nie Y, Jiang DG. [Reliving refractory pain of spinal metastasis patients with radiofrequency ablation through transforaminal endoscopy]. Zhonghua Yi Xue Za Zhi 2013; 93(29): 2321-3. [Reliving refractory pain of spinal metastasis patients with radiofrequency ablation through transforaminal endoscopy].
[PMID: 24300156]

[70]   Sairyo K, Kitagawa Y, Dezawa A. Percutaneous endoscopic discectomy and thermal annuloplasty for professional athletes. Asian J Endosc Surg 2013; 6(4): 292-7.
[http://dx.doi.org/10.1111/ases.12055] [PMID: 23968546]

[71]   Pereira P, Severo M, Monteiro P, *et al.* Results of Lumbar Endoscopic Adhesiolysis Using a Radiofrequency Catheter in Patients with Postoperative Fibrosis and Persistent or Recurrent Symptoms After Discectomy. Pain Pract 2016; 16(1): 67-79.
[http://dx.doi.org/10.1111/papr.12266] [PMID: 25470113]

[72]   Bellini M, Barbieri M. A comparison of non-endoscopic and endoscopic adhesiolysis of epidural fibrosis. Anaesthesiol Intensive Ther 2016; 48(4): 266-71.
[http://dx.doi.org/10.5603/AIT.a2016.0035] [PMID: 27595746]

[73] Choi G, Lee SH, Raiturker PP, Lee S, Chae YS. Percutaneous endoscopic interlaminar discectomy for intracanalicular disc herniations at L5-S1 using a rigid working channel endoscope. Neurosurgery 2006; 58(1) (Suppl.): ONS59-68.
[http://dx.doi.org/10.1227/01.NEU.0000362000.35742.3D] [PMID: 16479630]

[74] Choi G, Lee SH, Bhanot A, Raiturker PP, Chae YS. Percutaneous endoscopic discectomy for extraforaminal lumbar disc herniations: extraforaminal targeted fragmentectomy technique using working channel endoscope. Spine 2007; 32(2): E93-9.
[http://dx.doi.org/10.1097/01.brs.0000252093.31632.54] [PMID: 17224806]

[75] Kong L, Shang XF, Zhang WZ, *et al.* Percutaneous endoscopic lumbar discectomy and microsurgical laminotomy: A prospective, randomized controlled trial of patients with lumbar disc herniation and lateral recess stenosis. Orthopade 2018; •••
[http://dx.doi.org/10.1007/s00132-018-3610-z] [PMID: 30076437]

[76] Chen Z, Zhang L, Dong J, *et al.* Percutaneous transforaminal endoscopic discectomy compared with microendoscopic discectomy for lumbar disc herniation: 1-year results of an ongoing randomized controlled trial. J Neurosurg Spine 2018; 28(3): 300-10.
[http://dx.doi.org/10.3171/2017.7.SPINE161434] [PMID: 29303469]

[77] Choi KC, Lee JH, Kim JS, *et al.* Unsuccessful percutaneous endoscopic lumbar discectomy: a single-center experience of 10,228 cases. Neurosurgery 2015; 76(4): 372-80. discussion 380-1; quiz 381

[78] Choi KC, Kim JS, Kang BU, Lee CD, Lee SH. Changes in back pain after percutaneous endoscopic lumbar discectomy and annuloplasty for lumbar disc herniation: a prospective study. Pain Med 2011; 12(11): 1615-21.
[http://dx.doi.org/10.1111/j.1526-4637.2011.01250.x] [PMID: 21992543]

[79] Ahn Y, Lee SH, Park WM, Lee HY, Shin SW, Kang HY. Percutaneous endoscopic lumbar discectomy for recurrent disc herniation: surgical technique, outcome, and prognostic factors of 43 consecutive cases. Spine 2004; 29(16): E326-32.
[http://dx.doi.org/10.1097/01.BRS.0000134591.32462.98] [PMID: 15303041]

[80] Ahn Y, Lee SH, Lee SC, Shin SW, Chung SE. Factors predicting excellent outcome of percutaneous cervical discectomy: analysis of 111 consecutive cases. Neuroradiology 2004; 46(5): 378-84.
[http://dx.doi.org/10.1007/s00234-004-1197-z] [PMID: 15103434]

[81] Heo DH, Son SK, Eum JH, Park CK. Fully endoscopic lumbar interbody fusion using a percutaneous unilateral biportal endoscopic technique: technical note and preliminary clinical results. Neurosurg Focus 2017; 43(2): E8.
[http://dx.doi.org/10.3171/2017.5.FOCUS17146] [PMID: 28760038]

[82] Heo DH, Kim JS. Clinical and radiological outcomes of spinal endoscopic discectomy-assisted oblique lumbar interbody fusion: preliminary results. Neurosurg Focus 2017; 43(2): E13.
[http://dx.doi.org/10.3171/2017.5.FOCUS17196] [PMID: 28760027]

[83] Kim JS, Seong JH. Endoscope-assisted oblique lumbar interbody fusion for the treatment of cauda equina syndrome: a technical note. Eur Spine J 2017; 26(2): 397-403.
[http://dx.doi.org/10.1007/s00586-016-4902-9] [PMID: 27924416]

[84] Heo DH, Choi WS, Park CK, Kim JS. Minimally Invasive Oblique Lumbar Interbody Fusion with Spinal Endoscope Assistance: Technical Note. World Neurosurg 2016; 96: 530-6.
[http://dx.doi.org/10.1016/j.wneu.2016.09.033] [PMID: 27641264]

[85] De Antoni DJ, Claro ML, Poehling GG, Hughes SS. Translaminar lumbar epidural endoscopy: anatomy, technique, and indications. Arthroscopy 1996; 12(3): 330-4.
[http://dx.doi.org/10.1016/S0749-8063(96)90069-9] [PMID: 8783828]

[86] Destandau J. [Technical features of endoscopic surgery for lumbar disc herniation: 191 patients]. Neurochirurgie 2004; 50(1): 6-10.
[http://dx.doi.org/10.1016/S0028-3770(04)98300-2] [PMID: 15097915]

[87]   Akbary K, Kim JS, Park CW, Jun SG, Hwang JH. Biportal Endoscopic Decompression of Exiting and Traversing Nerve Roots Through a Single Interlaminar Window Using a Contralateral Approach: Technical Feasibilities and Morphometric Changes of the Lumbar Canal and Foramen. World Neurosurg 2018; 117: 153-61.
[http://dx.doi.org/10.1016/j.wneu.2018.05.111] [PMID: 29857220]

[88]   Choi KC, Shim HK, Hwang JS, *et al.* Comparison of Surgical Invasiveness Between Microdiscectomy and 3 Different Endoscopic Discectomy Techniques for Lumbar Disc Herniation. World Neurosurg 2018; 116: e750-8.
[http://dx.doi.org/10.1016/j.wneu.2018.05.085] [PMID: 29787880]

[89]   Hwa Eum J, Hwa Heo D, Son SK, Park CK. Percutaneous biportal endoscopic decompression for lumbar spinal stenosis: a technical note and preliminary clinical results. J Neurosurg Spine 2016; 24(4): 602-7.
[http://dx.doi.org/10.3171/2015.7.SPINE15304] [PMID: 26722954]

CHAPTER 2

Endoscopic Lumbar Discectomy – Anatomy, Indications and Techniques

Ji-Yeon Kim[1,*], Hyeun sung Kim[2], Kai-Uwe Lewandrowski[2,3,4] and Tae Jang[1]

[1] *Department of Neurosurgery, Nanoori Hospital, Seoul City, South Korea*

[2] *Center for Advanced Spine Care of Southern Arizona and Surgical Institute of Tucson, Tucson AZ, USA*

[3] *Associate Professor of Orthopaedic Surgery, Universidad Colsanitas, Bogota, Colombia, USA*

[4] *Visiting Professor, Department Orthopaedic Surgery, UNIRIO, Rio de Janeiro, Brazil*

Abstract: Various endoscopic spinal surgery techniques to remove herniated discs in the lumbar spine have gained popularity. The "inside-out" and "outside-in" transforaminal techniques have been employed extensively, and their clinical indications have expanded with the advances in video-imaging and endoscopic optical and surgical equipment. In this chapter, the authors review some of the relevant anatomical considerations the endoscopic spine surgeon should consider when scheduling a patient for endoscopic spinal surgery. The authors also present their most up-to-date knowledge of technological advances and new endoscopic surgery techniques to provide the reader with a snapshot of modern advancements of the established transforaminal "inside-out" and "outside-in" and interlaminar methods. This chapter sets the anatomical stage for many of the following chapters in this volume 2 of the Bentham text series on Contemporary Endoscopic Spinal Surgery.

Keywords: Endoscopic approaches & techniques, Foraminal anatomy.

INTRODUCTION

Until recently, microscopic lumbar discectomy has been a standard operation for lumbar disc surgery. Recently, percutaneous endoscopic lumbar discectomy has developed significantly [1 - 5]. Percutaneous endoscopic lumbar discectomy (PELD) can be classified into Transforaminal PELD [1, 6 - 15] and Interlaminar PELD [1, 16 - 21] according to the routes of access. And each method has its own advantages and disadvantages. In this chapter, the indications and anatomical considerations for various common clinical PELD scenario are discussed.

---

* **Corresponding author Ji-Yeon Kim:** Department of Neurosurgery, Nanoori Hospital, Seoul City, Republic of Korea; E-mail: soar1945@gmail.com

ANATOMICAL CONSIDERATIONS

Considering the anatomical aspect of transforaminal PELD, disc diseases can be divided into intra- and extracanalicular categories [22 - 25]. Among many surgical approaches, the surgeon should decide which nerve should be decompressed between exiting- or traversing nerve roots. The choice of preferred approach depends on the location and type of disc herniation. For example, extraforaminal disc herniation, foraminal disc herniation, and superior migrated disc herniation may be more accessible from the transforaminal approach. It may be more associated with higher postoperative dysesthesia rates and other neurologic complications than with interlaminar decompression of the traversing root [26]. Migrated disc may be challenging to remove using a rigid percutaneous endoscope. Because of these and other pertinent considerations, the endoscopic spine surgeon should be well and accurately informed about the operative field's anatomy.

Anatomical Classification of Percutaneous Endoscopic Approach (Fig. 1) [27]

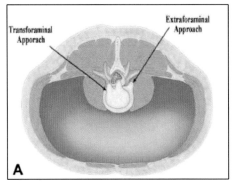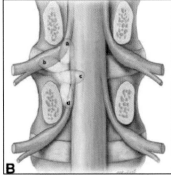

Fig. (1). Classification of percutaneous endoscopic lumbar discectomy. A. Anatomical, B. Neurological; a. superior migration, b. foraminal to far lateral, c. paracentral to central, d. inferior migration [32].

A. Extra-Foraminal Approach [2, 9, 28, 29]
  i. Far lateral Disc
B. Trans-foraminal Approach [6 - 15, 30, 31]
  i. Foraminal Disc
  ii. Superior Migration Disc
  iii. Inferior Migration Disc
  iv. Paracentral Disc
  v. Central Disc
C. Interlaminar Approach [16 - 21]
  1. Neurological Classification of Percutaneous Endoscopic Approach
    A. Exiting Root Approach

        i. Far Lateral Disc

        ii. Foraminal Disc

        iii. Superior Migration Disc

    B. Traversing Root Approach

        i. Paracentral Disc

        ii. Central

        iii. Inferior Migrated Disc

2. Surgery Related Classification of Percutaneous Endoscopic Approach (Fig. **2**)

    A. **Migration:** A migrated disc herniation was defined as a herniation, which was displaced away from the extrusion site, either above the endplate of the upper body, or below the endplate of the lower body.

        i. **High grade superior migration:** Far-upward From the inferior margin of upper pedicle to 3 mm below of the inferior margin of upper pedicle

        ii. **Low grade superior migration:** Near-upward From 3 mm below of the inferior margin of upper pedicle to the inferior margin of upper vertebral body

        iii. **Low grade inferior migration:** Near-downward From the superior margin of lower vertebral body to the center of lower pedicle

        iv. **High grade inferior migration:** Far-downward From the center to the inferior margin of lower pedicle

    B. **Canal Compromise:** Herniation exceeding 50% of the canal cross sectional area

        i. Mild

        ii. Severe

    C. **Iliac Crest:** lower part of upper vertebrae

        i. Low

        ii. High

    D. **Foraminal Stenosis:** Lateral flexion X-ray: between posterior margin of vertebrae to ventral margin of superior articular process of lower vertebrae

        i. Mild

        ii. Severe

        A. EQUIPMENT CONSIDERATION OF PELD

           1. Equipment of endoscope

              • Endoscope, working channel, suction-irrigation system, radiofrequency coagulator, video-endoscopy tower, stylet, guide needle, obturator, rongeur, forcep, punch, probe, drill, shaver [1, 13 - 15, 34 - 38].

           2. Working channel

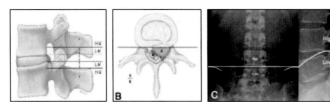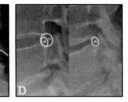

Fig. (2). Surgery related classification of percutaneous transforaminal lumbar discectomy [27 - 33]. A. migration (H-M: high-grade migration, L-M: low-grade migration), B. canal compromise: a, size of herniated disc; b, size of the spinal canal, C. iliac crest, D. foraminal stenosis: a; severe, b; mild.

Types of Percutaneous Endoscopic Lumbar Discectomy System Working Channel (Fig. 3)

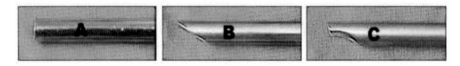

Fig. (3). Types of percutaneous endoscopic lumbar discectomy system working channel. A. Round type, B. Bevel type, C. Combination type.

A. Round type
- **Advantages**
  - Protection: Neural damage (Exiting / Traversing)
  - Protection: Structural encroaching (nerve / vessel / fat / muscle)
- **Disadvantages**
  - Difficulty in manipulation of the working channel
- **Indications**
  - Exiting root approach: Far lateral, foraminal, Superior migration
B. Bevel Type
- **Advantages**
  - Easy manipulation of the working channel after the learning curve is reached.
- **Disadvantages**
  - Learning curve:: foraminal work / working channel manipulation
  - Neural / Structural encroachment in operation field
- **Indication**
  - Traversing root approach
  - Interlaminar approach
C. Combination Type
- Easy for beginner: complex advantages of round type and bevel type

In the approach to decompress exiting nerve roots such as is used in the far lateral, foraminal, and superior migrated disc cases, a round working cannula is useful to protect the exiting nerve root and the easy exposure of the ruptured disc material. However, the other approach to decompress traversing nerve, especially for the highly inferior migrated or high canal compromised type cases, the bevel type working cannula is better than the round type because of easier working channel handling.

DIAGNOSIS

Thorough information about the pathological disc is necessary to succeed in PELD. More precise and detailed information about the pathologic disc can be acquired using the discogram combined with 3D reconstruction computerized tomography (CT) [30, 31]. It helps to check the radiological images during and immediately after surgery to remove the symptomatic surgical disc successfully (Figs. **4** - **8**).

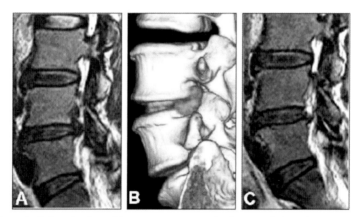

Fig. (4). L4-5 foraminal disc: In the exiting root approach, the far lateral disc, foraminal disc, and superior migration disc are usually accompanied by multiple fragmentations of the disc. A. Preoperative MRI, B. Images of 3D reconstruction CT with discogram, C. Postoperative MRI.

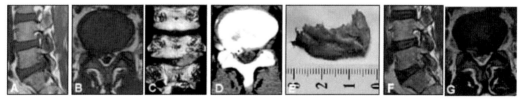

Fig. (5). L5-S1 Foraminal disc: In some cases, the foraminal disc looks smaller than expected, considering the severity of clinical symptoms. A, B. Preoperative MRI, C, D. Images of 3D reconstruction CT with discogram showing the large size of the ruptured disc, E, F, G. huge postoperative ruptured disc material and postoperative MRI.

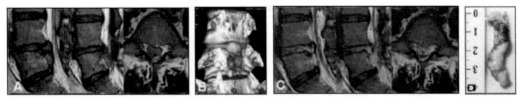

Fig. (6). L4-5 inferior migrated disc: **A.** Preoperative MRI, **B.** Images of 3D reconstruction CT with discogram showing an extensive un-fragmented ruptured disc material connected to the intervertebral disc space, **C, D.** Postoperative MRI, and huge ruptured disc material.

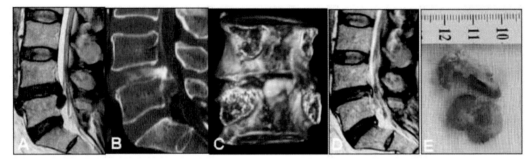

Fig. (7). L4-5 huge inferior migrated disc: In the cases of an inferior migrated disc, if the migrated disc material seems to be connected with the intervertebral space, migrated disc material should be checked more cautiously. **A.** Preoperative MRI: inferior migrated disc material appears to be associated with the intervertebral space, **B, C.** Images of a 3D reconstruction CT with a discogram showing the inferior migrated disc material which does not seem to be connected to the intervertebral disc space, **D.** Postoperative MRI, **E.** Postoperative extracted disc material reveal complete separation. If we finish the operation after taking the blood-tinged, huge, hard disc material, remained huge migrated disc material will induce remaining symptoms.

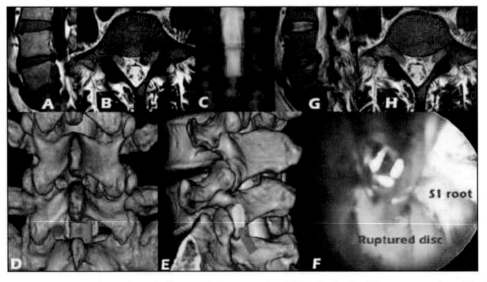

Fig. (8). L5-S1 superior migrated disc: **A,B.** Preoperative MRI, **C, D, E:** 3D reconstruction CT with myelogram, **F.** Intraoperative video image, **G, H.** Postoperative MRI.

PREPARATION

Set-up

In the operating room's standard set-up, we should check the relative positions of the surgeon, nurse, and instrument table position, and check the position of the X-ray and the video and image processing equipment (Fig. **9**).

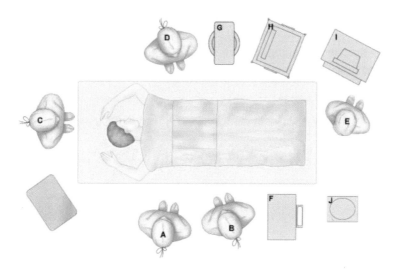

Fig. (9). Standard set-up of the operating room. **A.** Surgeon, **B.** Nurse, **C.** Anesthetist, **D.** X-ray technician, **E.** Technician, **F.** Instrument table, **G.** C-arc X-ray, **H.** Video equipment, **I.** Image processing, **J.** Suction irrigation equipment.

Position

Operation position in percutaneous endoscopic lumbar discectomy will be the prone position and recumbent position.

ANESTHESIA
< Anesthetic Methods for Percutaneous Endoscopic Lumbar Discectomy >

1. Local anesthesia
2. Interlaminar epidural anesthesia
   ○ Anesthetics: (levo) bupibacaine, lidocaine, mixed
   ○ Bleeding Control: Epinephrine
3. Transforaminal epidural anesthesia: Commonly used method

< Booster transforaminal epidural anesthetic method >

- **1ˢᵗ injection**
  - Transforaminal Space
  - Anesthetics: Lidocaine
  - Pain control
- **Additional injection**
  - 3~5 minutes after 1ˢᵗ injection
  - Anesthetics: epinephrine mixed Lidocaine
  - Additional pain control, Bleeding control
    1. General anesthesia

The protocols for general anesthesia applications are reviewed in other chapters of this Bentham three-volume series on contemporary spinal endoscopy techniques (Table **1**).

Table 1. Anesthetic methods for percutaneous endoscopic lumbar discectomy.

-	Local	Epidural		General
		Interlaminar	**Transforaminal**	
Pain Control	weak	moderate	moderate	strong
Neural Monitoring	good	moderate	moderate	weak

DISCUSSION

When considering an endoscopic decompression for a herniated disc, understanding the patient's anatomy is of utmost importance to effectively deploy modern endoscopic spinal surgery techniques and its associated equipment. In this chapter, the authors summarized the basics of the applied surgical anatomy the endoscopic spine surgeon should consider when selecting patients for the procedure. While there are many other chapters in this three-volume book series highlighting the technological advances that have prompted expansions of the surgical indications for endoscopic surgery of the spine, it remains undisputed that the underlying disease and the clinical decision making required to treat patients with the endoscopic surgery techniques successfully have remained unchanged. The problems clinicians face when treating patients with herniated disc and spinal stenosis in the central or lateral spinal canal are fundamentally the same as they apply to open and other forms of minimally invasive translaminar spine surgery. Endoscopic spine care focuses on diminishing the adverse side effects of traditional spine surgery related to tissue destruction, blood loss, postoperative pain, recovery from lengthy anesthesia, postoperative scarring, and instability of the spinal motion segment, to name a few. Other factors contributing to unfavorable long-term clinical outcomes with the open lumbar spine surgery may be related to arachnoiditis and the nerve roots' tethering *via* epidural fibrosis. In essence, endoscopic spine care is designed to accomplish neural element decompression at minimal short- and long-term burden to the patient. While this all seems obvious, the devil is in the detail, and understanding the anatomical factors at large whose appropriate treatment may be impacting clinical outcomes is of utmost importance. This team of authors has additional chapters in this volume 2 of the Bentham series on Contemporary Endoscopic Spinal Surgery, which carry the spirit of this anatomy, indications, and technical considerations chapter forward into discussing the specifics of the transforaminal and interlaminar endoscopic approaches to the lumbar spine.

CONCLUSION

The most practiced endoscopic surgical techniques to the lumbar spine are the inside-out and the outside-in approach. With the inside-out technique, the working cannular first is positioned into the intervertebral disc space. From there, it can be moved into the epidural space to accomplish further decompression. Annular windows and partial annular resections are practical tools to achieve this goal. The outside-in technique places the working cannula initially into the neuroforamen and thereby lateral to the dural sac. It requires a more reliable understanding of the applied endoscopic anatomy to carry the operation out safely. The endoscopic spine surgeon needs to acquire knowledge of the nerve roots' video endoscopic appearance to distinguish them from foraminal ligaments. The endoscopic view of a herniated disc, annular tears, bony stenosis stemming from osteophytosis of the facet joint, or the ring apophysis is distinctly different from the microsurgical visualization through the operating microscope. It takes some getting used to, mainly for the novice surgeon who does not have a lot of experience in endoscopy of other parts of the human body.

CONSENT FOR PUBLICATION

Not applicable.

CONFLICT OF INTEREST

The authors declare no conflict of interest, financial or otherwise.

ACKNOWLEDGEMENT

Declared none.

REFERENCES

[1]   Kim DH, Choi G, Lee SH. Endoscopic Spine Procedures. Thieme Medical Publishers 2011; p. 11.

[2]   Abdullah AF, Wolber PG, Warfield JR, Gunadi IK. Surgical management of extreme lateral lumbar disc herniations: review of 138 cases. Neurosurgery 1988; 22(4): 648-53.
[http://dx.doi.org/10.1227/00006123-198804000-00005] [PMID: 3374776]

[3]   Ahn Y, Lee SH, Park WM, Lee HY, Shin SW, Kang HY. Percutaneous endoscopic lumbar discectomy for recurrent disc herniation: surgical technique, outcome, and prognostic factors of 43 consecutive cases. Spine 2004; 29(16): E326-32.
[http://dx.doi.org/10.1097/01.BRS.0000134591.32462.98] [PMID: 15303041]

[4]   McCulloch JA. Principles of Microsurgery for Lumbar Disc Diseases. New York: Raven Press 1989.

[5]   Mekhail N, Kapural L. Intradiscal thermal annuloplasty for discogenic pain: an outcome study. Pain Pract 2004; 4(2): 84-90.
[http://dx.doi.org/10.1111/j.1533-2500.2004.04203.x] [PMID: 17166191]

[6]   Ditsworth DA. Endoscopic transforaminal lumbar discectomy and reconfiguration: a postero-lateral approach into the spinal canal. Surg Neurol 1998; 49(6): 588-97.
[http://dx.doi.org/10.1016/S0090-3019(98)00004-4] [PMID: 9637618]

[7]   Tsou PM, Yeung AT. Transforaminal endoscopic decompression for radiculopathy secondary to intracanal noncontained lumbar disc herniations: outcome and technique. Spine J 2002; 2(1): 41-8.
[http://dx.doi.org/10.1016/S1529-9430(01)00153-X] [PMID: 14588287]

[8]   Tsou PM, Alan Yeung C, Yeung AT. Posterolateral transforaminal selective endoscopic discectomy and thermal annuloplasty for chronic lumbar discogenic pain: a minimal access visualized intradiscal surgical procedure. Spine J 2004; 4(5): 564-73.
[http://dx.doi.org/10.1016/j.spinee.2004.01.014] [PMID: 15363430]

[9]   Ruetten S, Komp M, Godolias G. An extreme lateral access for the surgery of lumbar disc herniations inside the spinal canal using the full-endoscopic uniportal transforaminal approach-technique and prospective results of 463 patients. Spine 2005; 30(22): 2570-8.
[http://dx.doi.org/10.1097/01.brs.0000186327.21435.cc] [PMID: 16284597]

[10]   Jasper GP, Francisco GM, Telfeian AE. Endoscopic transforaminal discectomy for an extruded lumbar disc herniation. Pain Physician 2013; 16(1): E31-5.
[PMID: 23340542]

[11]   Eustacchio S, Flaschka G, Trummer M, Fuchs I, Unger F. Endoscopic percutaneous transforaminal treatment for herniated lumbar discs. Acta Neurochir (Wien) 2002; 144(10): 997-1004.
[http://dx.doi.org/10.1007/s00701-002-1003-9] [PMID: 12382128]

[12]   Gibson JN, Cowie JG, Iprenburg M. Transforaminal endoscopic spinal surgery: the future 'gold standard' for discectomy? - A review. Surgeon 2012; 10(5): 290-6.
[http://dx.doi.org/10.1016/j.surge.2012.05.001] [PMID: 22705355]

[13]   Yeung AT, Tsou PM. Posterolateral endoscopic excision for lumbar disc herniation: Surgical technique, outcome, and complications in 307 consecutive cases. Spine 2002; 27(7): 722-31.
[http://dx.doi.org/10.1097/00007632-200204010-00009] [PMID: 11923665]

[14]   Yeung AT, Yeung CA. Advances in endoscopic disc and spine surgery: foraminal approach. Surg Technol Int 2003; 11: 255-63.
[PMID: 12931309]

[15]   Yeung AT. The evolution of percutaneous spinal endoscopy and discectomy: state of the art. Mt Sinai J Med 2000; 67(4): 327-32.
[PMID: 11021785]

[16]   Maroon JC. Current concepts in minimally invasive discectomy. Neurosurgery 2002; 51(5) (Suppl.): S137-45.

[PMID: 12234441]

[17]   Kim HS, Park JY. Comparative assessment of different percutaneous endoscopic interlaminar lumbar discectomy (PEID) techniques. Pain Physician 2013; 16(4): 359-67.
[PMID: 23877452]

[18]   Choi G, Lee SH, Raiturker PP, Lee S, Chae YS. Percutaneous endoscopic interlaminar discectomy for intracanalicular disc herniations at L5-S1 using a rigid working channel endoscope. Neurosurgery 2006; 58(1) (Suppl.): ONS59-68.
[http://dx.doi.org/10.1227/01.NEU.0000362000.35742.3D] [PMID: 16479630]

[19]   Ruetten S, Komp M, Godolias G. A New full-endoscopic technique for the interlaminar operation of lumbar disc herniations using 6-mm endoscopes: prospective 2-year results of 331 patients. Minim Invasive Neurosurg 2006; 49(2): 80-7.
[http://dx.doi.org/10.1055/s-2006-932172] [PMID: 16708336]

[20]   Ruetten S, Komp M, Merk H, Godolias G. Use of newly developed instruments and endoscopes: full-endoscopic resection of lumbar disc herniations *via* the interlaminar and lateral transforaminal approach. J Neurosurg Spine 2007; 6(6): 521-30.
[http://dx.doi.org/10.3171/spi.2007.6.6.2] [PMID: 17561740]

[21]   Ruetten S, Komp M, Merk H, Godolias G. Full-endoscopic interlaminar and transforaminal lumbar discectomy *versus* conventional microsurgical technique: a prospective, randomized, controlled study. Spine 2008; 33(9): 931-9.
[http://dx.doi.org/10.1097/BRS.0b013e31816c8af7] [PMID: 18427312]

[22]   Soldner F, Hoelper BM, Wallenfang T, Behr R. The translaminar approach to canalicular and cranio-dorsolateral lumbar disc herniations. Acta Neurochir (Wien) 2002; 144(4): 315-20.
[http://dx.doi.org/10.1007/s007010200043] [PMID: 12021876]

[23]   Birbilis T, Koulalis D, Matis G, Theodoropoulou E, Papaparaskeva K. Microsurgical muscle-splitting approach for extracanalicular lumbar disc herniation: an analysis of 28 consecutive cases. Acta Orthop Belg 2009; 75(1): 70-4.
[PMID: 19358402]

[24]   Huber P, Reulen HJ. CT-observations of the intra- and extracanalicular disc herniation. Acta Neurochir (Wien) 1989; 100(1-2): 3-11.
[http://dx.doi.org/10.1007/BF01405267] [PMID: 2816531]

[25]   Reulen HJ, Pfaundler S, Ebeling U. The lateral microsurgical approach to the "extracanalicular" lumbar disc herniation. I: A technical note. Acta Neurochir (Wien) 1987; 84(1-2): 64-7.
[http://dx.doi.org/10.1007/BF01456353] [PMID: 3825610]

[26]   Min JH, Kang SH, Lee JB, Cho TH, Suh JK, Rhyu IJ. Morphometric analysis of the working zone for endoscopic lumbar discectomy. J Spinal Disord Tech 2005; 18(2): 132-5.
[http://dx.doi.org/10.1097/01.bsd.0000159034.97246.4f] [PMID: 15800429]

[27]   Choi G, Lee SH, Lokhande P, *et al.* Percutaneous endoscopic approach for highly migrated intracanal disc herniations by foraminoplastic technique using rigid working channel endoscope. Spine 2008; 33(15): E508-15.
[http://dx.doi.org/10.1097/BRS.0b013e31817bfa1a] [PMID: 18594449]

[28]   Choi G, Lee SH, Bhanot A, Raiturker PP, Chae YS. Percutaneous endoscopic discectomy for extraforaminal lumbar disc herniations: extraforaminal targeted fragmentectomy technique using working channel endoscope. Spine 2007; 32(2): E93-9.
[http://dx.doi.org/10.1097/01.brs.0000252093.31632.54] [PMID: 17224806]

[29]   Epimenio RO, Giancarlo D, Giuseppe T, Raffaelino R, Luigi F. Extraforaminal lumbar herniation: "far lateral" microinvasive approach retrospective study. J Spinal Disord Tech 2003; 16(6): 534-8.
[http://dx.doi.org/10.1097/00024720-200312000-00009] [PMID: 14657751]

[30]   Kim HS, Ju CI, Kim SW, Kim JG. Endoscopic transforaminal suprapedicular approach in high grade

inferior migrated lumbar disc herniation. J Korean Neurosurg Soc 2009; 45(2): 67-73.
[http://dx.doi.org/10.3340/jkns.2009.45.2.67] [PMID: 19274114]

[31]   Chae KH, Ju CI, Lee SM, Kim BW, Kim SY, Kim HS. Strategies for Noncontained Lumbar Disc Herniation by an Endoscopic Approach : Transforaminal Suprapedicular Approach, Semi-Rigid Flexible Curved Probe, and 3-Dimensional Reconstruction CT with Discogram. J Korean Neurosurg Soc 2009; 46(4): 312-6.
[http://dx.doi.org/10.3340/jkns.2009.46.4.312] [PMID: 19893718]

[32]   Ahn Y. Transforaminal percutaneous endoscopic lumbar discectomy: technical tips to prevent complications. Expert Rev Med Devices 2012; 9(4): 361-6.
[http://dx.doi.org/10.1586/erd.12.23] [PMID: 22905840]

[33]   Lee S, Kim SK, Lee SH, *et al.* Percutaneous endoscopic lumbar discectomy for migrated disc herniation: classification of disc migration and surgical approaches. Eur Spine J 2007; 16(3): 431-7.
[http://dx.doi.org/10.1007/s00586-006-0219-4] [PMID: 16972067]

[34]   Kambin P, Vaccaro A. Arthroscopic microdiscectomy. Spine J 2003; 3(3) (Suppl.): 60S-4S.
[http://dx.doi.org/10.1016/S1529-9430(02)00558-2] [PMID: 14589219]

[35]   Kambin P, Savitz MH. Arthroscopic microdiscectomy: an alternative to open disc surgery. Mt Sinai J Med 2000; 67(4): 283-7.
[PMID: 11021778]

[36]   Kambin P, O'Brien E, Zhou L, Schaffer JL. Arthroscopic microdiscectomy and selective fragmentectomy. Clin Orthop Relat Res 1998; (347): 150-67.
[PMID: 9520885]

[37]   Kambin P, Zhou L. Arthroscopic discectomy of the lumbar spine. Clin Orthop Relat Res 1997; 337: 49-57.
[http://dx.doi.org/10.1097/00003086-199704000-00007] [PMID: 9137176]

[38]   Kambin P, Zhou L. History and current status of percutaneous arthroscopic disc surgery. Spine 1996; 21(24) (Suppl.): 57S-61S.
[http://dx.doi.org/10.1097/00007632-199612151-00006] [PMID: 9112325]

CHAPTER 3

Patient Reported Outcome Measures, Nomenclature & Classifications in Clinical Research of Endoscopic Spine Surgery

Kai-Uwe Lewandrowski[1,2,3,*], **Álvaro Dowling**[4,5], **Said G Osman**[6], **Jin-Sung Kim**[7], **Stefan Hellinger**[8], **Nimar Salari**[9], **Rômulo Pedroza Pinheiro**[10], **Ramon Torres**[11] and **Anthony Yeung**[12]

[1] *Center for Advanced Spine Care of Southern Arizona and Surgical Institute of Tucson, Tucson AZ, USA*

[2] *Associate Professor of Orthopaedic Surgery, Universidad Colsanitas, Bogota, Colombia, USA*

[3] *Visiting Professor, Department Neurosurgery, UNIRIO, Rio de Janeiro, Brazil*

[4] *Endoscopic Spine Clinic, Santiago, Chile*

[5] *Department of Orthopaedic Surgery, USP, Ribeirão Preto, Brazil*

[6] *Sky Spine Endoscopy Institute 1003 W 7th St, Frederick, MD 21701, USA*

[7] *Professor, Spine Center, Department of Neurosurgery, Seoul St. Mary's Hospital, College of Medicine, The Catholic University of Korea 222 Banpo Daero, Seocho-gu, Seoul, 137-701, Korea*

[8] *Department of Orthopedic Surgery, Isar Hospital, Munich, Germany*

[9] *Desert Institute for Spine Care, Phoenix, AZ, USA*

[10] *Orthopeadic Spine Surgery Department of Orthopedics and Anestesiology, Ribeirão Preto Medical School, University of São Paulo. Ribeirão Preto - SP, Brazil*

[11] *Orthopedic Surgeon/ Spine Surgery Fellowship,, Universidad de Chile, Instituto Traumatologico, Santiago, Chile*

[12] *Clinical Professor, University of New Mexico School of Medicine, Albuquerque, New Mexico Desert Institute for Spine Care, Phoenix, AZ, USA*

Abstract: Uniform use of nomenclature and classification systems appears logical to anyone attempting to systematically study clinical outcomes with new emerging technology applications in spine surgery. At the introduction of spinal endoscopy into routine clinical practice, today's key opinion leaders introduced nomenclature conducive to the description of their innovations at the time. With endoscopy of the spine becoming more mainstream several authors have pushed classification systems

---

* Corresponding author Kai-Uwe Lewandrowski: Center for Advanced Spine Care of Southern Arizona and Surgical Institute of Tucson, Tucson, AZ, USA, Department of Orthopaedic Surgery, UNIRIO, Rio de Janeiro, Brazil and Department of Orthoapedic Surgery, Fundación Universitaria Sanitas, Bogotá, D.C., Colombia, USA; Tel: +1 520 204-1495; Fax: +1 623 218-1215; E-mail: business@tucsonspine.com

Kai-Uwe Lewandrowski, Jorge Felipe Ramírez León, Anthony Yeung, Hyeun-Sung Kim, Xifeng Zhang, Gun Choi, Stefan Hellinger and Álvaro Dowling (Eds.)
All rights reserved-© 2022 Bentham Science Publishers

for clinical outcome studies. Others have introduced terminology in hopes of them being adopted to further research and health care policy agendas. These nomenclature and classification systems' practicality in routine clinical practice may be debatable and perhaps be considered by some an academic exercise. However, the need for some common language and categorization of descriptors of painful pathology, confounding factors, and their treatments are accepted by most. This chapter summarizes the literature on nomenclature, terminology, and classification systems relevant to clinical outcome research in spinal endoscopy. It was motivated by the desire to formalize its clinical outcome research, bring it up to par with traditional translaminar spine surgery techniques, and, ultimately, incorporate it into clinical treatment and coverage guidelines formulated by spine societies and payors.

Keywords: Classification, Clinical outcome research, Nomenclature, Spinal endoscopy, Terminology.

INTRODUCTION

The pioneers of endoscopic spine surgery techniques started reporting their clinical outcomes in the late 1980s and early 1990s. At the time, there was not much interest in the procedure, and it was carried out by a few who fought an uphill battle against the proponents of traditional open spinal surgery techniques, which at the time itself were relatively new. Pedicle screws had just been introduced, and their widespread application was challenged in a class-action lawsuit in the early 1990ies. Ultimately, one of the pioneering physicians and President of the North American Spine Society at the time, Dr. Hansen Yuan, recognized the overwhelming benefit of this technology for patients and spearheaded the defense against the trial lawyers. He orchestrated the formulation of clinical treatment guidelines, which ultimately formed the basis for modern spinal surgery, based on alleviating pain by surgical freeing-up of compressed neural elements and stabilizing instability and deformity. The media attention was horrendous and spinal endoscopy appeared to be the stepchild of the public debate of indications and clinical outcomes with modern spine surgery. That debate intensified in the early 2000s, highlighting the need for more formalized outcome research to make a case for selective endoscopic treatment of validated pain generators rather than image-based treatment guidelines focusing on stenosis, instability, and deformity. The senior authors of this chapter lived through these tumultuous times and argued the case for spinal endoscopy in many debates in his local community and on a national and international level. He published the up to date most widely cited article on selective endoscopic lumbar discectomy in 2003. Some 20 years later, many of today's spinal endoscopy proponents benefit from these earlier arguments. However, the debate on whether it is appropriate to replace traditional open, translaminar, and other forms of minimally invasive spine surgeries with endoscopy continues.

WIDELY USED CLINICAL OUTCOME TOOLS

Patient-reported outcome measures (PROM) frequently used in spine outcome research include the visual analog score (VAS) [1 - 12] and the Oswestry Disability Index (ODI) [13 - 18]. Understanding the ability of these PROM scores to detect improvements in health status resulting from an intervention meaningful to the patient is critical to support conclusions in favor of one treatment over another. The VAS is a ten-digit integer score from 0 (no pain) to 10 (worst pain imaginable) [12]. The ODI is a ten-item composite instrument. It assesses pain intensity, personal care, and function, including walking, lifting, personal care, sitting, standing, sleeping, social interaction, and traveling [19 - 22]. Each ODI item is scored from 0 (no impairment) to 5 (worst impairment). Then, the scores are summed up and then multiplied by two to obtain the ODI index ranging from 0 to 100. The Macnab criteria are commonly used in spinal endoscopy outcome studies [23, 24]. Briefly, follow-up outcome results are classified as Excellent when the patient experiences little pain, and can perform desired activities with few limitations. Good Macnab outcomes are defined when the patient complains of occasional pain or dysesthesia but can perform daily activities with minor restrictions and did not need pain medication. Fair Macnab outcomes are assigned when the pain level is somewhat improved but a continued to need pain medication exists. Poor Macnab outcomes describe a patient with worse function or in need of additional surgery to address symptoms. Another way to best stratify clinical improvements in clinical research is the anchor-based approach by calculating a patient satisfaction index based on a modification of the Macnab criteria [23 - 25]. At each follow-up visit and final follow up, patients may be asked to determine whether the 1) the endoscopic surgery met their expectations, have little pain, and can perform desired activities with few limitations (Excellent), 2) the endoscopic surgery met their expectations, have occasional pain or sensory problems, but I can perform daily activities with minor restrictions and do not take pain medication (Good), 3) the endoscopic surgery met their expectations, with somewhat improved pain, but continue to need pain medication (Fair), and 4) their expectations were not met by the endoscopic surgery, and are worse off or needed additional surgery. (Poor). The patient satisfaction index can then be dichotomized considering patients with Excellent, Good, and Fair outcomes as "Improved" and with Poor outcomes as "Failed." Then, the dichotomization results can be used in the anchor approach in a receiver operating characteristic (ROC) analysis with the area under the curve (AUC) to assess the quality of the numerical ODI and VAS PROMs to measure patient satisfaction as a result of the transforaminal endoscopic decompression procedure.

Unquestionably, these PROMs are helpful to improve patients' participation in the management of their health issues. The judgment of such improvements or the lack thereof may be influenced by a patient's demographic, geographical, and cultural factors. Additional prejudice may come from differences in disease baseline severity, recall bias of the intrinsic nature of the patient's condition before the intervention. Instead of comparing the postoperative against the preoperative functional status, a moving goal post dynamic is frequently encountered as patients' often report their improvements by making a comparison to their present-day expectations [26], or the functional status of their "normal" peers [27] and fall victim to recall bias by failing to remember the prior extent of their intrinsic spinal disability honestly [28]. Hence, the retrospective VAS and ODI comparisons are inherently imprecise, and statistically significant differences in outcomes may, in fact, not be clinically meaningful or relevant. To circumvent these problems, Jaeschke developed the minimal clinically important difference score (MCID) in 1989 [29]. As outlined in the following, the MCID is determined as the threshold value of a spine care outcome instrument that spine surgeons and their patients perceive as clinically meaningful.

MINIMAL CLINICALLY IMPORTANT DIFFERENCE SCORE

The concept of a staged endoscopic management [30, 31] of lumbar degenerative spine disease has been employed by the authors and published in various clinical studies [32 - 35]. These studies demonstrated longer-lasting symptom relief when compared to non-surgical and pain management ablation options, which by their nature are intended as an intermediate step before considering surgery by providing a temporary reduction of symptoms [36]. These management concepts are distinctly different from the image-based threshold criteria employed by many traditionally trained spine surgeons who utilize them to define the surgical indication for correcting symptoms stemming from spinal stenosis, deformity, and instability. With these criteria, many patients received surgical treatment when the degenerative spine disease has reached its end-stage, at which point an aggressive instrumented fusion is often performed. An unbiased assessment of the outcome results is needed to prove the clinical advantage of an early and staged endoscopic spine care program. Therefore, this team of authors investigated the MCIDs with VAS and ODI in transforaminal endoscopic spinal surgery patients to validate these commonly used PROMs and to improve the clinicians' ability to identify those endoscopic treatments of common painful conditions of the lumbar spine associated with better clinical outcomes when directly compared with traditional open translaminar surgeries.

The MCID was defined by Jaeschke "…. The slightest difference in score in the domain of interest which patients perceive as beneficial and which would mandate, in the absence of troublesome side effects and high cost, a change in the patient's management" [29]. The MCID can be calculated in many ways. The shift in clinician reporting, disease state, clinical parameters, effect size, baseline, and postintervention data from patients may be anchored to external criteria such as the patient satisfaction index (PSI) employed by the authors (Table **1**). Alternatively, the outcome measurement may be anchored to another instrument's internal values (distribution approach). MCIDs are not static numbers and are heavily influenced by a myriad of patient demographic factors, the individual baseline severity of the disease, the dynamic of a recall bias of the intrinsic nature of their initial condition while comparing the current functional status against expectations which are heavily impacted by the performed procedure and the public perceptions about it. The severity or extent of the baseline symptoms [36], and differences between age, education, or socioeconomic status of study populations may also influence the MCID [37 - 39]. The impact of these variations may carry forward and play out in expectation-driven patient response measures and therefore render different MCID values and ranges for other spine procedures [36]. One of the most relevant and everyday problems, though, is patients' inability to understand the context of improvement [40]. This problem more complex or lengthy outcome instruments that consist of multiple questions with many multiple choice answers. The ODI, for example, is a ten-item instrument *versus* the VAS being a single integer instrument from 0 to 10. The more complex ODI can induce more recall bias than the simple VAS score. One could contemplate how patients' understanding of the proper context of improvement may be more impaired with lengthier instruments, such as the SF-36.

The authors' MCID data analysis studies on 406 lumbar endoscopic spine surgery patients were anchored in the dichotomized patient satisfaction index, which showed postoperative improvement in 92.9% of patients who underwent the transforaminal endoscopic decompression procedure (Table **1**). Our postintervention data from our postoperative endoscopic decompression patients were anchored to external Macnab criteria defined as the patient satisfaction index (PSI; Table **1**). Patients were deemed "improved" with *Excellent, Good*, and *Fair* Macnab outcomes, and deemed "failed" with *Poor* Macnab outcomes.

Table 1. Outcomes by modified Macnab criteria, and dichotomized PSI* (n = 406).

MacNab Outcomes	Frequency	Percent	Valid Percent	Cumulative Percent
Excellent	224	55.2	55.2	55.2
Good	112	27.6	27.6	92.9
Fair	41	10.1	10.1	65.3
Poor	29	7.1	7.1	100.0
Total	406	100.0	100.0	-

(Table 1) cont.....

MacNab Outcomes	Frequency	Percent	Valid Percent	Cumulative Percent
Dichotomized PSI	Frequency	Percent	Valid Percent	Cumulative Percent
Improved	377	92.9	92.9	92.9
Failed	29	7.1	7.1	100.0
Total	406	100.0	100.0	-

*PSI – Patient Satisfaction Index

The PROMs also showed statistically significant reductions (p < 0.0001) from a mean preoperative VAS of 8.0813 to a mean postoperative VAS score of 2.2463. The ODI reductions were equally significant (p < 0.0001) from a mean preoperative ODI of 47.46 to a mean postoperative ODI score of 13.98 (Table **2**).

Table 2. VAS and ODI Paired Samples Statistics (n = 406).

-	Mean	N	Std. Deviation	Std. Error Mean
Preoperative VAS	8.0813	406	1.46255	.07259
Postoperative VAS	2.2463	406	1.55823	.07733
Preoperative ODI	47.46	406	8.624	.428
Postoperative ODI	13.98	406	6.197	.308

Paired Differences		95% Confidence Interval of the Difference					
Mean	Std. Dev	Std. Error Mean	Lower	Upper	t	df	Sig. (2-tailed)
5.83498	2.09287	.10387	5.63079	6.03916	56.177	405	< .0001
33.478	10.659	.529	32.438	34.518	63.287	405	< .0001

The Receiver Operating Characteristic (ROC) curve plots for both the VAS and ODI PROMs corroborated this problem (Figs. **1** and **2**). The area under the curve (AUC) is proportional to the percentage of randomly drawn pairs, which were correctly identified as having a determined outcome or not. Employing previously published criteria [41], the AUC analysis for both PROMs of this study showed that the single integer VAS score had excellent accuracy (area 0.926) compared to the ODI, which produced only fair accuracy (area 0.751) in assessing MCID with the transforaminal endoscopic decompression procedure.

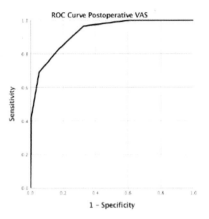

Fig. (1). Receiver operating characteristic (ROC) curve for postoperative <u>Visual Analog Scale</u> (VAS) scores given by patients who underwent outpatient transforaminal endoscopic decompression surgery. The area under the curve was 0.926 with an asymptotic 95% confidence interval lower limit of 0.882 and upper limit of 0.97.

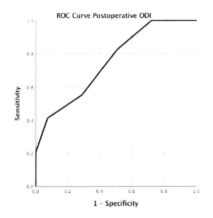

Fig. (2). Receiver operating characteristic (ROC) curve for postoperative <u>Oswestry Disablity Index</u> (ODI) scores given by patients who underwent outpatient transforaminal endoscopic decompression surgery. The area under the curve was 0.751 with an asymptotic 95% confidence interval lower limit of 0.663 and upper limit of 0.840.

The sought specificity and sensitivity dictate the MCID calculation. Therefore, reporting rigid MCID makes little sense [40]. Outcome instruments should have a sensitivity and a specificity of 1, translating into a false positive rate (1−specificity) of zero [40]. The ROC curve's upper left corner is typically closest to this situation (Figs. **1** and **2**). A Youden index may be calculated in cases where sensitivity and specificity are diagnostically equally important. The optimal cutoff or MCID threshold value is where the Youden index is closest to one as represented in the ROC-curve. Meaningful MCIDs for the VAS score reduction were determined between 2.5 to 3.5 and for ODI score reductions between 14 and 17. These VAS and ODI MCID numbers are known to be context-specific [28] to the transforaminal endoscopic procedure.

A recent meta-analysis on full endoscopic decompression for lumbar central and lateral recess stenosis using the interlaminar approach analyzed context-specific VAS and ODI MCIDs [42]. This meta-analysis could have overestimated the VAS and ODI reductions (ODI 41.71; 95% CI, 39.80-43.62, VAS leg 5.95; 95% CI, 5.70-6.21, and VAS back 4.22; 95% CI, 3.88-4.56) since they were statistically significantly higher than the MCIDs reported by its specific studies. The original studies employing other types of lumbar decompression procedures for sciatica-type low back and leg pain reported PROM reductions and MCIDs similar to ours. This MCID discussion highlights the need for context-driven analysis of the indications and appropriate timing of surgical spine care when employing the transforaminal endoscopic decompression surgery in patients who will report their improvements from their biased point of view with shifting expectations. Therefore, the MCID discussion with commonly used PROMS with the endoscopic spine care is timely and more relevant than ever.

ENDOSCOPIC CLASSIFICATION OF STENOSIS

The most common indication for spinal endoscopy in the lumbar spine is foraminal and lateral recess stenosis. Depending on the painful compressive pathology location, the patient may complain of sciatica in the dermatomal distribution of the traversing or exiting nerve root. Traversing nerve root pain syndromes are typically more common as exiting nerve root pain syndromes as the latter are primarily caused by extraforaminal herniations or facet joint cysts that may lead to chronic inflammation of the dorsal root ganglion. In such cases, symptoms may seemingly be out of proportion to the compressive pathology's extent on the corresponding advanced imaging studies. As discussed in other areas of this text, mechanical compression of neural elements is one of many reasons why patients may present with sciatica. Other pain generators that may escape detection by the routine MRI scan exist and should be considered in the differential diagnosis of sciatica-type low back and leg pain when assessing such patients for intervention. Examples of such poorly visualized pain generators frequently missed by the MRI scan include toxic annular tears, small facet cysts, intradiscal fissuring, cavitation, and end-stage degeneration with vacuum disc and vertical instability. Foraminal adhesions or tethering of the nerve roots from contracted foraminal ligaments or older burned-out inflammatory processes are other examples that demonstrated the need to stratify patients by the nature of the painful pathoanatomy. Attempting the reduce the medical necessity determination for intervention and surgery to just mechanical compression of the neural elements will fail many patients who are otherwise eligible for treatment and have a good chance for improvement if treated appropriately.

It is only logical for the endoscopic spine surgeon to associate what is seen during direct video endoscopic visualization in surgery with the MRI image correlate. Communicating and justifying the need for the endoscopic lumbar spine surgery in patients without prominent MRI findings takes this debate straight to the controversy's center. Experienced endoscopic spine surgeons understand the diagnostic gap with routine MRI scans whose current protocols are not sensitive enough to detect many pain generators responsive to endoscopic treatment. Nonetheless, reverting to MRI descriptors of spinal stenosis is essentially the only way to substantiate the endoscopic treatment of painful conditions of the lumbar spine since the MRI images compared to endoscopic views are well-understood by most surgeons. Therefore, many key opinion leaders of endoscopic spine surgery have published MRI descriptors of the surgical pathology. One example is Lee's foraminal stenosis classification within the neuroforamen. To stratify patients for the most straightforward endoscopic approach technique, Lee *et al*. divided the neuroforamen from medial to lateral into the entry (dura to pedicle; zone 1), middle (medial pedicle wall to center pedicle; zone 2), and exit zone (center pedicle to the lateral border of the facet joint; zone 3) [43]. Surgeons further classify foraminal and lateral recess stenosis according to the primary offending pathology as an extruded herniated disc or a disc bulge with or without associated stenosis from osteophytosis or ligament hypertrophy. The North American Spine Society has published their stenosis guidelines where a herniated disc classification is best described [44]. For the endoscopic spine surgeon, the disc herniation's size and direction are often more critical than any other factor since these two descriptors of a herniated disc may impact the surgeon's ability to reach this painful pathology with the endoscope. With these considerations in mind, Lee and Kim *et al*. studied their outcomes when they classified disc herniations as upward, downward, migrated, or centered around this disc space using a four-zone classification [46]. The authors treated near-migrated disc herniations classified as those within proximity to the disc space with what they coined as the "half-and-half" technique. This technique involves positioning a beveled working sheath across the disc space to the epidural space. Far-migrated discs, on the other hand, were preferentially treated with the "epiduroscopic" technique. The latter technique involves introducing the endoscope into the epidural space entirely. Employing these two endoscopic techniques, the authors achieved consistent clinical improvements in their 116 patients with lumbar disc herniations [45]. Besides the location of migrated disc herniations, Hasegawa analyzed foraminal and posterior disc height in cadaver dissections and posthumously correlated these numbers with observations on lumbar imaging studies and the former patients' clinical records [46]. Foraminal height of less than 15 mm and a posterior intervertebral disc height of less than 3 mm were considered evidence of spinal stenosis. The medical records review done by Hasegawa did confirm that the mere presence of spinal stenosis is not always associated with sciatica or claudication symptoms. However, the aforementioned cut-off parameters of reduced foraminal stenosis or posterior intervertebral disc height were associated with symptomatic spinal stenosis in some 80% of examined patients. The MRI classification system published by Pfirrmann *et al.* is routinely used to MRI appearance of disc degeneration [47]. However, it has found little use amongst endoscopic spine surgeon since their focus the endoscopic treatment of painful pathology and not of the MRI scan. No correlative analysis of endoscopic visualized intradiscal pathology with the MRI appearance of the various Pfirmann grades has been published to the author's knowledge and it seems unlikely that the Pfirmann classification will gain more traction amongst endoscopic spine surgeons when stratifying patients for endoscopic surgery. However, another MRI classification published by Lee *et al.* may be of more relevance since it is based on the assessment of exiting nerve root compression based on the MRI appearance of perineural fat [49]. In this classification, grade 0 refers to normal neuroforamen. Grade 1 constitutes mild foraminal stenosis when perineural fat obliteration is observed in two opposing directions. Grade 2 refers to moderate foraminal stenosis showing perineural fat obliteration in four directions, and Grade 3 is assigned in cases of severe foraminal stenosis as shown by morphologic changes in the nerve root itself [49].

Nearly every endoscopic spine surgeon will have to deal with the facet joint complex at one point or another. The lumbar motion segment's degenerative aging process also plays out at the facet joint complex, which is often hypertrophied and contributes to nerve root impingement as much as a herniated disc or hypertrophied ligamentum flavum. An arthritic facet joint can be painful and may give rise to cysts that can become highly inflammatory and extraordinarily painful. Hypertrophy of the facet joint's superior articular process may cause nerve root impingement in the foraminal exit zone [43]. An osteophyte underneath the pars interarticularis was considered a mid-zone problem. In contrast, subluxation of the inferior articular process often leads to entry-zone stenosis [17, 35, 48, 49]. What is clear from this thorough review of radiographically based classification systems is that there is a gap between those imaged-based medical necessity criteria for surgery and endoscopically visualized lumbar spinal pathology. Collaborative research efforts should be directed to fill this gap.

THE NOMENCLATURE MAZE

The AO Spine published a recent consensus paper on nomenclature for working-channel endoscopic spinal procedures with the intent of providing improved consensus definitions for clincal research with the various endoscopic techniques [50]. This group of 27 authors searched the PubMed database using query terms such as "spine," "full-endoscopic," "working-channel endoscope," "spine endoscopy," and "percutaneous", and identified studies that utilized the full-endoscopic visualized techniques. The authors proposed a systematic nomenclature by integrating the previously utilized nomenclature by surgical approach corridor, the mode of visualization, the spinal segment, and the type of procedure [50]. They grossly divided endoscopic spine surgery (ESS) into full endoscopic decompression surgery and endoscopically assisted surgery. The latter includes microendoscopic discectomy (MED) [51 - 53], the microendoscopic laminectomy (MEL) [54], the unilateral biportal endoscopy (UBE) [55], the tubular retractor system popularized by Destandeau [56 - 58], and the endoscopically assisted fusion versions of these procedures including the transforaminal endoscopic lumbar interbody fusion [59 - 62], the UBE fusion [63 - 68], and the endoscopic oblique lateral interbody fusion (OLIF) [69 - 72]. While the authors of the AO Spine article do categorize the currently used terminology for all areas of the spine based on a thorough analysis of the background literature, including a review of the goal of the operation and the rationale for the proposed nomenclature, the proposed lumbar spine nomenclature is of particular relevance to most endoscopic spine surgeons since the vast majority of endoscopic spinal decompressions are being carried out in the lumbar spine. Based on the prior published literature, the authors recommended the following nomenclature for the full-endoscopic lumbar discectomy procedures: Transforaminal endoscopic lumbar discectomy (TELD) [73 - 76], interlaminar endoscopic lumbar discectomy (IELD) [73, 74, 77], extraforaminal endoscopic lumbar discectomy (EELD) [78, 79]. Lumbar endoscopic foraminotomy procedures were categorized as transforaminal endoscopic lumbar foraminotomy (TELF) [80 - 83], interlaminar contralateral endoscopic lumbar foraminotomy (ICELF) [84 - 87]. The full-endoscopic lumbar lateral recess decompression was classified as transforaminal endoscopic lateral recess decompression (TE-LRD) [80, 88 - 92], and interlaminar endoscopic lateral recess decompression (IE-LRD) [93 - 96]. Lastly, the terminology of lumbar endoscopic unilateral laminotomy for bilateral decompression (LE-ULBD) including full-endoscopic laminotomy for bilateral decompression was proposed for the full-endoscopic laminotomy for bilateral decompression [97 - 104].

While the intention of this AO nomenclature to standardize the language used in investigating and communicating clinical outcome research results with endoscopic spine surgery is certainly rationale and appears helpful in front of the traditional educational backdrop for which the AO (Arbeitsgemeinschaft für Osteosynthesefragen) is known for, it remains to be seen whether or not this proposed terminology proves itself useful in factual clinical research. The authors of this chapter have not found any publication validating the usefulness of the AO terminology at the time of this chapter's writing. Future research will have to show whether this nomenclature will gain any traction amongst endoscopic spine surgeons or be outpaced by technology advances that drive the development of new clinical protocols to treat neural encroachment from stenosis or instability. The nomenclature suggested by the AOSpine for lumbar endoscopy is summarized in Table **3**.

Table 3. Proposed AOSpine Lumbar Endoscopic Spine Surgery Nomenclature.

Full-endoscopic Discectomy	Transforaminal endoscopic lumbar discectomy (TELD)
-	Interlaminar endoscopic lumbar discectomy (IELD)
-	Extraforaminal endoscopic lumbar discectomy (EELD)
Lumbar endoscopic foraminotomy	Transforaminal endoscopic lumbar foraminotomy (TELF)
-	Interlaminar contralateral endoscopic lumbar foraminotomy (ICELF)
Full-endoscopic lumbar lateral recess decompression	Transforaminal endoscopic lateral recess decompression (TE-LRD)
-	Interlaminar endoscopic lateral recess decompression (IE-LRD)
Full-endoscopic laminotomy for bilateral decompression	Lumbar endoscopic unilateral laminotomy for bilateral decompression (LE-ULBD)

LUMBAR DISEASE CLASSIFICATION FOR ENDOSCOPIC SPINE SURGERY

William Kirkaldy Willis first described the lumbar motion segment's degenerative cascade as it affects the three-joint complex formed by the intervertebral disc and the facet joints [105 - 107]. Spengler recognized that herniations may be grouped into protrusion, prolapse, and sequestrated [108]. Considering the disc herniation location within the spinal canal, they may be further classified as central, paracentral, intraformational, or extraforaminal. Pathria described four stages of lumbar facet degeneration [109], which was utilized by Fujiwara *et al.* [110] and Weishaupt *et al.* [111] in their MRI and CT studies of facet degeneration. These studies determined that facet arthropathy was more accurately assessed by CT scan and disc herniation by MRI instead [110, 111]. Thalgott *et al.* combined the MRI analysis of degenerative disc disease with plain X-rays and provocative discography analysis of the degenerative disc process in the anterior spinal column and the facet degeneration in the posterior spinal column [112]. The clinical context at the time was lumbar disc replacement surgery since understanding the degree of facet joint disease was critical to the success of disc arthroplasty. Rauschning performed high-quality cryosections of fresh-frozen cadavers allowing correlation sagittal, coronal, oblique, and axial CT-scan images to the corresponding pathoanatomy [113]. Yeung published on correlating the advanced CT and MRI image- and discography findings with directly videoendoscopically visualized pathology [114 - 116]. The recognized need to extract prognosticators of favorable clinical outcomes with endscopic decompression of offending painful pathoanatomy from the preoperative MRI and CT scan was the impetus for Osman *et al.* to propose a detailed CT and MRI classification of the spinal motion-segment's degenerative disease severity by grading each component. The structural elements identified in the Osman classification are the disc, the facet joints, and the spinal alignment. The severity of the disease is graded from 0 to 4. Consequently, D0, D1, D2, D3, and D4 describe the disc degeneration, with D0 being normal and the D4 showing a collapsed disc with posterior osteophytes. The facet is graded F0, F1, F2, F3, and F4. The ligament flavum is classified as L0, L1, L2, L3, L4, and the alignment is classified as A0, A1, A2, A3, and A4. The details of each of the 5 grades are listed in Table **4** and illustrated in Fig. (**3**).

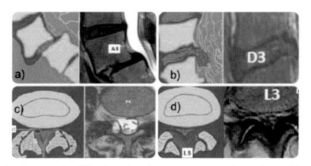

Fig. (3). Excerpts of the Osman classification showing an example of a patient with a degenerative disease severity grading of A3DL3F4.

Table 4. Grading of disease severity of the lumbar motion segment by MRI / CT appearance of spinal alignment, intervertebral disc disease, facet degeneration and ligamentum flavum (LF).

A = Alignment	D = Disc	F = Facet Joint	L = Ligamentum Flavum (LF)
A0 = Normal A1= Retrolisthesis A2 = Grade I spondylolisthesis A3 = Grade II spondylolisthesis A4= Grade 3 & 4 Spondylolisthesis	D0 = Normal disc D1 = Global bulging disc D2 = Contained herniation D3 = Free frag herniation D4 = Disc osteophytes (in canal)	F0 = Normal facet F1 = IAP hypertrophy F2 = SAP hypertrophy F3 = IAP & SAP hypertrophy F4 = IAP & SAP hypertrophy & synovial cyst.	L0 = Normal L1= Minimal hypertrophy of LF L2= Moderate hypertrophy of the LF L3= Severe hypertrophy of the LF L4 = Calcified/ossified

IAP = Inferior Articular Process SAP = Superior Articular Process

The crosstabulation of these four categories allows for 494 theoretical combinations. The authors published the graphic depiction of a few common combinations in their 2013 article, some of which are shown here for demonstrative purposes. Employing a retrospective study of lumbar MRI, including 220 lumbar spinal motion-segments of 54 patients, the authors determined the most prevalent combinations between degenerative disease stages of the disc, facet joints, ligamentum flavum hypertrophy, and spinal alignment (Table **5**). The age range of these patients was 16 to 87 years (mean age 47.3 years). There were 30 male and 24 female patients.

Table 5. Ten most common grading combinations observed in the Osman retrospective lumbar MRI grading study of the spinal motion segment's disease severity.

Pathology Combination	Percentage	Pathologic Process
D0A0L0F0	33.3	Normal disc, normal alignment, normal ligamentum flavum, normal facet joint
D1A0L0F0	8.8	Degenerative global bulging disc, normal alignment, normal LF, and normal facet joint
D2A0L0F2	6.9	Intra-annular disc herniation, normal alignment, normal LF, and hypertrophy of superior articular process
D1A0L1F3	6.4	Global bulging disc, normal alignment, mild hypertrophy LF, hypertrophic superior & inferior articular processes
D1A0L1F0	3.9	Global disc bulge, normal alignment, mild hypertrophy of LF, normal facet joint
D1A1L1F1	3	Global disc bulge, retrolisthesis, mile LF hypertrophy, superior and inferior process hypertrophy
D1A2L1F3	3	Global disc bulge, grade I spondylolisthesis, mild LF hypertrophy, superior and inferior process hypertrophy
D2A0L1F0	2.5	Intra-articular disc herniation, normal alignment, mild hypertrophy of LF,
D3A0L0F0	2.5	Extra-annular disc herniation, normal alignment, normal LF, normal facet joint
D1A0L0F3	2	Global disc bulge, normal alignment, normal LF, Superior and inferior articular processes

LF – ligamentum flavum

Osman *et al.* need to be credited for organizing the information extracted from the MRI and CT scan by reaching a higher level of detail than typically provided with the MRI report [117 - 121]. Their intent was to identify common combinations of pathoanatomic abnormalities to research the clinical consequences of their presence on advanced MRI and CT imaging studies. However, the level of detail can be overwhelming and frankly impractical in routine clinical use. The authors themselves have published no additional clinical research studies that validate their classification system beyond the scope of their initial feasibility study of 54 patients and 220 levels. Nonetheless, they did identify 14 common patterns - 10 of which are listed in Table **5**. Ideally, additional clinical research was to be conducted on a simplified version of the Osman classification system to be more conducive to routine clinical practice. For example, the various D-A-L-F subtypes could be reduced into 3 to 4 subtypes to be determined by clinical outcomes with endoscopic spinal surgery treatments that are directed at the underlying pathology for each of the graded structures and factors at the surgical level: the disc, alignment/instability, facet joints, and ligamentum flavum. Such a simplified system may find better acceptance amongst spine surgeons since the Osman classification does not take into account additional well-accepted image-based medical necessity criteria for surgery including global coronal and sagittal alignment, positive spinal balance, multilevel instability and deformity patterns. Reducing endoscopic spine care to validated pain generators with staged management strategies [30] is preferred clinical practice for most endoscopic spine surgeons in an attempt to simplify spine care [114, 120, 122 - 124]. These concepts are still relatively new to most traditionally trained spine surgeons, thus, making the case for a simplified easy-to-understand classification.

DISCUSSION

The use of sensitive patient-reported outcome measures (PROMs) and reliable and easy-to-use nomenclatures & classifications categories in clinical research of endoscopic spine surgery is pertinent to any meaningful clinical outcome research that is aimed at demonstrating equality or superiority of the endoscopic spinal surgery when compared to traditional open spinal surgery protocols that it is attempting to replace. In this chapter, the authors focused on illustrating the current state-of-the-art concerning suggested nomenclature, classification, and PROMs by recognizing confident key opinion leaders (KOLs) [17, 31, 43, 45, 116, 125 - 127] and active clinical research groups, the AOSpine group [50]. While there clearly is a need to communicate clinical observations in uniform terms and categories, and to employ standardized PROMs with reliable statistical performance characteristics to conduct clinical research [126], many classification and nomenclature systems have found little meaningful clinical application primarily because of rapid technological advances that render the need for them less relevant because the field has simply moved on and replaced the procedures that prompted the development of classifications with others. The Osman approach of employing an anatomical classification concept seems more survivable since the underlying disease process dynamics do not change too much [125]. Technology- or approach-driven classifications such as the AOSpine show a current snapshot in time, but will they remain relevant as technology advances are implemented? The burden of proof lies with its authors to provide sufficient clinical evidence to justify its broader acceptance by endoscopic spine surgeons worldwide.

The extraction of better front-end prognosticators of favorable clinical outcomes with the endoscopic spinal surgery procedure for common clinical problems such as herniated disc and spinal stenosis for now largely rests on radiographic advanced imaging studies. This chapter briefly reviewed the radiographic MRI- and CT-based classifications of a herniated disc and spinal stenosis. Many of these classifications account for the location and extent of the offending pathology [17, 35, 48, 49]. The diagnostic gap between MRI reporting and what is seen during direct video endoscopic visualization has been recognized by several authors [117, 128] who proposed additional protocols with diagnostic injections to predict the outcome more accurately the endoscopic spine surgery [129]. Detecting clinical improvements and superiority of one procedure over another hinge on employing outcome tools with reliable statistical performance characteristics by leaving little room for bias [130]. Hindsight bias is a common problem that plagues many clinical outcome studies using complex multi-tier questionnaires as patients measure their progress with any spine intervention not by recalling their functional status before surgery but by comparing their postoperative function with their new expectations driven by the comparison to the functional status of their peers, relatives, and friends [131]. Simpler numerical outcome tools such as the VAS score system have been proven to be less sensitive to these recall biases [126].

CONCLUSION

Demonstrating equivalency and, in some cases, the superiority of the endoscopic spinal surgery with traditional open spine surgeries and other forms of minimally invasive spine surgery is the primary motivator for any clinical outcome study. This goal can only be achieved by conducting clinical outcome research employing the same standards used in the study of traditional spine surgery protocols endoscopic spine surgery is attempting to replace. The authors of this chapter have contributed to this debate with many of their clinical outcome studies to make precisely that case. The illustration of the current state-of-the-art in endoscopic nomenclature and classification and the proper utility of validated patient self-reported outcome tools brought the reader to the forefront of the debate that will likely continue as the endoscopic procedure advances.

CONSENT FOR PUBLICATION

Not Applicable.

CONFLICT OF INTEREST

The authors declare no conflict of interest, financial or otherwise.

ACKNOWLEDGEMENT

Declared none.

REFEERENCES

[1]   Lewandrowski KU. Readmissions After Outpatient Transforaminal Decompression for Lumbar Foraminal and Lateral Recess Stenosis. Int J Spine Surg 2018; 12(3): 342-51.
[http://dx.doi.org/10.14444/5040] [PMID: 30276091]

[2]   Lewandrowski KU. Incidence, Management, and Cost of Complications After Transforaminal Endoscopic Decompression Surgery for Lumbar Foraminal and Lateral Recess Stenosis: A Value Proposition for Outpatient Ambulatory Surgery. Int J Spine Surg 2019; 13(1): 53-67.
[http://dx.doi.org/10.14444/6008] [PMID: 30805287]

[3]   Lewandrowski KU, Gresser JD, Wise DL, White RL, Trantolo DJ. Osteoconductivity of an injectable and bioresorbable poly(propylene glycol-co-fumaric acid) bone cement. Biomaterials 2000; 21(3): 293-8.
[http://dx.doi.org/10.1016/S0142-9612(99)00180-5] [PMID: 10646946]

[4]   Markovic M, Zivkovic N, Spaic M, *et al.* Full-endoscopic interlaminar operations in lumbar compressive lesions surgery: prospective study of 350 patients. "Endos" study. J Neurosurg Sci 2016; •••: 2016.
[PMID: 27362665]

[5]   Ruetten S, Hahn P, Oezdemir S, *et al.* The full-endoscopic uniportal technique for decompression of the anterior craniocervical junction using the retropharyngeal approach: an anatomical feasibility study in human cadavers and review of the literature. J Neurosurg Spine 2018; 29(6): 615-21.
[http://dx.doi.org/10.3171/2018.4.SPINE171156] [PMID: 30192216]

[6]   Ruetten S, Komp M, Merk H, Godolias G. Use of newly developed instruments and endoscopes: full-endoscopic resection of lumbar disc herniations *via* the interlaminar and lateral transforaminal approach. J Neurosurg Spine 2007; 6(6): 521-30.
[http://dx.doi.org/10.3171/spi.2007.6.6.2] [PMID: 17561740]

[7]   Shahidi B, Hubbard JC, Gibbons MC, *et al.* Lumbar multifidus muscle degenerates in individuals with chronic degenerative lumbar spine pathology. J Orthop Res 2017; 35(12): 2700-6.
[http://dx.doi.org/10.1002/jor.23597] [PMID: 28480978]

[8]   Tabaraee E, Ahn J, Bohl DD, *et al.* Quantification of Multifidus Atrophy and Fatty Infiltration Following a Minimally Invasive Microdiscectomy. Int J Spine Surg 2015; 9: 25.
[http://dx.doi.org/10.14444/2025]

[9]   Tsou PM, Yeung AT. Transforaminal endoscopic decompression for radiculopathy secondary to intracanal noncontained lumbar disc herniations: outcome and technique. Spine J 2002; 2(1): 41-8.
[http://dx.doi.org/10.1016/S1529-9430(01)00153-X] [PMID: 14588287]

[10]   Yeung A, Kotheeranurak V. Transforaminal Endoscopic Decompression of the Lumbar Spine for Stable Isthmic Spondylolisthesis as the Least Invasive Surgical Treatment Using the YESS Surgery Technique. Int J Spine Surg 2018; 12(3): 408-14.

[http://dx.doi.org/10.14444/5048] [PMID: 30276099]

[11] Yeung AT, Yeung CA. Minimally invasive techniques for the management of lumbar disc herniation. Orthop Clin North Am 2007; 38(3): 363-72.
[http://dx.doi.org/10.1016/j.ocl.2007.04.005] [PMID: 17629984]

[12] Reed CC, Wolf WA, Cotton CC, Dellon ES. A visual analogue scale and a Likert scale are simple and responsive tools for assessing dysphagia in eosinophilic oesophagitis. Aliment Pharmacol Ther 2017; 45(11): 1443-8.
[http://dx.doi.org/10.1111/apt.14061] [PMID: 28370355]

[13] Choi G, Prada N, Modi HN, Vasavada NB, Kim JS, Lee SH. Percutaneous endoscopic lumbar herniectomy for high-grade down-migrated L4-L5 disc through an L5-S1 interlaminar approach: a technical note. Minim Invasive Neurosurg 2010; 53(3): 147-52.
[http://dx.doi.org/10.1055/s-0030-1254145] [PMID: 20809458]

[14] Erçalık T, Gencer Atalay K, Şanal Toprak C, Gündüz OH. Outcome measurement in patients with low back pain undergoing epidural steroid injection. Turk J Phys Med Rehabil 2019; 65(2): 154-9.
[http://dx.doi.org/10.5606/tftrd.2019.2350] [PMID: 31453556]

[15] Hermansen E, Myklebust TA, Austevoll IM, *et al.* Clinical outcome after surgery for lumbar spinal stenosis in patients with insignificant lower extremity pain. A prospective cohort study from the Norwegian registry for spine surgery. BMC Musculoskelet Disord 2019; 20-36.
[http://dx.doi.org/10.1186/s12891-019-2407-5]

[16] Hong X, Shi R, Wang YT, Liu L, Bao JP, Wu XT. Lumbar disc herniation treated by microendoscopic discectomy : Prognostic predictors of long-term postoperative outcome. Orthopade 2018; 47(12): 993-1002.
[http://dx.doi.org/10.1007/s00132-018-3624-6] [PMID: 30171289]

[17] Lewandrowski KU. "Outside-in" technique, clinical results, and indications with transforaminal lumbar endoscopic surgery: a retrospective study on 220 patients on applied radiographic classification of foraminal spinal stenosis. Int J Spine Surg 2014; 8
[http://dx.doi.org/10.14444/1026]

[18] Lewandrowski KU. Endoscopic Transforaminal and Lateral Recess Decompression After Previous Spinal Surgery. Int J Spine Surg 2018; 12(2): 98-111.
[http://dx.doi.org/10.14444/5016] [PMID: 30276068]

[19] Fairbank J. Use of Oswestry Disability Index (ODI). Spine 1995; 20(13): 1535-7.
[http://dx.doi.org/10.1097/00007632-199507000-00020] [PMID: 8623078]

[20] Fairbank JC, Pynsent PB. The Oswestry Disability Index. Spine 2000; 25(22): 2940-52.
[http://dx.doi.org/10.1097/00007632-200011150-00017] [PMID: 11074683]

[21] van Hooff ML, Spruit M, Fairbank JC, van Limbeek J, Jacobs WC. The Oswestry Disability Index (version 2.1a): validation of a Dutch language version. Spine 2015; 40(2): E83-90.
[http://dx.doi.org/10.1097/BRS.0000000000000683] [PMID: 25575092]

[22] van Hooff ML, Mannion AF, Staub LP, Ostelo RW, Fairbank JC. Determination of the Oswestry Disability Index score equivalent to a "satisfactory symptom state" in patients undergoing surgery for degenerative disorders of the lumbar spine-a Spine Tango registry-based study. Spine J 2016; 16(10): 1221-30.
[http://dx.doi.org/10.1016/j.spinee.2016.06.010] [PMID: 27343730]

[23] Macnab I. The surgery of lumbar disc degeneration. Surg Annu 1976; 8(8): 447-80.
[PMID: 936011]

[24] Macnab I. Negative disc exploration. An analysis of the causes of nerve-root involvement in sixty-eight patients. J Bone Joint Surg Am 1971; 53(5): 891-903.
[http://dx.doi.org/10.2106/00004623-197153050-00004] [PMID: 4326746]

[25] Macnab I, St Louis EL, Grabias SL, Jacob R. Selective ascending lumbosacral venography in the

assessment of lumbar-disc herniation. An anatomical study and clinical experience. J Bone Joint Surg Am 1976; 58(8): 1093-8.
[http://dx.doi.org/10.2106/00004623-197658080-00009] [PMID: 794071]

[26] Mancuso CA, Salvati EA, Johanson NA, Peterson MG, Charlson ME. Patients' expectations and satisfaction with total hip arthroplasty. J Arthroplasty 1997; 12(4): 387-96.
[http://dx.doi.org/10.1016/S0883-5403(97)90194-7] [PMID: 9195314]

[27] Hajiro T, Nishimura K. Minimal clinically significant difference in health status: the thorny path of health status measures? Eur Respir J 2002; 19(3): 390-1.
[http://dx.doi.org/10.1183/09031936.02.00283402] [PMID: 11936512]

[28] Beaton DE, Boers M, Wells GA. Many faces of the minimal clinically important difference (MCID): a literature review and directions for future research. Curr Opin Rheumatol 2002; 14(2): 109-14.
[http://dx.doi.org/10.1097/00002281-200203000-00006] [PMID: 11845014]

[29] Jaeschke R, Singer J, Guyatt GH. Measurement of health status. Ascertaining the minimal clinically important difference. Control Clin Trials 1989; 10(4): 407-15.
[http://dx.doi.org/10.1016/0197-2456(89)90005-6] [PMID: 2691207]

[30] Yeung A, Lewandrowski KU. Early and staged endoscopic management of common pain generators in the spine. J Spine Surg 2020; 6(6) (Suppl. 1): S1-5.
[http://dx.doi.org/10.21037/jss.2019.09.03] [PMID: 32195407]

[31] Lewandrowski K-U, Yeung A. Meaningful outcome research to validate endoscopic treatment of common lumbar pain generators with durability analysis. J Spine Surg 2020; 6(S1) (Suppl. 1): S6-S13.
[http://dx.doi.org/10.21037/jss.2019.09.07] [PMID: 32195408]

[32] Lewandrowski KU, Ransom NA. Five-year clinical outcomes with endoscopic transforaminal outside-in foraminoplasty techniques for symptomatic degenerative conditions of the lumbar spine. J Spine Surg 2020; 6(6) (Suppl. 1): S54-65.
[http://dx.doi.org/10.21037/jss.2019.07.03] [PMID: 32195416]

[33] Lewandrowski KU, Ransom NA, Yeung A. Return to work and recovery time analysis after outpatient endoscopic lumbar transforaminal decompression surgery. J Spine Surg 2020; 6(6) (Suppl. 1): S100-15.
[http://dx.doi.org/10.21037/jss.2019.10.01] [PMID: 32195419]

[34] Lewandrowski KU, Yeung A. Lumbar Endoscopic Bony and Soft Tissue Decompression With the Hybridized Inside-Out Approach: A Review And Technical Note. Neurospine 2020; 17(17) (Suppl. 1): S34-43.
[http://dx.doi.org/10.14245/ns.2040160.080] [PMID: 32746516]

[35] Yeung A, Lewandrowski KU. Five-year clinical outcomes with endoscopic transforaminal foraminoplasty for symptomatic degenerative conditions of the lumbar spine: a comparative study of *inside-out* versus *outside-in* techniques. J Spine Surg 2020; 6(6) (Suppl. 1): S66-83.
[http://dx.doi.org/10.21037/jss.2019.06.08] [PMID: 32195417]

[36] Lauridsen HH, Hartvigsen J, Manniche C, *et al.* Responsiveness and minimal clinically important difference for pain and disability instruments in low back pain patients. BMC Musculoskelet Disord 2006; 7
[http://dx.doi.org/10.1186/1471-2474-7-82]

[37] Chung AS, Copay AG, Olmscheid N, Campbell D, Walker JB, Chutkan N. Minimum Clinically Important Difference: Current Trends in the Spine Literature. Spine 2017; 42(14): 1096-105.
[http://dx.doi.org/10.1097/BRS.0000000000001990] [PMID: 27870805]

[38] Copay AG, Chung AS, Eyberg B, *et al.* Minimum Clinically Important Difference: Current Trends in the Orthopaedic Literature, Part I: Upper Extremity: A Systematic Review. JBJS Rev 2018; 6: e1.
[http://dx.doi.org/10.2106/JBJS.RVW.17.00159]

[39] Copay AG, Eyberg B, Chung AS, *et al.* Minimum Clinically Important Difference: Current Trends in

the Orthopaedic Literature, Part II: Lower Extremity: A Systematic Review. JBJS Rev 2018; 6: e2.
[http://dx.doi.org/10.2106/JBJS.RVW.17.00160]

[40] Cook CE. Clinimetrics Corner: The Minimal Clinically Important Change Score (MCID): A Necessary Pretense. J Manual Manip Ther 2008; 16(4): E82-3.
[http://dx.doi.org/10.1179/jmt.2008.16.4.82E] [PMID: 19771185]

[41] Metz CE. Basic principles of ROC analysis. Semin Nucl Med 1978; 8(4): 283-98.
[http://dx.doi.org/10.1016/S0001-2998(78)80014-2] [PMID: 112681]

[42] Lee CH, Choi M, Ryu DS, *et al.* Efficacy and Safety of Full-endoscopic Decompression *via* Interlaminar Approach for Central or Lateral Recess Spinal Stenosis of the Lumbar Spine: A Meta-analysis. Spine 2018; 43(24): 1756-64.
[http://dx.doi.org/10.1097/BRS.0000000000002708] [PMID: 29794584]

[43] Lee CK, Rauschning W, Glenn W. Lateral lumbar spinal canal stenosis: classification, pathologic anatomy and surgical decompression. Spine 1988; 13(3): 313-20.
[http://dx.doi.org/10.1097/00007632-198803000-00015] [PMID: 3388117]

[44] Haig AJ. Diagnostic tests the NASS stenosis guidelines. Spine J 2014; 14(1): 200-1.
[http://dx.doi.org/10.1016/j.spinee.2013.08.008] [PMID: 24332322]

[45] Lee S, Kim SK, Lee SH, *et al.* Percutaneous endoscopic lumbar discectomy for migrated disc herniation: classification of disc migration and surgical approaches. Eur Spine J 2007; 16(3): 431-7.
[http://dx.doi.org/10.1007/s00586-006-0219-4] [PMID: 16972067]

[46] Hasegawa T, An HS, Haughton VM, Nowicki BH. Lumbar foraminal stenosis: critical heights of the intervertebral discs and foramina. A cryomicrotome study in cadavera. J Bone Joint Surg Am 1995; 77(1): 32-8.
[http://dx.doi.org/10.2106/00004623-199501000-00005] [PMID: 7822353]

[47] Pfirrmann CW, Metzdorf A, Zanetti M, Hodler J, Boos N. Magnetic resonance classification of lumbar intervertebral disc degeneration. Spine 2001; 26(17): 1873-8.
[http://dx.doi.org/10.1097/00007632-200109010-00011] [PMID: 11568697]

[48] Kim HS, Adsul N, Kapoor A, *et al.* A Mobile Outside-in Technique of Transforaminal Lumbar Endoscopy for Lumbar Disc Herniations. J Vis Exp 2018; 2018(138)
[http://dx.doi.org/10.3791/57999] [PMID: 30148483]

[49] Liu KC, Yang SK, Ou BR, *et al.* Using Percutaneous Endoscopic Outside-In Technique to Treat Selected Patients with Refractory Discogenic Low Back Pain. Pain Physician 2019; 22(2): 187-98.
[PMID: 30921984]

[50] Hofstetter CP, Ahn Y, Choi G, *et al.* AOSpine Consensus Paper on Nomenclature for Working-Channel Endoscopic Spinal Procedures. Global Spine J 2020; 10(2) (Suppl.): 111S-21S.
[http://dx.doi.org/10.1177/2192568219887364] [PMID: 32528794]

[51] Liu X, Yuan S, Tian Y, *et al.* Comparison of percutaneous endoscopic transforaminal discectomy, microendoscopic discectomy, and microdiscectomy for symptomatic lumbar disc herniation: minimum 2-year follow-up results. J Neurosurg Spine 2018; 28(3): 317-25.
[http://dx.doi.org/10.3171/2017.6.SPINE172] [PMID: 29303471]

[52] Marappan K, Jothi R, Paul Raj S. Microendoscopic discectomy (MED) for lumbar disc herniation: comparison of learning curve of the surgery and outcome with other established case studies. J Spine Surg 2018; 4(3): 630-7.
[http://dx.doi.org/10.21037/jss.2018.06.14] [PMID: 30547129]

[53] Ahn Y. Devices for minimally-invasive microdiscectomy: current status and future prospects. Expert Rev Med Devices 2020; 17(2): 131-8.
[http://dx.doi.org/10.1080/17434440.2020.1708189] [PMID: 31865755]

[54] Iwai H, Inanami H, Koga H. Comparative study between full-endoscopic laminectomy and microendoscopic laminectomy for the treatment of lumbar spinal canal stenosis. J Spine Surg 2020;

6(2): E3-E11.
[http://dx.doi.org/10.21037/jss-20-620] [PMID: 32656392]

[55]   Ito Z, Shibayama M, Nakamura S, *et al.* Clinical Comparison of Unilateral Biportal Endoscopic Laminectomy *versus* Microendoscopic Laminectomy for Single-Level Laminectomy: A Single-Center, Retrospective Analysis. World Neurosurg 2021; 148: e581-8.
[http://dx.doi.org/10.1016/j.wneu.2021.01.031] [PMID: 33476779]

[56]   Destandau J. A special device for endoscopic surgery of lumbar disc herniation. Neurol Res 1999; 21(1): 39-42.
[http://dx.doi.org/10.1080/01616412.1999.11740889] [PMID: 10048052]

[57]   Destandau J. [Technical features of endoscopic surgery for lumbar disc herniation: 191 patients]. Neurochirurgie 2004; 50(1): 6-10.
[http://dx.doi.org/10.1016/S0028-3770(04)98300-2] [PMID: 15097915]

[58]   Xu B, Xu H, Destandau J, *et al.* Anatomic investigation of lumbar transforaminal fenestration approach and its clinical application in far lateral disc herniation. Medicine (Baltimore) 2017; 96: e7542.
[http://dx.doi.org/10.1097/MD.0000000000007542]

[59]   Kim JE, Choi DJ. Biportal Endoscopic Transforaminal Lumbar Interbody Fusion with Arthroscopy. Clin Orthop Surg 2018; 10(2): 248-52.
[http://dx.doi.org/10.4055/cios.2018.10.2.248] [PMID: 29854350]

[60]   Ahn Y, Youn MS, Heo DH. Endoscopic transforaminal lumbar interbody fusion: a comprehensive review. Expert Rev Med Devices 2019; 16(5): 373-80.
[http://dx.doi.org/10.1080/17434440.2019.1610388] [PMID: 31044627]

[61]   Heo DH, Park CK. Clinical results of percutaneous biportal endoscopic lumbar interbody fusion with application of enhanced recovery after surgery. Neurosurg Focus 2019; 46: E18.
[http://dx.doi.org/10.3171/2019.1.FOCUS18695]

[62]   Kolcun JPG, Brusko GD, Wang MY. Endoscopic transforaminal lumbar interbody fusion without general anesthesia: technical innovations and outcomes. Ann Transl Med 2019; 7: S167.
[http://dx.doi.org/10.21037/atm.2019.07.92]

[63]   Park MK, Park SA, Son SK, *et al.* Correction to: Clinical and radiological outcomes of unilateral biportal endoscopic lumbar interbody fusion (ULIF) compared with conventional posterior lumbar interbody fusion (PLIF): 1-year follow-up. Neurosurg Rev 2019; 42: 763.
[http://dx.doi.org/10.1007/s10143-019-01131-2]

[64]   Park MK, Park SA, Son SK, Park WW, Choi SH. Clinical and radiological outcomes of unilateral biportal endoscopic lumbar interbody fusion (ULIF) compared with conventional posterior lumbar interbody fusion (PLIF): 1-year follow-up. Neurosurg Rev 2019; 42(3): 753-61.
[http://dx.doi.org/10.1007/s10143-019-01114-3] [PMID: 31144195]

[65]   Kim KR, Park JY. The Technical Feasibility of Unilateral Biportal Endoscopic Decompression for The Unpredicted Complication Following Minimally Invasive Transforaminal Lumbar Interbody Fusion: Case Report. Neurospine 2020; 17(17) (Suppl. 1): S154-9.
[http://dx.doi.org/10.14245/ns.2040174.087] [PMID: 32746529]

[66]   Quillo-Olvera J, Quillo-Reséndiz J, Quillo-Olvera D, Barrera-Arreola M, Kim JS. Ten-Step Biportal Endoscopic Transforaminal Lumbar Interbody Fusion Under Computed Tomography-Based Intraoperative Navigation: Technical Report and Preliminary Outcomes in Mexico. Oper Neurosurg (Hagerstown) 2020; 19(5): 608-18.
[http://dx.doi.org/10.1093/ons/opaa226] [PMID: 32726423]

[67]   Heo DH, Eum JH, Jo JY, Chung H. Modified far lateral endoscopic transforaminal lumbar interbody fusion using a biportal endoscopic approach: technical report and preliminary results. Acta Neurochir (Wien) 2021; 163(4): 1205-9.
[http://dx.doi.org/10.1007/s00701-021-04758-7] [PMID: 33606101]

[68] Kang MS, Chung HJ, Jung HJ, Park HJ. How I do it? Extraforaminal lumbar interbody fusion assisted with biportal endoscopic technique. Acta Neurochir (Wien) 2021; 163(1): 295-9.
[http://dx.doi.org/10.1007/s00701-020-04435-1] [PMID: 32514621]

[69] Katzell J. Endoscopic foraminal decompression preceding oblique lateral lumbar interbody fusion to decrease the incidence of post operative dysaesthesia. Int J Spine Surg 2014; 8
[http://dx.doi.org/10.14444/1019]

[70] Heo DH, Kim JS. Clinical and radiological outcomes of spinal endoscopic discectomy-assisted oblique lumbar interbody fusion: preliminary results. Neurosurg Focus 2017; 43: E13.
[http://dx.doi.org/10.3171/2017.5.FOCUS17196]

[71] Ling Q, He E, Zhang H, Lin H, Huang W. A novel narrow surface cage for full endoscopic oblique lateral lumbar interbody fusion: A finite element study. J Orthop Sci 2019; 24(6): 991-8.
[http://dx.doi.org/10.1016/j.jos.2019.08.013] [PMID: 31519402]

[72] Yang Z, Chang J, Sun L, *et al.* Comparing Oblique Lumbar Interbody Fusion with Lateral Screw Fixation and Transforaminal Full-Endoscopic Lumbar Discectomy (OLIF-TELD) and Posterior Lumbar Interbody Fusion (PLIF) for the Treatment of Adjacent Segment Disease. Biomed Res Int 2020.
[http://dx.doi.org/10.1155/2020/4610128]

[73] Wu C, Lee CY, Chen SC, *et al.* Functional outcomes of full-endoscopic spine surgery for high-grade migrated lumbar disc herniation: a prospective registry-based cohort study with more than 5 years of follow-up. BMC Musculoskelet Disord 2021; 22: 58.
[http://dx.doi.org/10.1186/s12891-020-03891-1]

[74] Huang K, Chen G, Lu S, *et al.* Early Clinical Outcomes of Percutaneous Endoscopic Lumbar Discectomy for L4-5 Highly Down-Migrated Disc Herniation: Interlaminar Approach *Versus* Transforaminal Approach. World Neurosurg 2021; 146(146): e413-8.
[http://dx.doi.org/10.1016/j.wneu.2020.10.105] [PMID: 33353758]

[75] Krzok G. Transforaminal Endoscopic Surgery: Outside-In Technique. Neurospine 2020; 17(17) (Suppl. 1): S44-57.
[http://dx.doi.org/10.14245/ns.2040128.064] [PMID: 32746517]

[76] Chen KT, Wei ST, Tseng C, Ou SW, Sun LW, Chen CM. Transforaminal Endoscopic Lumbar Discectomy for L5-S1 Disc Herniation With High Iliac Crest: Technical Note and Preliminary Series. Neurospine 2020; 17(17) (Suppl. 1): S81-7.
[http://dx.doi.org/10.14245/ns.2040166.060] [PMID: 32746521]

[77] Shim HK, Choi KC, Cha KH, Lee DC, Park CK. Interlaminar Endoscopic Lumbar Discectomy Using a New 8.4-mm Endoscope and Nerve Root Retractor. Clin Spine Surg 2020; 33(7): 265-70.
[http://dx.doi.org/10.1097/BSD.0000000000000878] [PMID: 31490243]

[78] Yoshikane K, Kikuchi K, Okazaki K. Posterolateral Transforaminal Full-Endoscopic Lumbar Discectomy for Foraminal or Extraforaminal Lumbar Disc Herniations. World Neurosurg 2021; 146(146): e1278-86.
[http://dx.doi.org/10.1016/j.wneu.2020.11.141] [PMID: 33276171]

[79] Aydın AL, Sasani M, Sasani H, *et al.* Comparison of Two Minimally Invasive Techniques with Endoscopy and Microscopy for Extraforaminal Disc Herniations. World Neurosurg 2020; 144(144): e612-21.
[http://dx.doi.org/10.1016/j.wneu.2020.09.022] [PMID: 32916351]

[80] Zou HJ, Hu Y, Liu JB, Wu J. Percutaneous Endoscopic Transforaminal Lumbar Discectomy *via* Eccentric Trepan foraminoplasty Technology for Unilateral Stenosed Serve Root Canals. Orthop Surg 2020; 12(4): 1205-11.
[http://dx.doi.org/10.1111/os.12739] [PMID: 32857925]

[81] Sakti YM, Mafaza A, Lanodiyu ZA, Sakadewa GP, Magetsari R. Management of distal adjacent

segment disease due to central subsidence of PLIF using local anesthetic transforaminal foraminotomy and lumbar discectomy. Int J Surg Case Rep 2020; 77(77): 269-75.
[http://dx.doi.org/10.1016/j.ijscr.2020.10.089] [PMID: 33189009]

[82]　Hussain I, Rapoport BI, Krause K, Kinney G, Hofstetter CP, Elowitz E. Transforaminal Endoscopic Lumbar Discectomy and Foraminotomy with Modified Radiofrequency Nerve Stimulator and Continuous Electromyography Under General Anesthesia. World Neurosurg 2020; 137(137): 102-10.
[http://dx.doi.org/10.1016/j.wneu.2020.01.186] [PMID: 32036064]

[83]　Ahn Y, Keum HJ, Son S. Percutaneous Endoscopic Lumbar Foraminotomy for Foraminal Stenosis with Postlaminectomy Syndrome in Geriatric Patients. World Neurosurg 2019; 130(130): e1070-6.
[http://dx.doi.org/10.1016/j.wneu.2019.07.087] [PMID: 31323406]

[84]　Kim HS, Kim JY, Wu PH, Jang IT. Effect of Dorsal Root Ganglion Retraction in Endoscopic Lumbar Decompressive Surgery for Foraminal Pathology: A Retrospective Cohort Study of Interlaminar Contralateral Endoscopic Lumbar Foraminotomy and Discectomy *versus* Transforaminal Endoscopic Lumbar Foraminotomy and Discectomy. World Neurosurg 2021; 148: e101-14.
[http://dx.doi.org/10.1016/j.wneu.2020.12.176] [PMID: 33444831]

[85]　Kashlan ON, Kim HS, Khalsa SSS, *et al.* Percutaneous Endoscopic Contralateral Lumbar Foraminal Decompression *via* an Interlaminar Approach: 2-Dimensional Operative Video. Oper Neurosurg (Hagerstown) 2020; 18(4): E118-9.
[http://dx.doi.org/10.1093/ons/opz162] [PMID: 31232437]

[86]　Chen KT, Song MS, Kim JS. How I do it? Interlaminar contralateral endoscopic lumbar foraminotomy assisted with the O-arm navigation. Acta Neurochir (Wien) 2020; 162(1): 121-5.
[http://dx.doi.org/10.1007/s00701-019-04104-y] [PMID: 31811466]

[87]　Kim HS, Singh R, Adsul NM, Oh SW, Noh JH, Jang IT. Management of Root-Level Double Crush: Case Report with Technical Notes on Contralateral Interlaminar Foraminotomy with Full Endoscopic Uniportal Approach. World Neurosurg 2019; 122(122): 505-7.
[http://dx.doi.org/10.1016/j.wneu.2018.11.110] [PMID: 30476660]

[88]　Xie P, Feng F, Chen Z, *et al.* Percutaneous transforaminal full endoscopic decompression for the treatment of lumbar spinal stenosis. BMC Musculoskelet Disord 2020; 21: 546.
[http://dx.doi.org/10.1186/s12891-020-03566-x]

[89]　Wu B, Xiong C, Huang B, *et al.* Clinical outcomes of transforaminal endoscopic lateral recess decompression by using the visualized drilled foraminoplasty and visualized reamed foraminoplasty: a comparison study. BMC Musculoskelet Disord 2020; 21: 829.
[http://dx.doi.org/10.1186/s12891-020-03849-3]

[90]　Sugiura K, Yamashita K, Manabe H, *et al.* Prompt Return to Work after Bilateral Transforaminal Full-endoscopic Lateral Recess Decompression under Local Anesthesia: A Case Report. J Neurol Surg A Cent Eur Neurosurg 2020; 2020
[http://dx.doi.org/10.1055/s-0040-1712463] [PMID: 33352609]

[91]　Li X, Liu T, Fan J, *et al.* Outcome of lumbar lateral recess stenosis with percutaneous endoscopic transforaminal decompression in patients 65 years of age or older and in younger patients. Medicine (Baltimore) 2020; 99: e21049.
[http://dx.doi.org/10.1097/MD.0000000000021049]

[92]　Dowling Á, Bárcenas JGH, Lewandrowski KU. Transforaminal endoscopic decompression and uninstrumented allograft lumbar interbody fusion: A feasibility study in patients with end-stage vacuum degenerative disc disease. Clin Neurol Neurosurg 2020; 196: 106002.
[http://dx.doi.org/10.1016/j.clineuro.2020.106002]

[93]　Wagner R, Haefner M. Indications and Contraindications of Full-Endoscopic Interlaminar Lumbar Decompression. World Neurosurg 2021; 145(145): 657-62.
[http://dx.doi.org/10.1016/j.wneu.2020.08.042] [PMID: 32810629]

[94]　Chen KT, Choi KC, Song MS, Jabri H, Lokanath YK, Kim JS. Hybrid Interlaminar Endoscopic

Lumbar Decompression in Disc Herniation Combined With Spinal Stenosis. Oper Neurosurg (Hagerstown) 2021; 20(3): E168-74.
[http://dx.doi.org/10.1093/ons/opaa360] [PMID: 33294926]

[95] Xin Z, Huang P, Zheng G, Liao W, Zhang X, Wang Y. Using a percutaneous spinal endoscopy unilateral posterior interlaminar approach to perform bilateral decompression for patients with lumbar lateral recess stenosis. Asian J Surg 2020; 43(5): 593-602.
[http://dx.doi.org/10.1016/j.asjsur.2019.08.010] [PMID: 31594687]

[96] Dowling Á, Lewandrowski KU, da Silva FHP, Parra JAA, Portillo DM, Giménez YCP. Patient selection protocols for endoscopic transforaminal, interlaminar, and translaminar decompression of lumbar spinal stenosis. J Spine Surg 2020; 6(6) (Suppl. 1): S120-32.
[http://dx.doi.org/10.21037/jss.2019.11.07] [PMID: 32195421]

[97] Zhao XB, Ma HJ, Geng B, Zhou HG, Xia YY. Percutaneous Endoscopic Unilateral Laminotomy and Bilateral Decompression for Lumbar Spinal Stenosis. Orthop Surg 2021; 13(2): 641-50.
[http://dx.doi.org/10.1111/os.12925] [PMID: 33565271]

[98] Wu MH, Wu PC, Lee CY, *et al.* Outcome analysis of lumbar endoscopic unilateral laminotomy for bilateral decompression in patients with degenerative lumbar central canal stenosis. Spine J 2021; 21(1): 122-33.
[http://dx.doi.org/10.1016/j.spinee.2020.08.010] [PMID: 32871276]

[99] Lim KT, Meceda EJA, Park CK. Inside-Out Approach of Lumbar Endoscopic Unilateral Laminotomy for Bilateral Decompression: A Detailed Technical Description, Rationale and Outcomes. Neurospine 2020; 17(17) (Suppl. 1): S88-98.
[http://dx.doi.org/10.14245/ns.2040196.098] [PMID: 32746522]

[100] Kim HS, Wu PH, Jang IT. Lumbar Endoscopic Unilateral Laminotomy for Bilateral Decompression Outside-In Approach: A Proctorship Guideline With 12 Steps of Effectiveness and Safety. Neurospine 2020; 17(17) (Suppl. 1): S99-S109.
[http://dx.doi.org/10.14245/ns.2040078.039] [PMID: 32746523]

[101] Kim HS, Choi SH, Shim DM, Lee IS, Oh YK, Woo YH. Advantages of New Endoscopic Unilateral Laminectomy for Bilateral Decompression (ULBD) over Conventional Microscopic ULBD. Clin Orthop Surg 2020; 12(3): 330-6.
[http://dx.doi.org/10.4055/cios19136] [PMID: 32904063]

[102] Hua W, Wang B, Ke W, *et al.* Comparison of lumbar endoscopic unilateral laminotomy bilateral decompression and minimally invasive surgery transforaminal lumbar interbody fusion for one-level lumbar spinal stenosis. BMC Musculoskelet Disord 2020; 21: 785.
[http://dx.doi.org/10.1186/s12891-020-03820-2]

[103] Ho TY, Lin CW, Chang CC, *et al.* Percutaneous endoscopic unilateral laminotomy and bilateral decompression under 3D real-time image-guided navigation for spinal stenosis in degenerative lumbar kyphoscoliosis patients: an innovative preliminary study. BMC Musculoskelet Disord 2020; 21: 734.
[http://dx.doi.org/10.1186/s12891-020-03745-w]

[104] Carr DA, Abecassis IJ, Hofstetter CP. Full endoscopic unilateral laminotomy for bilateral decompression of the cervical spine: surgical technique and early experience. J Spine Surg 2020; 6(2): 447-56.
[http://dx.doi.org/10.21037/jss.2020.01.03] [PMID: 32656382]

[105] Kirkaldy-Willis WH, Wedge JH, Yong-Hing K, Tchang S, de Korompay V, Shannon R. Lumbar spinal nerve lateral entrapment. Clin Orthop Relat Res 1982; (169): 171-8.
[PMID: 7105575]

[106] Kirkaldy-Willis WH, Farfan HF. Instability of the lumbar spine. Clin Orthop Relat Res 1982; (165): 110-23.
[PMID: 6210480]

[107] Keim HA, Kirkaldy-Willis WH. Low back pain. Clin Symp 1987; 39(6): 1-32.

[PMID: 2963721]

[108]   Spengler DM, Ouellette EA, Battié M, Zeh J. Elective discectomy for herniation of a lumbar disc. Additional experience with an objective method. J Bone Joint Surg Am 1990; 72(2): 230-7.
[http://dx.doi.org/10.2106/00004623-199072020-00010] [PMID: 2303509]

[109]   Pathria M, Sartoris DJ, Resnick D. Osteoarthritis of the facet joints: accuracy of oblique radiographic assessment. Radiology 1987; 164(1): 227-30.
[http://dx.doi.org/10.1148/radiology.164.1.3588910] [PMID: 3588910]

[110]   Fujiwara A, Tamai K, Yamato M, *et al.* The relationship between facet joint osteoarthritis and disc degeneration of the lumbar spine: an MRI study. Eur Spine J 1999; 8(5): 396-401.
[http://dx.doi.org/10.1007/s005860050193] [PMID: 10552323]

[111]   Weishaupt D, Zanetti M, Boos N, Hodler J. MR imaging and CT in osteoarthritis of the lumbar facet joints. Skeletal Radiol 1999; 28(4): 215-9.
[http://dx.doi.org/10.1007/s002560050503] [PMID: 10384992]

[112]   Thalgott JS, Albert TJ, Vaccaro AR, *et al.* A new classification system for degenerative disc disease of the lumbar spine based on magnetic resonance imaging, provocative discography, plain radiographs and anatomic considerations. Spine J 2004; 4(6) (Suppl.): 167S-72S.
[http://dx.doi.org/10.1016/j.spinee.2004.07.001] [PMID: 15541662]

[113]   Rauschning W. Computed tomography and cryomicrotomy of lumbar spine specimens. A new technique for multiplanar anatomic correlation. Spine 1983; 8(2): 170-80.
[http://dx.doi.org/10.1097/00007632-198303000-00008] [PMID: 6857388]

[114]   Tsou PM, Alan Yeung C, Yeung AT. Posterolateral transforaminal selective endoscopic discectomy and thermal annuloplasty for chronic lumbar discogenic pain: a minimal access visualized intradiscal surgical procedure. Spine J 2004; 4(5): 564-73.
[http://dx.doi.org/10.1016/j.spinee.2004.01.014] [PMID: 15363430]

[115]   Yeung A, Gore S. Endoscopically guided foraminal and dorsal rhizotomy for chronic axial back pain based on cadaver and endoscopically visualized anatomic study. Int J Spine Surg 2014; 8.
[http://dx.doi.org/10.14444/1023]

[116]   Yeung A, Roberts A, Zhu L, Qi L, Zhang J, Lewandrowski KU. Treatment of Soft Tissue and Bony Spinal Stenosis by a Visualized Endoscopic Transforaminal Technique Under Local Anesthesia. Neurospine 2019; 16(1): 52-62.
[http://dx.doi.org/10.14245/ns.1938038.019] [PMID: 30943707]

[117]   Lewandrowski KU. Retrospective analysis of accuracy and positive predictive value of preoperative lumbar MRI grading after successful outcome following outpatient endoscopic decompression for lumbar foraminal and lateral recess stenosis. Clin Neurol Neurosurg 2019; 179(179): 74-80.
[http://dx.doi.org/10.1016/j.clineuro.2019.02.019] [PMID: 30870712]

[118]   Lewandrowski KU, Muraleedharan N, Eddy SA, *et al.* Artificial Intelligence Comparison of the Radiologist Report With Endoscopic Predictors of Successful Transforaminal Decompression for Painful Conditions of the Lumber Spine: Application of Deep Learning Algorithm Interpretation of Routine Lumbar Magnetic Resonance Imaging Scan. Int J Spine Surg 2020; 14(s3): S75-85.
[http://dx.doi.org/10.14444/7130] [PMID: 33208388]

[119]   Lewandrowski KU, Muraleedharan N, Eddy SA, *et al.* Reliability Analysis of Deep Learning Algorithms for Reporting of Routine Lumbar MRI Scans. Int J Spine Surg 2020; 14(s3): S98-S107.
[http://dx.doi.org/10.14444/7131] [PMID: 33122182]

[120]   Lewandrowski KU, Yeung A. Meaningful outcome research to validate endoscopic treatment of common lumbar pain generators with durability analysis. J Spine Surg 2020; 6(6) (Suppl. 1): S6-S13.
[http://dx.doi.org/10.21037/jss.2019.09.07] [PMID: 32195408]

[121]   LewandrowskI KU, Muraleedharan N, Eddy SA, *et al.* Feasibility of Deep Learning Algorithms for Reporting in Routine Spine Magnetic Resonance Imaging. Int J Spine Surg 2020; 14(s3): S86-97.

[http://dx.doi.org/10.14444/7131] [PMID: 33298549]

[122] Lewandrowski KU. The strategies behind "inside-out" and "outside-in" endoscopy of the lumbar spine: treating the pain generator. J Spine Surg 2020; 6(6) (Suppl. 1): S35-9.
[http://dx.doi.org/10.21037/jss.2019.06.06] [PMID: 32195412]

[123] Yeung AT, Gore S. *In-vivo* Endoscopic Visualization of Patho-anatomy in Symptomatic Degenerative Conditions of the Lumbar Spine II: Intradiscal, Foraminal, and Central Canal Decompression. Surg Technol Int 2011; 21(21): 299-319.
[PMID: 22505004]

[124] Gore S, Yeung A. The "inside out" transforaminal technique to treat lumbar spinal pain in an awake and aware patient under local anesthesia: results and a review of the literature. Int J Spine Surg 2014; 8.
[http://dx.doi.org/10.14444/1028]

[125] Osman SG, Narayanan M, Malik A, *et al.* Anatomic Treatment-based Classification of Diseased Lumbar Spinal Motion-segment. International Journal of Neuro & Spinal Sciences 2013; 1: 1-10.

[126] Lewandrowski KU, DE Carvalho PST, DE Carvalho P Jr, Yeung A. Minimal Clinically Important Difference in Patient-Reported Outcome Measures with the Transforaminal Endoscopic Decompression for Lateral Recess and Foraminal Stenosis. Int J Spine Surg 2020; 14(2): 254-66.
[http://dx.doi.org/10.14444/7034] [PMID: 32355633]

[127] Lee S, Lee JW, Yeom JS, *et al.* A practical MRI grading system for lumbar foraminal stenosis. AJR Am J Roentgenol 2010; 194(4): 1095-8.
[http://dx.doi.org/10.2214/AJR.09.2772] [PMID: 20308517]

[128] Yeung AT, Lewandrowski KU. Retrospective analysis of accuracy and positive predictive value of preoperative lumbar MRI grading after successful outcome following outpatient endoscopic decompression for lumbar foraminal and lateral recess stenosis. Clin Neurol Neurosurg 2019; 181: 52.
[http://dx.doi.org/10.1016/j.clineuro.2019.03.011]

[129] Lewandrowski KU. Successful outcome after outpatient transforaminal decompression for lumbar foraminal and lateral recess stenosis: The positive predictive value of diagnostic epidural steroid injection. Clin Neurol Neurosurg 2018; 173(173): 38-45.
[http://dx.doi.org/10.1016/j.clineuro.2018.07.015] [PMID: 30075346]

[130] Zwaan L, Monteiro S, Sherbino J, Ilgen J, Howey B, Norman G. Is bias in the eye of the beholder? A vignette study to assess recognition of cognitive biases in clinical case workups. BMJ Qual Saf 2017; 26(2): 104-10.
[http://dx.doi.org/10.1136/bmjqs-2015-005014] [PMID: 26825476]

[131] Henriksen K, Kaplan H. Hindsight bias, outcome knowledge and adaptive learning. Qual Saf Health Care 2003; 12(12) (Suppl. 2): ii46-50.
[http://dx.doi.org/10.1136/qhc.12.suppl_2.ii46] [PMID: 14645895]

CHAPTER 4

Transforaminal Percutaneous Endoscopic Lumbar Discectomy

Ji-Yeon Kim[1,*]**, Hyeun sung Kim**[1]**, Kai-Uwe Lewandrowski**[2,3,4] **and Il-Tae Jang**[1]

[1] *Department of Neurosurgery, Nanoori Hospital, Seoul City, South Korea*

[2] *Center for Advanced Spine Care of Southern Arizona and Surgical Institute of Tucson, Tucson AZ, USA*

[3] *Associate Professor Department of Orthopaedics, Fundación Universitaria Sanitas, Bogotá, D.C., Colombia, USA*

[4] *Visiting Professor, Department Orthopaedic Surgery, UNIRIO, Rio de Janeiro, Brazil*

Abstract: The transforaminal spinal surgery technique is the most commonly performed way of endoscopic discectomy. Initial placement of the working cannula may determine the sequence of procedural steps. Commonly applied variations of the technique include the "inside-out" and "outside-in" techniques. In this up-to-date chapter, the authors describe the necessary procedure steps of the transforaminal endoscopic discectomy procedure, focusing on downward migrated disc herniations as these may push the endoscopic spine surgeon to the limits of his or her skill set. Therefore, the authors describe the limitations of the technique and assess adequate neural element decompression in great detail.

Keywords: Lumbar disc herniation, Transforaminal approach.

INTRODUCTION

The transforaminal technique is one of the most commonly employed endoscopic spinal surgery methods in the treatment of lumbar disc herniation [1 - 5]. Percutaneous endoscopic lumbar discectomy (PELD) can be classified into Transforaminal PELD [1, 6 - 15] and Interlaminar PELD [1, 16 - 21] by way of the primary access to the compressive pathology. In this chapter, the authors highlight the anatomical and surgical tips of the transforaminal approach.

---

[*] **Corresponding author Ji-Yeon Kim:** Department of Neurosurgery, Nanoori Hospital, Seoul City, Republic of Korea; E-mail: soar1945@gmail.com

Kai-Uwe Lewandrowski, Jorge Felipe Ramírez León, Anthony Yeung, Hyeun-Sung Kim, Xifeng Zhang, Gun Choi, Stefan Hellinger and Álvaro Dowling (Eds.)

INDICATIONS AND APPLICATIONS

Recently, the techniques and devices used in percutaneous endoscopic lumbar discectomy have developed significantly.

Therefore, nearly all kinds of lumbar disc disease can be operated on using percutaneous endoscopic lumbar discectomy. Percutaneous endoscopic lumbar discectomy is not easy to perform due to the steep learning curve, especially in difficult and complicated cases. Some of these cases are presented in this chapter for the purpose of discussing the most modern applications of endoscopic spinal surgery technology.

1. Common Indications for Percutaneous Endoscopic Lumbar Discectomy

- Paramedian disc herniations with predominant leg pain
- Subligamentous ruptured or extruded disc with migration less than the height of the disc space
- Central disc herniation with predominant back pain
- Annular tears that cause chemical sciatica
- Lateral and extreme lateral disc herniation
- Foraminal disc herniation
- Synovial cysts of the facet joint
- Discal cyst [22]

2. Indications for Difficult Cases of Percutaneous Endoscopic Lumbar Discectomy

- Huge central protruded disc: high canal compromise
- Sequestrated disc that has migrated: superior migration, inferior migration
- Recurred Disc
    ○ after open lumbar discectomy
    ○ after percutaneous endoscopic lumbar discectomy
- Calcified disc
- Lateral recess stenosis
- Multi-level herniated disc

1. General Structural Anatomy: Posterolateral PELD Approach

According to anatomical consideration, to achieve an excellent clinical result using percutaneous endoscopic transforaminal discectomy, understanding the confines of Kambin's triangle formed by the exiting, and the traversing nerve root, and the inferior pedicle (Table **1**) [23 - 26]. The segmental artery commonly passes under the exiting nerve root (Figs. **1** - **3**). Therefore, this segmental artery may be associated with postoperative retroperitoneal hematoma [27 - 29].

Table 1. General anatomical structures in the PELD.

1) Kambin's triangular working zone
2) Exiting nerve root
3) Traversing nerve root
4) Annulus
5) Posterior longitudinal ligament (PLL)
6) Dura
7) Sympathetic nerve and sinuvertebral nerve
8) Iliolumbar vasculature and segmental artery
9) Viscera in the retroperitoneal space

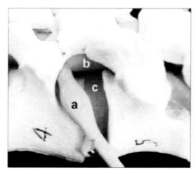

Fig. (1). Anatomical relationship of the transforaminal approach. **a.** exiting nerve root, **b.** traversing nerve root, **c.** Kambin's triangle.

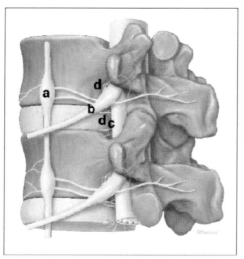

Fig. (2). Neurological relationship of the transforaminal approach. **a.** sympathetic trunk and ganglia, **b.** exiting nerve, **c.** traversing nerve, **d.** sinuvertebral nerves.

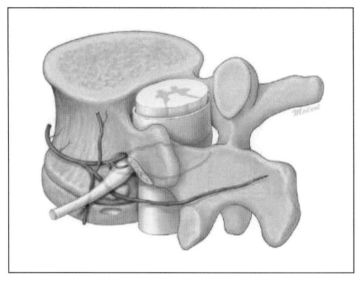

Fig. (3). Relationships of the segmental artery in the transforaminal approach. The segmental artery passes under the exiting nerve root. Therefore, when using the PELD for the exiting nerve root approach in cases of far lateral, foraminal, and superior migration discs, attention should be paid to prevent segmental artery injury. This can result in a serious retroperitoneal hematoma [30 - 32].

2. General Operative Anatomy: Posterolateral PELD Approach

The endoscopic spine surgeon should keep in mind the transforaminal anatomy when employing the endoscope (Fig. **4**). At the time of the first insertion of the endoscope, the surgeon can check the foraminal ligament, epidural fat, and annulus using the out-and-in approach (Fig. **5**).

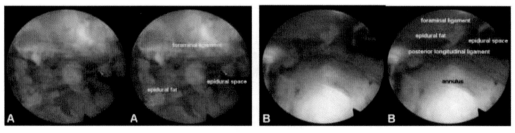

Fig. (4). Intraoperative images before **(A)** and after clearing **(B)** through a well-positioned working cannula are shown during the outside-in technique. The structures encountered during PELD are listed in Table **2**. .

After resection of the annulus, the posterior longitudinal ligament, annulus, epidural fat, and epidural space should be inspected to assess the decompression.

Operative Anatomical Structures in PELD

1. Annulus
2. Posterior longitudinal ligament
3. Dura
4. Exiting Nerve Root
5. Traversing Nerve Root
6. Ruptured Disc
7. Suprapedicular Route
8. Foraminal ligament
9. Epidural fat

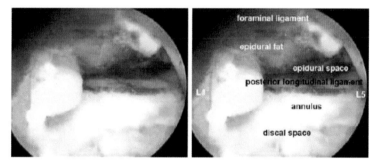

Fig. (5). Intraoperative image of well-positioned working cannula opening into the transforaminal space initially employing the inside-out approach and after annulotomy performed with outside-in methods.

3. Special Operative Anatomy: Posterolateral PELD Approach

In the advanced procedures of PELD, the patient's anatomy, such as the exiting nerve root, ruptured disc of the exiting nerve root, should be carefully examined. The suprapedicular area and the traversing nerve root approach's epidural space should also be thoroughly investigated.

Table 2. Special Operative Structures in the PELD.

-	Exiting Nerve Root Approach	Traversing Nerve Root Approach
Categories	• Far Lateral HNP • Foraminal HNP • Superior Migrated HNP	• Central HNP • Paracentral HNP • Inferior Migrated HNP
Important Structures	• Exiting nerve root • Segmental artery • Axillar area • Epidural space • Foraminal ligament	• Traversing nerve root • Epidural space • Suprapedicular area • Inferior migrated disc

4. Exiting Nerve Root Approach

The exiting nerve root should be protected while performing the exiting root approach. The exiting nerve root should be retracted by the working channel. It is also essential to identify the remnant disc by exposing the axilla area located rostral to the disc (Fig. **6**).

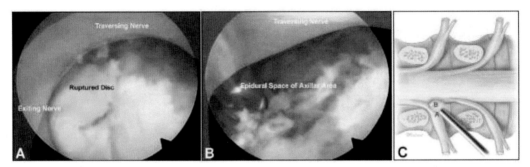

Fig. (6). Video images of the exiting root approach: After exiting root retraction **(A)** and an approach into the axilla area **(B)**. Illustrated image **(C)** A. image A, B. image B. To protect the exiting root during the exiting root approach, such as in far lateral, foraminal and superior migration HNP, displacement of the exiting root should be carefully performed.

5. Traversing Nerve Root Approach

In the traversing nerve root approach, it is critical to open the epidural space sufficiently to decompress the traversing nerve root. When the hard bony foraminal space is wide enough, it is easy to expose the epidural space by using the half-and-half approach (Fig. **7**) [33]. On the other hand, when the hard bony space is narrow, it is difficult to directly expose the epidural space by focusing on the suprapedicular area (Fig. **8**).

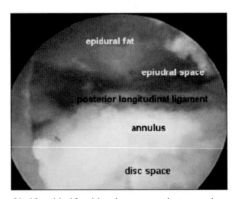

Fig. (7). Intraoperative image of half and half epidural exposure in traversing root approach.

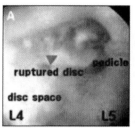 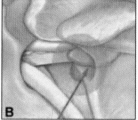 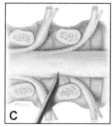 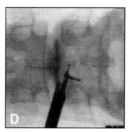

Fig. (8). Intraoperative **(A)** and illustrated **(B, C)** images of the suprapedicular area in the traversing root approach. For the approach to the inferior migrated area's epidural space, this suprapedicular point will give easy exposure to the epidural space—intraoperative image **(D)**.

6. Operative Safety Zone Anatomy

According to anatomical considerations, Kambin's triangle can change concerning the approach trajectory of the 1) conventional posterolateral approach, 2) less angled lateral approach, 3) exiting nerve root approach, and 4) suprapedicular approach (Fig. **8**). As an example of this change, the size of Kambin's triangle may decrease significantly under the less angled lateral approach than the conventional posterolateral approach. This decreased Kambin's triangle size may damage the exiting nerve root (Figs. **9** and **10**) [34 - 37].

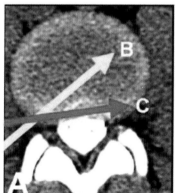 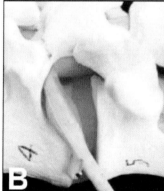 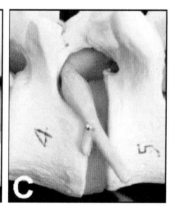

Fig. (9). Volume change of Kambin's safety triangle and exiting nerve root based on the transverse axis approach angle. A. Transverse axis approach, B. Conventional posterolateral approach, C. Less angled lateral approach.

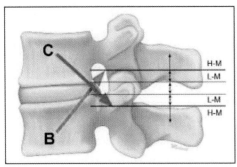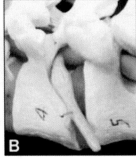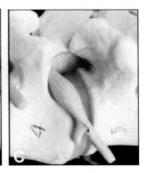

Fig. (10). Volume change of Kambin's safety triangle and exiting nerve root based on the longitudinal axis approach angle. A. Longitudinal axis approach, B. Exiting Nerve Root approach, C. Suprapedicular approach.

In the exiting nerve root approach, it is useful to use the round type working channel, preventing the exiting root from encroaching onto the working channel. It can reduce intraoperative injury to the nerve root caused by radiofrequency or forceps. Inferiorly migrated discs may cause severe pain because it is usually located right next to the pedicle causing a traversing nerve root pain syndrome. Therefore, it is important to open the perpendicular epidural space when approaching the inferior migration disc. While performing this maneuver, access to the epidural space to the suprapedicular area can be quickly achieved [39, 40].

7. SURGICAL PITFALLS

7.1. Position of the Working Cannula

We employed both the outside-in and the inside-out transforaminal approach for endoscopic lumbar discectomy. The outside-in approach may be more difficult for beginners. Nonetheless, it is more advantageous to remove high-grade inferior migrated disc cases (Table **3**; (Fig. **11**)).

Table 3. Characteristics of the Inside-out and outside-in approach.

-	Insight-out	Outside-In
Definition	• Insert the working cannula into the intradiscal space directly under the fluoroscopic guide annulus fenestration. • After then, change the working cannula target toward the disc fragment.	• Insert the working cannula into the transforaminal space before fenestration of the annulus. • After then, change the working cannula target toward the disc fragment.

(Table 3) cont.....

-	Insight-out	Outside-In
Advantages	• Easy • Safe for neural structures	• Preserving the anatomical structures: Ruptured disc • Easy for epidural exposure • Easy for working cannula manipulation • Decreasing the discal injury
Disadvantages	• Painful: Annulus fenestration • Distortion: Anatomical structures / ruptured disc • Discal injury	• Learning curve

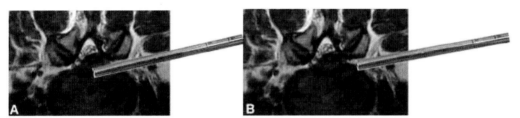

Fig. (11). Working Cannula Approach. A. Inside-out approach, B. Outside-In approach.

7.2. Anatomical Limitation

The anatomical relationship between the surgical neuroforamen and the iliac crest should be carefully evaluated before performing the transforaminal approach. This is because in the cases associated with a narrow foramen or a shallow suprapedicular area or a high iliac crest, or transitional anatomy, or vertical collapse of the lumbar spine due to advanced degeneration there will be the difficulty in approaching the target point [41 - 43]. Illustrative examples are shown in Figs. (**12 - 14**).

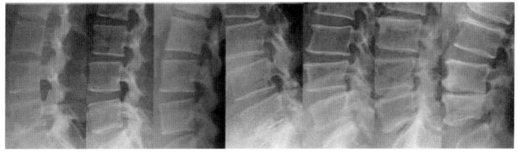

Fig. (12). Common clinical scenarios of foraminal stenosis that may raise the degree of difficulty during the transforaminal approach.

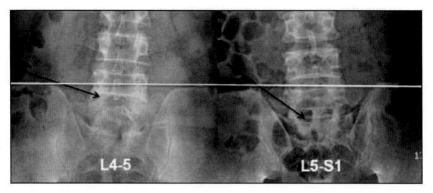

Fig. (13). High iliac crest compared to the target neuroforamen. In this situation, it is difficult to move toward the intraspinal target point to accomplish an epidural decompression.

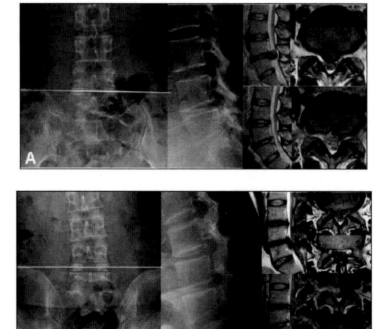

Fig. (14). An example of an unobliterated access to the L4/5 neuroforamen. Herniated disc material can usually be extracted despite a severely compromised canal (A) or highly inferior migrated cases (B).

• Foraminal Space

The condition of the foramina must be checked with a preoperative X-ray. When the foraminal space is narrow, another surgical method should be considered. In this situation, if the surgeon performs foraminal work with a drill or shaver, one can reach the target disc more conveniently (Fig. **12**).

• Iliac Crest

The iliac crest is essential for determining the direction of the working channel. If the iliac crest is high, it isn't easy to move upward from the intraspinal space and open the epidural space. When the iliac crest is at approximately the same level as the target disc, the endoscopic discectomy should not be difficult (Figs. **13 - 15**).

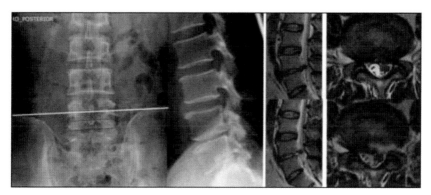

Fig. (15). In cases of narrow foramen at the surgical level and access obliteration by the iliac crest, removal of even small disc herniations may be difficult.

8. Accessible Surgical Access Area

A rigid endoscopic working cannula can cover a limited area for several disc levels in the transforaminal approach, including the paracentral level, superior migrated level, and some parts of the inferior migrated level. A moderate to highly inferior migrated disc may not be sufficiently accessible during the conventional posterolateral approach. Therefore, an inferior migrated disc will need a more advanced technique (Fig. **16**) [32].

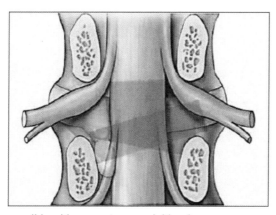

Fig. (16). Coverage area accessible with a percutaneous rigid endoscope.

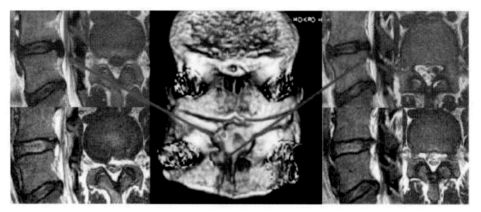

Fig. (17). In the cases of a disc fragment migrated inferior to the accessible coverage area illustrated in Fig. (**16**) the surgeon should consider an alternative translaminar approach.

9. TECHNIQUES FOR AN INFERIOR MIGRATED DISC

9.1. Epidural Exposure

Inferiorly migrated herniated discs can only be retrieved with the spinal endoscope if additional access to the epidural space is developed. The anatomical limitations to retrieve an inferior migrated disc with PELD at L4-5 are dictated by its relationship to the pedicle, iliac crest, and the foraminal width. Several approaches have been published to overcome difficulty dictated by anatomical restrictions:

9.1.1. Extreme Lateral Approach [2]

Dr. Ruetten introduced the extreme lateral approach as the first approach for the direct epidural space using a rigid endoscope. It approached the target point from a far lateral distance from the midline to the epidural space. Therefore, it inevitably had a low approach angle [9].

• Half-an-Half Technique and the Epiduroscopic Approach [41] In 2007, Lee *et al.* introduced the epiduroscopic approach, a half and half technique for migrated discs. Using this technique, the epidural space can be accessed more quickly [41].

9.1.2. Suprapedicular Approach

The suprapedicular approach was introduced in 2009 by Dr. Kim and used for high-grade inferior migrated discs. Entering the epidural space *via* the suprapedicular area will facilitate the transforaminal decompression (Fig. **17**) [17].

9.1.3. Foraminoplastic Technique

In cases of highly inferior migrated discs, disc removal using the rigid endoscope is not easy. The foraminoplastic technique introduced by Dr. Gun Choi, 2008 for the highly migrated disc, using the reamer or drill [38].

• L5-S1 interlaminar approach for L4-5 highly inferior migrated disc [27]

In 2010, Dr. Gun Choi, introduced the L5-S1 interlaminar approach for high grade down migrated L4-5 discs [44].

9.1.4. Contralateral approach [45]

In 2011, Dr. Kim and Yeom introduced the contra-lateral approach for high grade inferiorly migrated discs [45, 46].

Central canal stenosis may not pose an unsurmountable problem if foraminal configuration is sizable and the iliac crest does not obliterate access to the surgical neuroforamen. In those cases, the authors recommend PELD.

9.2. Entry Point

Checking the working channel's entry point is essential for performing a successful disc removal while minimizing damage to the exiting nerve root and other structures nearby; namely the abdominal organs.

9.2.1. MRI Length Measurement Method

In this method, the distance between the midline and the approaching target is measured on the preoperative MRI. It must be noted that the landmark on the skin can change position during surgery (Fig. **18**).

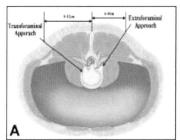 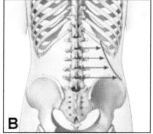 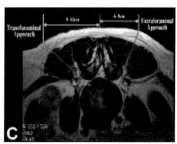

Fig. (18). MRI length measurement method. A. Anatomical sectional image, B. Surface image of approach length, C. MRI image of length measurement.

9.2.2. MRI Marker Method

Lee *et al.* recommend a preoperative MRI scan with markers placed on the patient's skin to determine the optimum skin insertion point for the working cannula (Fig. **19**).

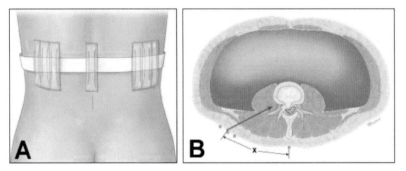

Fig. (19). MRI Marker Method illustrated **(A)** by placement of skin markers placed around the surgical level to determine the distance and best access angle on the preoperative MRI scan **(B)**.

10. INTRAOPERATIVE EXAMINATION METHOD

In addition, to measurements on preoperative advanced imaging studies, the endoscopic spine surgeon has the ability to measure best access trajectories and angles to the surgical neuroforamen. For this purpose, the surgeon should

1. Outline the borders of the posterior spinal musculature with its dorsal and ventral borders, to
2. Place a skin incision most appropriate for each patient's body habitus (Fig. **20**). This method has also been described in another chapter in volume 2 of this book series on the hybridized use of the "inside-out" and the "outside-in" technique.

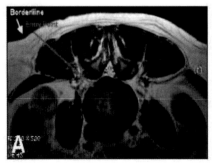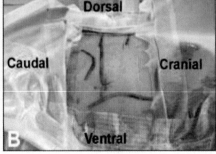

Fig. (20). Anatomical examination method. A. MRI Image, B. Surgical Surface Image.

11. PROCEDURAL STEPS

Endoscopic transforaminal lumbar discectomy is usually performed following the same choreography: Patient positioning, skin marking, making a skin incision administering local anesthesia, insertion of the needle and conducting provocative chromodiscography, working cannula insertion, decompressive discectomy, repositioning of the cannula and removal of the disc and finally, confirmation of the free exiting or traversing root. The steps of the transforaminal decompression surgery can by summarized as follows:

- Positioning & skin marking
- Anesthesia & Skin incision
- Needle insertion and provocative chromodiscography
- Working cannula insertion
- Decompressive discectomy
- Repositioning of the cannula & removal of disc
- Confirmation of the free exiting root or traversing root

11.1. Positioning & Skin Marking

- The first step of trans-foraminal PELD will be the marking of the insertion point. A fluoroscopic C-arm has always been a useful guide for identifying anatomical structures.
- The entry trajectory to the target level should be determine using data obtained from CT or MRI scans before the start of operation.
- Skin entry point commonly needed approximately 10 to 15 cm from the midline on the L4-5 level. And skin entry point from the midline decrease related to the above approach level (Fig. **20**).

11.2. Skin Incision & Anesthesia

- After local anesthetics infiltration in the operation field, the skin incision is made based on the preoperatively or intraoperatively estimated point.

11.3. Needle Insertion & Provocative Chromodiscography

- At this step, it is critical for good results of the targeted fragmentectomy to make a correct insertion point on the skin and to stick the needle straight into the target, which reduces injuries to the segmental arteries and nerves. Targeting should be performed using the safety Kambin's triangle method [22 - 26].
- This step is the most important step of PELD. When this step is performed

successfully, the rest of the procedure will proceed without much difficulty.

- After needle insertion, evocative chromodiscogram can apply for check the degenerated disc or lesional disc using the indigocarmin dye.

11.4. Guide Needle Insertion

- Guide needle insertion is usually carried out under local anesthesia. Fluoroscopic imaging is used to assess placement of the needle tip, the needle tip is advanced towards the more caudal and dorsal part of Kambin's triangle (Fig. **21**).
- To reduce the neural injury, guide needle target to the bony structures of facet(superior articular process) in the first step. After contact to the safe bony structures, guide needle repositioning to the safe Kambin's triange.

11.5. Evocative Chromodiscography

- After guide needle insertion, to identify the degenerated, surgical disc during procedure, Indigocarmin dye inject in the discal space.

11.6. Working Cannula Insertion

- After positioning and making the skin incision, the next step will be needle insertion into the correct and safe Kambin's triangle as soon as possible, toward the lowest part of Kambin's triangle that is located in the immediate upper part of the lower vertebrae (Fig. **21**).

The steps of the skin marking, needle insertion, and chromodiscography are summarized in the following videos:

Video-MIS Text 01-Video 01a-skin marking

Video-MIS Text 02-Video 01b-Needle Insertion, Chromodiscography

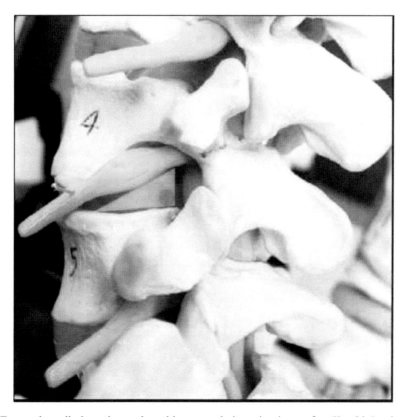

Fig. (21). Targeted needle insertion and working cannula insertion into safety Kambin's triangle. Needle insertion into the red circle area will provide the best targeting.

11.7. Working Cannula Placement

11.7.1. Outside-In Approach

The working cannula is inserted into the transforaminal space following the guidewire that is placed through a spinal needle that is advanced into the neuroforamen. Acceptable placement of this working cannula before entering the disc space *via* annulus fenestration (see inside-out technique) will be 1) at the medial interpedicular line formed by the ipsilateral pedicles on the fluoroscopic AP view, and 2) the most posterior part of the disc on the fluoroscopic lateral view. The working cannula will be located in the space between the exiting nerve root and the traversing nerve root (Fig. **22**).

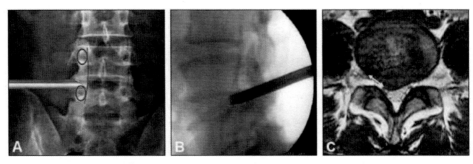

Fig. (22). A, B. Good placement of the working cannula in the foraminal space (out-and-in approach). C. Working cannula will pass through between exiting and traversing nerve root.

11.7.2. Inside-Out Approach

The working cannula is insert into the targeted intradiscal space after penetration through the annulus and *via* annulus fenestration. The working cannula may be advanced *via* the guidewire or serial dilators. Ideally, the working cannula is located close to the targeted disc fragment.

11.8. Decompressive Discectomy

11.8.1. Foraminal Work

From the aspect of the outside-in approach, the endoscope is inserted into the foraminal space through the working channel. In this situation, the surgeon should be able to enter the epidural space using decompressive endoscopic instruments with adjunctive use of the radiofrequency coagulation. The individual steps of the foraminal decompression procedural steps are summarized in the following videos.

Video-MIS Text 03-Video 02a-Foraminal Work-01: General

Video-MIS Text 04-Video 02b-Foraminal Work-02: Abundant Fatty Tissue-01

Video-MIS Text 05-Video 02c-Foraminal Work-03: Abundant Fatty Tissue-02

Video-MIS Text 06-Video 02d-Foraminal Work-04: Huge blood tinged

Video-MIS Text 07-Video 02e-Foraminal Work-05: Massive bleeding

11.8.2. Annulus Fenestration

The annular fenestration technique is required to position the working cannula inside the intervertebral disc space. Equipment needs and the procedural steps for annulus fenestration, including punch and endoscopic probe, are summarized in the following videos:

Video-MIS Text 08-Video 03a-Annulus Opening Technique-01-punch

Video-MIS Text 09-Video 03b-Annulus Opening Technique-02-punch

Video-MIS Text 10-Video 03c-Annulus Opening Technique-03-after decompression

11.8.3. Discectomy

After these previous procedural steps, the surgeon can commence the decompressive discectomy. The authors recommend that the endoscopic surgeon stop the "inside-out" intradiscal decompression before reaching the contralateral pedicle on the posteroanterior (PA) view (Fig. **23**). This precaution is intended to protect the anterior dural sac and the contralateral traversing root from injury. The decompression and the position of the endoscopic instruments should also be checked in the lateral projection to avoid anterior penetration of the annuls and, thus, vascular injury in the abdomen.

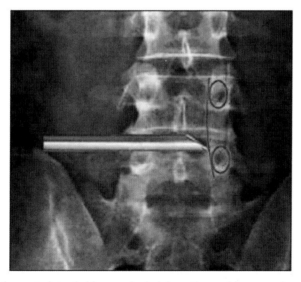

Fig. (23). To prevent the contralateral side neurologic injury, the working cannula and the working forceps should not over pass the contralateral side of pedicle inner margin.

The individual steps of the intradiscal decompression procedural steps are summarized in the following video.

Video-MIS Text 11-Video 04-decompression

11.9. Assessing the Decompression

The decompression of the neural elements can be best be assessed by repositioning of the working cannula. There are several ways to examine the decompression as frequently practiced by the authors:

11.9.1. Exiting Root Approach

In the superior exiting nerve root approach, a round type working cannula will give a safer and better clinical result. To prevent injury, the exiting root should be exposed by motions of gentle pushing with a round working channel. When the exiting root is identified, the working cannula should be introduced into the axilla area (Fig. **24**). The exiting root approach is shown in the following video.

Video-MIS Text 12-Video 05a-00-repositioning-exiting root approach

11.9.2. Epidural Central Approach

For cases of the high canal compromised type, epidural exposure will be the most important point for achieving the successful removal of the symptomatic disc disc herniation (Fig. **24**). The epidural central approach is shown in the following videos.

Video-MIS Text 13-Video 05b-repositioning-01-lateral annulus opening-01

Video-MIS Text 14-Video 05c-repositioning-02-epidural central approach-02

11.9.3. Epidural Inferior Approach

For cases of a highly inferior migrated disc, epidural exposure around the suprapedicular area will be helpful to expose the epidural space. This suprapedicular area is usually covered with abundant fatty tissue. After removal of the fatty tissue and clearing of this area, you can expose the ruptured, inferior migrated disc and traversing nerve root through this suprapedicular space (Fig. **24**). In the difficult situation of insertion of forceps or working instrument into the epidural space due to the barrier of the bony structures, foraminoplastic widening using the high speed drill or reamer will be helpful.

11.9.4. Major Concerns in the PELD for Inferior Migrated Disc

- Bleeding control
- Extraction of migrated disc material
- Confirmation of decompressed ventral epidural space

Video-MIS Text 15-Video 05-repositioning-03-epidural inferior approach-0--repositioning

Video-MIS Text 16-Video 05-repositioning-03-epidural inferior approach-0--clearing

Video-MIS Text 17-Video 05-repositioning-03-epidural inferior approach-03-disc extraction

Video-MIS Text 18-Video 05-repositioning-04-epidural inferior approach-0--direct exposure

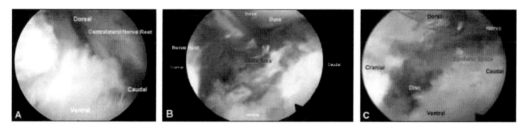

Fig. (24). Final confirmation of free nerve root. A. Contralateral approach, B. Superior approach, C. Inferior approach.

Video-MIS Text 19-Video 06-Confirmation-superior

Video-MIS Text 20-Video 06-Confirmation-contralateral

Video-MIS Text 21-Video 06-Confirmation-inferior migration

DISCUSSION

The transforaminal endoscopic discectomy is the workhorse procedure of spinal endoscopy. There are many variations of this time-proven technique. The novice endoscopic spine surgeon should take the procedural steps introduced by the authors of this chapter as a recommendation as to how to perform this procedure. The authors have arrived at the described protocols by performing the transforaminal endoscopic surgery techniques for over 15 years. Their concepts and protocols are based on their observations in their patients' operating room and clinical follow-up. The problems highlighted with downward migrated herniated discs focus on the authors' clinical practice as it can catch the inexperienced endoscopic spine surgeon off guard. As with any new surgical procedure, advanced postgraduate training by experienced master surgeons is recommended as the transforaminal endoscopy learning curve is steep. It may take more than a few cases to perfect the technique, particularly if the aspiring endoscopic spine surgeon has no experience with endoscopes of any sorts commonly used in other human joints or organ systems. The endoscopic view is distinctly different from the microsurgical view through the operating microscope. The authors hope that the reader of this chapter has found it helpful in advancing their understanding of common problems encountered during transforaminal endoscopic surgery.

CONCLUSION

The transforaminal endoscopic approach to the lumbar spine is the most widely used endoscopic spinal surgery technique. It is a time-proven and enables the endoscopic spine surgeon to address most herniated discs in the lumbar spine. The patient selection criteria, surgical indications, and other procedural related problems are well described in other chapters in this book series. In this chapter, the authors wanted to describe the necessary procedural steps to enable beginner surgeons to understand the procedure and aid them in their postgraduate endoscopic spine surgery training.

CONSENT FOR PUBLICATION

Not applicable.

CONFLICT OF INTEREST

The authors declare no conflict of interest, financial or otherwise.

ACKNOWLEDGEMENTS

Declared None.

REFERENCES

[1]   Kim DH, Choi G, Lee SH. Endoscopic Spine Procedures. Thieme Medical Publishers 2011; p. 11.

[2]   Abdullah AF, Wolber PG, Warfield JR, Gunadi IK. Surgical management of extreme lateral lumbar disc herniations: review of 138 cases. Neurosurgery 1988; 22(4): 648-53.
       [http://dx.doi.org/10.1227/00006123-198804000-00005] [PMID: 3374776]

[3]   Ahn Y, Lee SH, Park WM, Lee HY, Shin SW, Kang HY. Percutaneous endoscopic lumbar discectomy for recurrent disc herniation: surgical technique, outcome, and prognostic factors of 43 consecutive cases. Spine 2004; 29(16): E326-32.
       [http://dx.doi.org/10.1097/01.BRS.0000134591.32462.98] [PMID: 15303041]

[4]   McCulloch JA. Principles of Microsurgery for Lumbar Disc Diseases. New York: Raven Press 1989.

[5]   Mekhail N, Kapural L. Intradiscal thermal annuloplasty for discogenic pain: an outcome study. Pain Pract 2004; 4(2): 84-90.
       [http://dx.doi.org/10.1111/j.1533-2500.2004.04203.x] [PMID: 17166191]

[6]   Ditsworth DA. Endoscopic transforaminal lumbar discectomy and reconfiguration: a postero-lateral approach into the spinal canal. Surg Neurol 1998; 49(6): 588-97.
       [http://dx.doi.org/10.1016/S0090-3019(98)00004-4] [PMID: 9637618]

[7]   Tsou PM, Yeung AT. Transforaminal endoscopic decompression for radiculopathy secondary to intracanal noncontained lumbar disc herniations: outcome and technique. Spine J 2002; 2(1): 41-8.
        [http://dx.doi.org/10.1016/S1529-9430(01)00153-X] [PMID: 14588287]

[8]   Tsou PM, Alan Yeung C, Yeung AT. Posterolateral transforaminal selective endoscopic discectomy and thermal annuloplasty for chronic lumbar discogenic pain: a minimal access visualized intradiscal surgical procedure. Spine J 2004; 4(5): 564-73.
        [http://dx.doi.org/10.1016/j.spinee.2004.01.014] [PMID: 15363430]

[9]   Ruetten S, Komp M, Godolias G. An extreme lateral access for the surgery of lumbar disc herniations inside the spinal canal using the full-endoscopic uniportal transforaminal approach-technique and prospective results of 463 patients. Spine 2005; 30(22): 2570-8.
        [http://dx.doi.org/10.1097/01.brs.0000186327.21435.cc] [PMID: 16284597]

[10]   Jasper GP, Francisco GM, Telfeian AE. Endoscopic transforaminal discectomy for an extruded lumbar disc herniation. Pain Physician 2013; 16(1): E31-5.
        [PMID: 23340542]

[11]   Eustacchio S, Flaschka G, Trummer M, Fuchs I, Unger F. Endoscopic percutaneous transforaminal treatment for herniated lumbar discs. Acta Neurochir (Wien) 2002; 144(10): 997-1004.
        [http://dx.doi.org/10.1007/s00701-002-1003-9] [PMID: 12382128]

[12]   Gibson JN, Cowie JG, Iprenburg M. Transforaminal endoscopic spinal surgery: the future 'gold standard' for discectomy? - A review. Surgeon 2012; 10(5): 290-6.
        [http://dx.doi.org/10.1016/j.surge.2012.05.001] [PMID: 22705355]

[13]   Yeung AT, Tsou PM. Posterolateral endoscopic excision for lumbar disc herniation: Surgical technique, outcome, and complications in 307 consecutive cases. Spine 2002; 27(7): 722-31.
        [http://dx.doi.org/10.1097/00007632-200204010-00009] [PMID: 11923665]

[14]   Yeung AT, Yeung CA. Advances in endoscopic disc and spine surgery: foraminal approach. Surg Technol Int 2003; 11: 255-63.
        [PMID: 12931309]

[15]   Yeung AT. The evolution of percutaneous spinal endoscopy and discectomy: state of the art. Mt Sinai J Med 2000; 67(4): 327-32.
        [PMID: 11021785]

[16]   Maroon JC. Current concepts in minimally invasive discectomy. Neurosurgery 2002; 51(5) (Suppl.): S137-45.
        [PMID: 12234441]

[17]   Kim HS, Park JY. Comparative assessment of different percutaneous endoscopic interlaminar lumbar discectomy (PEID) techniques. Pain Physician 2013; 16(4): 359-67.
        [PMID: 23877452]

[18]   Choi G, Lee SH, Raiturker PP, Lee S, Chae YS. Percutaneous endoscopic interlaminar discectomy for intracanalicular disc herniations at L5-S1 using a rigid working channel endoscope. Neurosurgery 2006; 58(1) (Suppl.): ONS59-68.
        [http://dx.doi.org/10.1227/01.NEU.0000362000.35742.3D] [PMID: 16479630]

[19]   Ruetten S, Komp M, Godolias G. A New full-endoscopic technique for the interlaminar operation of lumbar disc herniations using 6-mm endoscopes: prospective 2-year results of 331 patients. Minim Invasive Neurosurg 2006; 49(2): 80-7.
        [http://dx.doi.org/10.1055/s-2006-932172] [PMID: 16708336]

[20]   Ruetten S, Komp M, Merk H, Godolias G. Use of newly developed instruments and endoscopes: full-endoscopic resection of lumbar disc herniations *via* the interlaminar and lateral transforaminal approach. J Neurosurg Spine 2007; 6(6): 521-30.
        [http://dx.doi.org/10.3171/spi.2007.6.6.2] [PMID: 17561740]

[21]   Ruetten S, Komp M, Merk H, Godolias G. Full-endoscopic interlaminar and transforaminal lumbar

discectomy *versus* conventional microsurgical technique: a prospective, randomized, controlled study. Spine 2008; 33(9): 931-9.
[http://dx.doi.org/10.1097/BRS.0b013e31816c8af7] [PMID: 18427312]

[22]   Kambin P, Zhou L. History and current status of percutaneous arthroscopic disc surgery. Spine 1996; 21(24) (Suppl.): 57S-61S.
[http://dx.doi.org/10.1097/00007632-199612151-00006] [PMID: 9112325]

[23]   Kambin P, Vaccaro A. Arthroscopic microdiscectomy. Spine J 2003; 3(3) (Suppl.): 60S-4S.
[http://dx.doi.org/10.1016/S1529-9430(02)00558-2] [PMID: 14589219]

[24]   Kambin P, Savitz MH. Arthroscopic microdiscectomy: an alternative to open disc surgery. Mt Sinai J Med 2000; 67(4): 283-7.
[PMID: 11021778]

[25]   Kambin P, O'Brien E, Zhou L, Schaffer JL. Arthroscopic microdiscectomy and selective fragmentectomy. Clin Orthop Relat Res 1998; (347): 150-67.
[PMID: 9520885]

[26]   Kambin P, Zhou L. Arthroscopic discectomy of the lumbar spine. Clin Orthop Relat Res 1997; 337: 49-57.
[http://dx.doi.org/10.1097/00003086-199704000-00007] [PMID: 9137176]

[27]   Kim HS, Ju CI, Kim SW, Kim JG. Huge Psoas Muscle Hematoma due to Lumbar Segmental Vessel Injury Following Percutaneous Endoscopic Lumbar Discectomy. J Korean Neurosurg Soc 2009; 45(3): 192-5.
[http://dx.doi.org/10.3340/jkns.2009.45.3.192] [PMID: 19352485]

[28]   Ahn Y, Kim JU, Lee BH, Lee SH, Park JD, Hong DH. Massive Retroperitoneal Hematoma after Transforaminal Percutaneous Endoscopic Lumbar Discectomy: Reoprt of Two Cases. Rachis 2008; (4): 10-1.

[29]   Ahn Y, Kim JU, Lee BH, *et al.* Postoperative retroperitoneal hematoma following transforaminal percutaneous endoscopic lumbar discectomy. J Neurosurg Spine 2009; 10(6): 595-602.
[http://dx.doi.org/10.3171/2009.2.SPINE08227] [PMID: 19558294]

[30]   Choi G, Lee SH, Bhanot A, Raiturker PP, Chae YS. Percutaneous endoscopic discectomy for extraforaminal lumbar disc herniations: extraforaminal targeted fragmentectomy technique using working channel endoscope. Spine 2007; 32(2): E93-9.
[http://dx.doi.org/10.1097/01.brs.0000252093.31632.54] [PMID: 17224806]

[31]   Epimenio RO, Giancarlo D, Giuseppe T, Raffaelino R, Luigi F. Extraforaminal lumbar herniation: "far lateral" microinvasive approach retrospective study. J Spinal Disord Tech 2003; 16(6): 534-8.
[http://dx.doi.org/10.1097/00024720-200312000-00009] [PMID: 14657751]

[32]   Kim HS, Ju CI, Kim SW, Kim JG. Endoscopic transforaminal suprapedicular approach in high grade inferior migrated lumbar disc herniation. J Korean Neurosurg Soc 2009; 45(2): 67-73.
[http://dx.doi.org/10.3340/jkns.2009.45.2.67] [PMID: 19274114]

[33]   Soldner F, Hoelper BM, Wallenfang T, Behr R. The translaminar approach to canalicular and cranio-dorsolateral lumbar disc herniations. Acta Neurochir (Wien) 2002; 144(4): 315-20.
[http://dx.doi.org/10.1007/s007010200043] [PMID: 12021876]

[34]   Birbilis T, Koulalis D, Matis G, Theodoropoulou E, Papaparaskeva K. Microsurgical muscle-splitting approach for extracanalicular lumbar disc herniation: an analysis of 28 consecutive cases. Acta Orthop Belg 2009; 75(1): 70-4.
[PMID: 19358402]

[35]   Huber P, Reulen HJ. CT-observations of the intra- and extracanalicular disc herniation. Acta Neurochir (Wien) 1989; 100(1-2): 3-11.
[http://dx.doi.org/10.1007/BF01405267] [PMID: 2816531]

[36]   Reulen HJ, Pfaundler S, Ebeling U. The lateral microsurgical approach to the "extracanalicular"

lumbar disc herniation. I: A technical note. Acta Neurochir (Wien) 1987; 84(1-2): 64-7.
[http://dx.doi.org/10.1007/BF01456353] [PMID: 3825610]

[37]   Min JH, Kang SH, Lee JB, Cho TH, Suh JK, Rhyu IJ. Morphometric analysis of the working zone for endoscopic lumbar discectomy. J Spinal Disord Tech 2005; 18(2): 132-5.
[http://dx.doi.org/10.1097/01.bsd.0000159034.97246.4f] [PMID: 15800429]

[38]   Choi G, Lee SH, Lokhande P, *et al.* Percutaneous endoscopic approach for highly migrated intracanal disc herniations by foraminoplastic technique using rigid working channel endoscope. Spine 2008; 33(15): E508-15.
[http://dx.doi.org/10.1097/BRS.0b013e31817bfa1a] [PMID: 18594449]

[39]   Chae KH, Ju CI, Lee SM, Kim BW, Kim SY, Kim HS. Strategies for Noncontained Lumbar Disc Herniation by an Endoscopic Approach : Transforaminal Suprapedicular Approach, Semi-Rigid Flexible Curved Probe, and 3-Dimensional Reconstruction CT with Discogram. J Korean Neurosurg Soc 2009; 46(4): 312-6.
[http://dx.doi.org/10.3340/jkns.2009.46.4.312] [PMID: 19893718]

[40]   Ahn Y. Transforaminal percutaneous endoscopic lumbar discectomy: technical tips to prevent complications. Expert Rev Med Devices 2012; 9(4): 361-6.
[http://dx.doi.org/10.1586/erd.12.23] [PMID: 22905840]

[41]   Lee S, Kim SK, Lee SH, *et al.* Percutaneous endoscopic lumbar discectomy for migrated disc herniation: classification of disc migration and surgical approaches. Eur Spine J 2007; 16(3): 431-7.
[http://dx.doi.org/10.1007/s00586-006-0219-4] [PMID: 16972067]

[42]   Ha SW, Ju CI, Kim SW, Lee S, Kim YH, Kim HS. Clinical outcomes of percutaneous endoscopic surgery for lumbar discal cyst. J Korean Neurosurg Soc 2012; 51(4): 208-14.
[http://dx.doi.org/10.3340/jkns.2012.51.4.208] [PMID: 22737300]

[43]   Choi I, Ahn JO, So WS, Lee SJ, Choi IJ, Kim H. Exiting root injury in transforaminal endoscopic discectomy: preoperative image considerations for safety. Eur Spine J 2013; 22(11): 2481-7. Epub ahead of print
[http://dx.doi.org/10.1007/s00586-013-2849-7] [PMID: 23754603]

[44]   Choi G, Prada N, Modi HN, Vasavada NB, Kim JS, Lee SH. Percutaneous endoscopic lumbar herniectomy for high-grade down-migrated L4-L5 disc through an L5-S1 interlaminar approach: a technical note. Minim Invasive Neurosurg 2010; 53(3): 147-52.
[http://dx.doi.org/10.1055/s-0030-1254145] [PMID: 20809458]

[45]   Yeom KS, Choi YS. Full endoscopic contralateral transforaminal discectomy for distally migrated lumbar disc herniation. J Orthop Sci 2011; 16(3): 263-9.
[http://dx.doi.org/10.1007/s00776-011-0048-0] [PMID: 21442187]

[46]   Kim JS, Choi G, Lee SH. Percutaneous endoscopic lumbar discectomy *via* contralateral approach: a technical case report. Spine 2011; 36(17): E1173-8.
[http://dx.doi.org/10.1097/BRS.0b013e3182264458] [PMID: 21785301]

CHAPTER 5

Structural Preservation Interlaminar Endoscopic Lumbar Discectomy (IELD) For L5-S1 Herniated Disc

Ravindra Singh[1], **Hyeun Sung Kim**[2,*] and **Il-Tae Jang**[2]

[1] *Department of Neurosurgery, Halifax Infirmary Hospital, Dalhousie University, Nova Scotia, Canada*

[2] *Department of Neurosurgery, Nanoori Hospital, Gangnam, Seoul, South Korea*

Abstract: Endoscopic spine surgeries are gradually evolving and being accepted by spine surgeons globally. Transforaminal approach discectomy is one of the initial surgeries done with a fully endoscopic approach. The transforaminal approach has various advantages. Nevertheless, it has certain limitations too, and a high lying iliac crest anatomically impeding access is one of them. An Interlaminar approach for L5-S1 herniated disc exploiting a wide interlaminar window is a phenomenal endoscopic approach to this common clinical problem.

Keywords: Endoscopic approach, Interlaminar Endoscopic Lumbar Discectomy, L5-S1 Herniated Disc, Transforaminal approach.

INTRODUCTION

Initial efforts in endoscopic spine surgeries included blind percutaneous discectomy performed under fluoroscopic guidance. Later on, with the pioneering work by Kambin *et al.* a full endoscopic discectomy became a reality. Percutaneous endoscopic discectomy has been improvised by many workers in due course of time and is getting acceptance globally among spine surgeons with results equivalent or superior to conventional surgeries [1, 2]. Despite the various advantages, the endoscopic discectomy has certain limitations, and the approach to L5-S1 disc, limited by anatomy of the iliac crest, transverse process, and foramen are a few of them [1, 3]. Spine surgeons are conventionally well-versed in the interlaminar approach utilizing the interlaminar window to access thecal sac and intervertebral disc space. The same interlaminar window can be used for the

---

* **Corresponding author Hyeun Sung Kim:** Department of Neurosurgery, Nanoori Hospital, Gangnam, Seoul, Republic of Korea; Tel: +82-10-2440-2631; E-mail: neurospinekim@gmail.com

access of the L5-S1 intervertebral disc in endoscopic surgery, bypassing the iliac crest and obviating the limitations of the transforaminal approach [2 - 7]. In this chapter, readers will be introduced to the interlaminar approach's rationale and techniques to the L5-S1 disc. The authors provide a concise description of the indications and surgical procedure, including intraoperative landmarks for skin incision, endoscope, and discectomy.

ANATOMY & RATIONALE

The interlaminar approach for endoscopic surgeries is easily possible due to a wide interlaminar window available due to the spacing of pedicles, lateral recesses, and superior and inferior laminae at the L5-S1 level [8, 9]. Knowledge of the radiographic anatomy of the L5-S1 spine is important for the interlaminar approach. The landmark for the approach are spinous process (L5 & S1), superior lamina for S1 vertebra, inferior lamina of L5 vertebra, superior articular process (SAP) of S1, inferior articular process (IAP) of L5, L5-S1 intervertebral disc, and lateral recesses [2, 6, 7, 10 - 12]. Middle sacral vessels right, and left iliac vessels are important structures lying anterior to the L5 and S1 vertebral bodies. Anatomically, they are far enough from the approach and surgical field, but care should be exerted not to injure them accidentally [10]. Recent advances in endoscopy techniques allow the transforaminal approach a great deal of flexibility, and most of the limitations of earlier techniques have been overcome. However, a high lying iliac crest, L5-S1 level, and sagittal plane deformity are still posing limitation to the transforaminal approach [1, 13, 14].

THE CONCEPT OF V-POINTS

For beginners, understanding the docking points from the start of the procedure and through intermediate steps to the conclusion is fundamental. The interlaminar approach surgery though docking points'. These docking points are typically described as 'V-Points (Fig. **1**) [5, 15, 16]. The ipsilateral V-Point is the first docking point and is defined as the junction of the most lateral points of the superior lamina of the S1 vertebra and the inferior lamina of L5 on the side skin incision is made. Midline 'V-Point' (Cranial) is the junction of the most cranial point on the ventral aspect of the L5 spinous process to the nearest point on the inferior lamina of the L5, also called cranial spinolaminar junction [5, 15, 16].

A similar midline 'V-Point' can be recognized caudally at the S1 spinous process's junction and superior S1 lamina (Fig. **1**). The contralateral 'V-point' is defined as the junction of the most lateral aspect of the superior lamina of the S1and the most caudal point of the medial part of the SAP of S1 on the opposite side. These V-points are important landmarks during surgery and guide the surgeon during the procedure. V-points are often used by the surgeon to orient them in the endoscopic space.

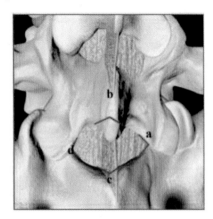

Fig. (1). "V-Points" **(a)** Ipsilateral for Right Approach **(b, c)** Cranial and Caudal Midline (Spinolaminar Junction) **(d)** Contralateral.

PRESERVATION OF THE MOTION SEGMENT

The motion segment consists of two adjacent vertebrae with the intervertebral disc and facet joints between them and their ligaments. Removal of one facet renders the motion segment unstable [17 - 19]. Interlaminar endoscopy can deal with spinal pathology with minimal resection of facets. This is also important for endoscopic discectomy at the L5-S1 level. Less facet resection translates into a decreased risk of iatrogenic instability of the motion segment [19, 20].

SURGICAL STEPS

Ipsilateral Discectomy Technique

Indications

Central, lateral, and lateral recess herniation

Anaesthesia

General anaesthesia, epidural anaesthesia

Position

Prone with hips and knees fixed. Preferably on Wilson™ (Mizuho OSI) frame.

Discography

L5-S1 discography with 0.8% Indigo Carmine (Carmine, Korea United

Pharmaceutical, Yoenki, Korea) mixed with Iobrix injection (Taejoon Pharma, Korea) is done through transforaminal route [2, 5, 15, 16]. This will ensure easy visualization of the disc (Fig. **2**).

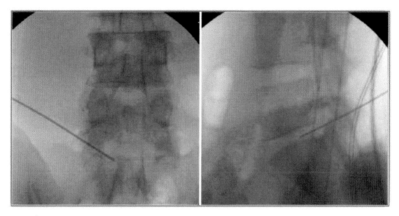

Fig. (2). Discography.

Skin Incision & Markings

The skin incision is marked under fluoroscopy guidance and placed over the most lateral aspect of the interlaminar window. Ipsilateral 'V-Point' is an important fluoroscopic landmark for the skin incision [5, 15, 16] (Fig. **3**).

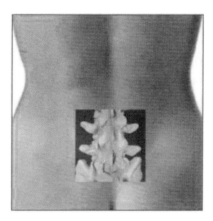

Fig. (3). Skin Incision.

Docking of Working Channel and Endosope

The endoscope author used is TESSYS^R (Joimax GmbH, Germany). This system has a working tube with outer diameter of 7.5 mm and bevelled tip. The endoscope has 6.5 mm outer diameter and 3.7 mm inner working channel. The viewing angle of the endoscope is 30°. Through the skin incision a thick and blunt tipped guiding rod is inserted and docked on the ipsilateral 'V-Point'. Dilator is inserted on this guide rod. The working channel is inserted over the final dilator which is removed then. The working tube is docked with the bevel end facing medially to protect thecal sheath. An endoscope is inserted through the working tube and obstructing structures (*e.g.* muscles and fat) are dissected and ligamentum flavum is exposed clearly [5, 15, 16] (Fig. **4**).

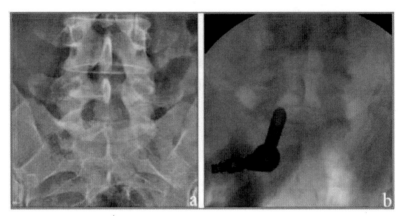

Fig. (4). Ipsilateral Approach **(a)** "V-Point" and **(b)** Docking of the Working Tube.

Splitting of Lgamentum Flavum

The ligamentum flavum is split vertically with dissector, and the gap thus formed is enlarged with the help of the bevel of the working tube by moving the bevel end clockwise to protect the exiting nerve root (Right side and the direction of the rotation will be opposite on the left side). In the epidural space thecal sac, nerve root and fat are identified. The epidural fat is dissected with a radiofrequency probe [Ellman's bipolar radiofrequency electro coagulator (Elliquence, Baldwin, New York, USA)] [5, 6, 15, 16] (Fig. **5**).

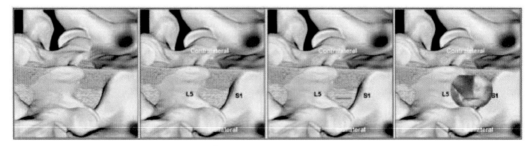

Fig. (5). Stages of Ligamentum Flavum Splitting.

Discectomy

If extruded disc material is seen in epidural space, it is removed with forceps. The herniated disc is located using clues from MRI images and retracting thecal and root with the rotational movement of the working channel. An annular cutter, punch, or dissector can be used to increase the opening on the annulus and discectomy is completed [2, 5 - 7, 15, 16, 18] (Figs. **6** and **7**).

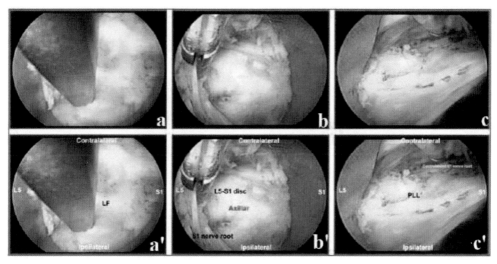

Fig. (6). Endoscopic Views (a, a') Ligamentum Flavum (b, b') Disc and Nerve Root (c, c') Contralateral Nerve Root, Posterior Longitudinal Ligament (PLL).

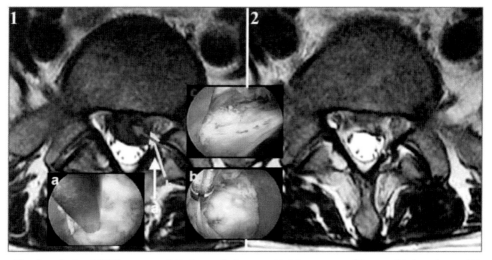

Fig. (7). Correlating MRI Images and Endoscopic Images **(a)** Ligamentum Flavum **(b)** Annulus and Nerve Root **(c)** Disc. 1 Preoperative MRI Image Showing Disc Herniation. 2 Postoperative MRI Image Showing Discectomy.

Annular Sealing

Following discectomy, the annular opening is closed using the coagulation function of bipolar radiofrequency. The coagulation is done at the periphery first near intact annular fibers first and proceeds further toward the centre of the annular defect [5] (Fig. **8**).

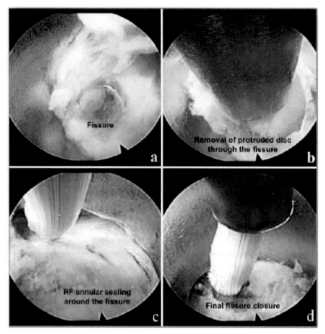

Fig. (8). Annular Sealing **(a)** Fissure, **(b)** Removal of the Disc and **(c, d)** Annular Sealing using RF Probe.

Skin Closure

Remove the working channel and endoscope and close the skin with Proline or Nylon sutures. The split fibers of the ligamentum flavum fall back together and need no closure. The intact ligamentum flavum prevents fibrosis (Fig. **9**).

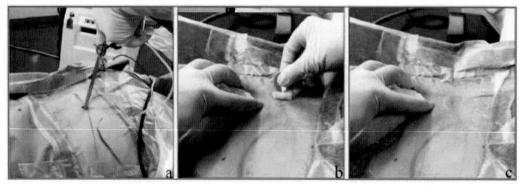

Fig. (9). Incision **(a)** Incision with Workig Tube and Endoscope, **(b)** Incision Closure, **(c)** Incision After Closure.

Contraleteral Discectomy Technique

Indications

Far lateral, foraminal or extraforaminal disc herniation

Anaesthesia

General anaesthesia, epidural anaesthesia

Position

Prone with hips and knees fixed. Preferably on Wilson™ (Mizuho OSI) frame.

Discography

L5-S1 discography with Indigo Carmine mixed radiopaque dye is done through the transforaminal route (see above).

Skin Incision & Markings

The skin incision is placed at 2-3 cm lateral to the midline in order to develop an approach angle of 45° [16].

Docking of Working Channel and Endoscope

Under fluoroscopy guidance, 18 gauge spine needle was inserted from a point approximately 3 cm lateral to the midline on the side opposite to the pathology approximately at 45° angle and docked on the medial aspect of the L5 inferior articular process (IAP). A guide-wire is then inserted and skin incision is made centred on it. This is followed by the insertion of the obturator and working channel. Obturator is replaced with the endoscope. Intervening muscles and other soft tissues are dissected and ligamentum flavum is exposed (Fig. **10**).

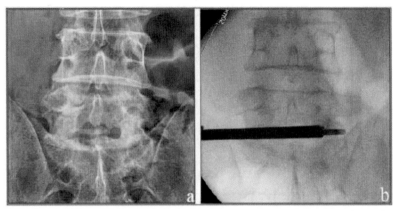

Fig. (10). L5-S1 Interlaminar Contralateral Approach **(a)** Contralateral "V-Point" for Left approach, **(b)** Probe in Right Foramen with Left Approach.

Ligamentum Flavum Splitting

The midline is approached with the rotational movement of the working channel. The ligamentum flavum is split off the interspinous ligament and the contralateral side of the canal and ligamentum flavum is exposed.

The contralateral foramen region is approached and keeping the MRI images in mind, the ligamentum flavum is split and the opening widened with rotational movement of the working channel. The thecal sac and nerve roots are identified and preserved by retracting away with the help of the working channel [16].

Discectomy

If extruded disc material is seen in epidural space, it is removed with forceps. The herniated disc is located using clues from MRI images and retracting thecal and root with the rotational movement of the working channel. Annular cutter, punch or dissector can be used to increase the opening on the annulus and discectomy is completed [2, 5].

Annular Sealing

Following discectomy, the annular opening is closed using the coagulation function of bipolar radiofrequency. The coagulation is done at the periphery first near intact annular fibers first and proceeds further toward the centre of the annular defect (See above).

Skin Closure

Skin closure is done as described in the ipsilateral discectomy technique.

POTENTIAL RISKS

Dural Tear

This is a potential complication. Care should be taken while widening the ligamentum flavum opening and any fibrosis or calcification between flavum and the dura should be dealt with caution. Similarly, fibrosis or calcification between dura and disc should be approached with utmost care. 1-4% incidence of the dura tear has been reported in the literature with a higher incidence in the revision surgery [2, 5, 21, 22].

Incomplete Discectomy

In 2 to 11% of the surgeries, the removal disc may be incomplete with a higher probability of failure in high canal compromised and badly migrated discs [22 - 24].

Nerve Root Injury

The endoscopic interlaminar approach is relatively safe for nerve root and cord. Transient and reversible root injuries have been reported, with incidences varying from 1 to 17% [5, 6, 21 - 23, 25, 26].

Epidural Hematoma

Intraoperative bleeding may sometimes be difficult to control and switching over to microscopic open technique to postoperative epidural hematoma has been reported [5, 6, 21 - 23, 25, 26].

Infection

Infection is not a common complication in endoscopic surgery. A very low incidence (<1%) has been reported and can be treated with a course of antibiotics or open surgical debridement [2, 5, 21 - 23, 26, 27].

Recurrence

Literature shows 1-7% cases may recur after endoscopic discectomy. Reported revision rate for conventional discectomy is 2-18%, with few studies showing a higher recurrence with conventional procedures [2, 4, 5, 7, 21, 22]. Higher recurrence rate is reported when the procedure is done under general anaesthesia vis-a-vis local anaesthesia [27].

Other risk factors are male gender, age, aging, weight-bearing, obesity, inappropriate patient selection and surgeon's experience [22, 26, 28, 29]. Sometimes recurrence may warrant nerve block postoperatively [6].

Less Common Complications

Different authors have reported various complications associated with interlaminar endoscopy which is uncommon and inconsistently reported in various studies. These include bladder and bowel dysfunction, transient muscle weakness, chronic pain syndrome, converting endoscopic to open surgery among others [13, 21, 23, 25, 27].

POSTOPERATIVE AND REHABILITATION PROTOCOL

Postoperative protocol is similar to the standard microscopic discectomy. Patients are encouraged mobilization immediate postoperative. Physiotherapist's guidance may be necessary initially. Gradual progression to the normal physical activity over few weeks is followed and usually patients are expected to return to their usual activities in a month [4 - 6, 15, 17].

CLINICAL SERIES

The authors published a case series of L5-S1 interlaminar discectomy, including 80 patients with 51 male and 29 female. Mean age of the study population was 40 ± 12 (range 18-73) years and mean follow-up 13 ± 6 (range 6 to 18) months. The mean visual analogue score (VAS) improved from 7.91±0.73 pre-operative to 1.15±0.62 at final follow-up (leg pain), and 5.15±0.71 pre-operative to 1.19± 0.75 at final follow-up (back pain). 96.25% had a good to excellent outcome and 3.75% had fair to poor outcome. Other than 2.5% recurrence the case series had no complication [5]. Two cases are represented in Figs. (**2 - 5**) show the discectomy done with the interlaminar approach at the L5-S1 level.

DISCUSSION

Endoscopic spine surgery has seen tremendous progress in recent years [1, 2, 5]. In terms of operative time, surgical outcome and complications, the interlaminar endoscopy and conventional techniques are comparable and at times, endoscopic surgery has proven better [2, 6, 7, 30, 31]. Interlaminar endoscopy can be performed under local anaesthesia with reduced hospital stay or day care procedure [31].

Three approaches for ligamentum flavum are described in the literature [1, 2, 5]:

1. Excising the ligamentum flavum to create a hole.

2. Sequential dilation of the ligamentum flavum with serial dilators inserted over a guide wire.
3. Ligamentum flavum splitting under direct endoscopic vision.

The third approach has advantages of direct visualisation, least traumatic and preventing epidural fibrosis postoperatively [1, 2, 5].

Annular sealing is very important technique for structural preservation [1, 2, 4, 5]. The area around the annular defect is coagulated with the radiofrequency probe which shrinks the tissue and seals the defect [1, 2, 5]. Reducing or if possible, completely sealing the annular defects is important because it may weaken the degenerated disc and contribute to the recurrence of herniation [1, 2, 5, 32, 33].

TECHNICAL PEARLS

1. At L5-S1 level interlaminar approach can be used for central, lateral recess and foraminal/ extraforaminal disc (contralateral IELD).
2. IELD exploits interlaminar space with minimal bone resection.
3. Splitting of ligamentum flavum (LF) under endoscopic vision preserves the LF.
4. Annular sealing helps prevent recurrence.
5. Surgical outcome are comparable to the conventional surgery with significant reduction in operative time.

CONCLUSION

L5-S1 discectomy with interlaminar approach full endoscopic technique is increasingly evolving with certain authors reporting results comparable or better than conventional technique. The endoscopic technique has added advantage of a potential day care procedure and crucial structure in the spine can be preserved.

CONSENT FOR PUBLICATION

Not applicable.

CONFLICT OF INTEREST

The authors declare no conflict of interest, financial or otherwise.

ACKNOWLEDGEMENT

Declared none.

REFERENCES

[1]   S.K. Hyeun, D.R. Harshavardhan, H.W. Pang, J.Y. Yeon, Tae Jang. Il. Evolution of endoscopic transforaminal lumbar approach for degenerative lumbar disease. 2020; 6
[http://dx.doi.org/10.21037/jss.2019.11.05]

[2]   Hyeun Sung Kim, Ravish Pate, Byapak Paude, Jee-Soo Jang, Il-Tae Jang, Seong-Hoon Oh, Jae Eun Park, Sol Lee. Early Outcomes of Endoscopic Contralateral Foraminal and Lateral Recess Decompression via an Interlaminar Approach in Patients with Unilateral Radiculopathy from Unilateral Foraminal Stenosis. World Neurosurg 2017; Vol. 108: pp. 763-73.
[http://dx.doi.org/10.1016/j.wneu.2017.09.018]

[3]   Kai Wu, Yuwei Zhao, Zhiyun Feng, Xiaojian Hu, Zhong Chen, Yue Wang. Stepwise Local Anesthesia for Percutaneous Endoscopic Interlaminar Discectomy Technique Strategy and Clinical Outcomes. World Neurosurg 2020; pp. e346-52.
[http://dx.doi.org/10.1016/j.wneu.2019.10.061]

[4]   Hyeun Sung Kim, Jeong Yoon Park. Comparative Assessment of Different Percutaneous Endoscopic Interlaminar Lumbar Discectomy (PEID) Techniques Pain Physician 2013; 16: 359-67.
[PMID: 23877452]

[5]   Jung-Sup Lee, Hyeun-Sung Kim, Jee-Soo Jang, Il-Tae Jang; Structural Preservation Percutaneous Endoscopic Lumbar Interlaminar Discectomy for L5-S1 Herniated Nucleus Pulposus. BioMed Research International. s.l: Hindawi Publishing Corporation 2016; p. 9.
[http://dx.doi.org/10.1155/2016/6250247]

[6]   Modified Interlaminar Endoscopic Lumbar Discectomy for Highly Upmigrated Disc Herniation. Neurospine 2020; 17: S66-73.
[http://dx.doi.org/10.14245/ns.2040264.132] [PMID: 32746519]

[7]   Hyeong-Ki Shim, Kyung-Chul Choi, Kyung Han Cha, Dong Chan Lee, Choon-Keun Park. Interlaminar Endoscopic Lumbar Discectomy Using a New 8.4-mm Endoscope and Nerve Root Retractor. Clin Spine Surg 2020; 33: 265-70.

[8]   Radiologic Anatomy of the Lumbar Interlaminar Window and Surgical Considerations for Lumbar Interlaminar Endoscopic and Microsurgical Disc Surgery. Zakir Sakci, Mehmet Resid Onen, Elif Fidan, Yunus Yasar, Hikmet Ulug, Sait Naderi 115. World Neurosurg 2018; pp. e22-6.
[http://dx.doi.org/10.1016/j.wneu.2018.03.049]

[9]   F. Ali, V. Reddy, A.B. Dublin. Anatomy, Back, Anterior Spinal Artery Treasure Island (FL): StatPearls 2020.
[PMID: 30422558]

[10]   The Vascular Anatomy Anterior to the L5–S1 Disk Space. Spine 2001; 26: 1205-8.
[http://dx.doi.org/10.1097/00007632-200106010-00007] [PMID: 11389384]

[11]   Paul Houle, Albert E. Telfeian, Ralf Wagner, Junseok Bae. Interspinous endoscopic lumbar decompression: technical note 40. AME Case Rep 2019; Vol. 3.
[http://dx.doi.org/10.21037/acr.2019.09.07]

[12]   Son S, Ahn Y, Lee SG, Kim WK. Learning curve of percutaneous endoscopic interlaminar lumbar discectomy *versus* open lumbar microdiscectomy at the L5–S1 level. Seong SonID, Yong Ahn, Sang Gu Lee, Woo Kyung Kim. 7. PLoS One 2020; 15(7): e0236296.
[http://dx.doi.org/10.1371/journal.pone.0236296]

[13]   Percutaneous Endoscopic Lumbar Discectomy. Med Sci Monit 2020; 26: e922777.
[http://dx.doi.org/10.12659/MSM.922777] [PMID: 32506068]

[14]   Yongjing Huang, Jianjian Yin, Zhenzhong Sun, Sheng Song, Yin Zhuang, Xueguang Liu, Shihao Du, Yongjun Rui. Percutaneous endoscopic lumbar discectomy for LDH via a transforaminal approach versus an interlaminar approach: a meta-analysis. Orthopäde 2020; 49: 338-49.
[http://dx.doi.org/10.1007/s00132-019-03710-z]

[15]   Hyeun Sung Kim, Byapak Paude, Ji Soo Jang, Seong Hoon Oh, Sol Lee, Jae Eun Park, Il Tae Jang. Percutaneous Full Endoscopic Bilateral Lumbar Decompression of Spinal Stenosis Through Uniportal-Contralateral Approach Techniques and Preliminary Results. World Neurosurg 2017; Vol. 103: pp. 201-9.
        [http://dx.doi.org/10.1016/j.wneu.2017.03.130]

[16]   Keun Lee, Hyeun-Sung Kim, Jee-Soo Jang, Yong-Hun Pee, Jin-Uk Kim, Jun-Ho Lee, Il-Tae Jang. Percutaneous Endoscopic Lumbar Discectomy for L5-S1 Foraminal Disc Herniation with Superior Migration using Contralateral Interlaminar Approach: A Technical Case Report. JMISST 2016; Vol. 1: pp. 40-3.
        [http://dx.doi.org/10.21182/jmisst.2016.00059]

[17]   Dmitriev AE. The Textbook of Spinal Surgery. In: L. Ronald, Keith H Dewald, III Bridwell, Eds. Philadelphia 2011; I: pp. 166-70.

[18]   H.-J. Wilke, S. T. Krischak, K. H. Wenger, L. E. Claes. Load-displacement properties of the thoracolumbar calf spine: experimental results and comparison to known human data. Eur Spine J 1997; 6: 129-37.

[19]   Kuniyoshi Abumi, Manohar M Punjabi, Kenneth M Kramer, Joanne Duranceau, Thomas Oxland, Joseph J Crisco. Biomechanical evaluation of lumbar spinal stability after graded facetectomies. Spine 1990; 15: 1142-7.

[20]   Siri Sahib Khalsa, Hyeun Sung Kim, Ravindra Singh, Osama Nezar Kashlan. 5. Radiographic outcomes of endoscopic decompression for lumbar spinal stenosis. Neurosurg Focus 2019; 46: E10.https://thejns.org/doi/abs/10.3171/2019.2.FOCUS18617

[21]   Full-Endoscopic ILD. Kanthika Wasinpongwanich, Krit Pongpirul, Khin Myat Myat Lwin, Withawin Kesornsak, Verapan Kuansongtham, Sebastian Ruetten. Retrospective Review of Clinical Results and Complications in 545 International Patients. World Neurosurg 2019; Vol. 132: pp. e922-8.
        [http://dx.doi.org/10.1016/j.wneu.2019.07.101]

[22]   Mingming Pan, Qifan Li, Sucheng Li, Haiqing Mao, Bin Meng, Feng Zhou, Huilin Yang. Percutaneous Endoscopic Lumbar Discectomy: Indications and Complications. Pain Physician 2020; 23: 49-56.

[23]   K.C. Choi, J.H. Lee, J.S. Kim, *et al.* Unsuccessful percutaneous endoscopic lumbar discectomy: A single-center experience of 10,228 cases. Neurosurgery 2015; 76: 372-81.

[24]   S.H. Lee, B.U. Kang, Y. Ahn, *et al.* Operative failure of percutaneous endoscopic lumbar discectomy: A radiologic analysis of 55 cases. Spine (Phila Pa 1976) 2006; 31: E285-90.

[25]   Chuanli Zhou, Guoqing Zhang, Ripul R. Panchal, Xianfeng Ren, Hongfei Xiang, Ma Xuexiao. Unique Complications of Percutaneous Endoscopic Lumbar Discectomy and Percutaneous Endoscopic Interlaminar Discectomy 1. Pain Physician 212018; : E105-12.

[26]   Transforaminal percutaneous endoscopic lumbar discectomy: Technical tips to prevent complications. Y, Ahn. Expert Rev Med Devices 2012; 9: 361-6.

[27]   Hsien-Te Chen, Chun-Hao Tsai, Shao-Ching Chao, Ting-Hsien Kao, Yen-Jen Chen, Horng-Chaung Hsu *et al.* Endoscopic discectomy of L5–S1 disc herniation via an interlaminar approach: Prospective controlled study under local and general anesthesia 93. Surgical Neurology International 2011; Vol. 2.
        [http://dx.doi.org/10.4103/2152-7806.82570]

[28]   . Y. Yao, H. Liu, H. Zhang, *et al.* Risk factors for recurrent herniation after percutaneous endoscopic lumbar discectomy. World Neurosury 2017; 100: 1-6.

[29]   Wang H, Zhou Y, Li C, Xiang L. Risk factors for failure of single-level percutaneous endoscopic lumbar discectomy. J Neurosurg Spine 2015; 23: 320-5.

[30]   Sebastian Ruetten, Martin Komp, Harry Merk, Georgios Godolias. Use of newly developed instruments and endoscopes: full endoscopic resection of lumbar disc herniations via the interlaminar

and lateral transforaminal approach. J Neurosurg Spine 2007; 6: 521-30.

[31]   Xue-Fei Ye, Sheng Wang, Ai-Min Wu, Lin-Zheng Xie, Xiang-Yang Wang, Jiao-Xiang Chen, Hui Xu, Sun-Ren Sheng. Comparison of the effects of general and local anesthesia in lumbar interlaminar endoscopic surgery. Ann Palliat Med 2020; Vol. 3: pp. 1103-8.
[http://dx.doi.org/10.21037/apm-20-623]

[32]   Chang-Jung Chiang, Cheng-Kung Cheng, Jui-Sheng Sun, Chun-Jen Liao, Yao-Horng Wang, Yang-Hwei Tsuang. The Effect of a New Anular Repair After Discectomy in Intervertebral Disc Degeneration An Experimental Study Using a Porcine Spine Model. SPINE 2011; Vol. 36: pp. 761-9.
[http://dx.doi.org/10.1097/BRS.0b013e3181e08f01]

[33]   R. N. Nataraja, G. B. J. Andersson, A. G. Patwardhan, S. Verma. Effect of Annular Incision Type on the Change in Biomechanical Properties in a Herniated Lumbar Intervertebral Disc. Journal of Biomechanical Engineering 2002; 24: 229-36.
[http://dx.doi.org/10.1115/1.1449906]

CHAPTER 6

Hybridized Inside-Out/Outside-In Approach for Treatment of Endstage Vacuum Degenerative Lumbar Disc Disease

Kai-Uwe Lewandrowski[1,2,3,*] and **Anthony Yeung**[4]

[1] *Center for Advanced Spine Care of Southern Arizona and Surgical Institute of Tucson, Tucson AZ, USA*

[2] *Associate Professor of Orthopaedic Surgery, Universidad Colsanitas, Bogota, Colombia, USA*

[3] *Visiting Professor, Department Orthopaedic Surgery, UNIRIO, Rio de Janeiro, Brazil*

[4] *Clinical Professor of Endoscopic Surgery, University of New Mexico School of Medicine Department of Neurosurgery Albuquerque, New Mexico, Associate, Desert Institute for Spine Care, Phoenix, AZ, USA*

Abstract: Commonly employed transforaminal decompression techniques may use the "inside-out" and "outside-in" technique, not as a standalone technique, but as a combined technique that considers different surgical philosophies. The inside-out technique calls for an initial emphasis on visualization of the intradiscal cavity with the endoscope by advancing the working cannula inside the lumbar intervertebral disc for intradiscal examination when appropriate. In contrast, the outside-in approach places it initially into the neuroforamen and lateral recess. The authors present an illustrative case series of 411 patients in whom they employed a hybridization of these two techniques because they found it to be more reliable in cases of end-stage degenerative vacuum disc disease. The study group consisted of 192 (46.7%) females and 219 (53.3%) males with an average age of 54.84 ± 16.32. The average follow-up of 43.2 ± 26.53 months. Patients underwent surgery for herniated disc (135/411;32.8%), foraminal spinal stenosis (101/411;24.6%), a combination of the latter two conditions (162/411;39.4%), or low-grade spondylolisthesis (13/411;3.2%).

Results of our clinical series showed a significant reduction of preoperative ODI and VAS for leg pain of 49.8 ± 17.65, and 7.9 ± 1.55 to postoperatively 12.2 ± 9.34, and 2.41 ±5 1.55 at final follow-up (p 0.0001), respectively. Macnab outcomes were Excellent in 134 (32.6%), Good in 228 (55.5%), Fair in 40 (9.7%), and Poor in 9 (2.2%) patients, respectively. There was end-stage degenerative vacuum disc disease in 304 (74%) of the 411 patients; 37.5% had Excellent and 50% Good Macnab outcomes.

⁎ **Corresponding author Kai-Uwe Lewandrowski:** Center for Advanced Spine Care of Southern Arizona and Surgical Institute of Tucson, Tucson, AZ, USA, Department of Orthopaedic Surgery, UNIRIO, Rio de Janeiro, Brazil and Department of Orthopaedic Surgery, Fundación Universitaria Sanitas, Bogotá, D.C., Colombia, USA; Tel: +1 520 204-1495; Fax: +1 623 218-1215; E-mail:business@tucsonspine.com

Patients without vacuum discs had Excellent and Good 18.7% and 71.% of the time. With our hybridized technique, patients with end-stage degenerative vacuum disc disease did very well with the endoscopic decompression procedure. Improved clinical outcomes may be obtained with the direct visualization of pain generators in the epidural- and intradiscal space. It is the authors' preferred transforaminal decompression technique.

Keywords: Clinical outcomes, Inside-out, Outside-In, Transforaminal endoscopy.

INTRODUCTION

Spinal stenosis related operations are on the rise creating the demand for less costly, and less complicated surgical treatments that allow patients to stay out of hospitals and return to their demanding lives sooner with fewer disruptions in the postoperative recovery [1, 2]. The increased demand for these simplified spinal decompression of procedures will become more relevant to all stakeholders of the healthcare delivery equation as older patients seek medical attention for stenosis related problems. Simplified solutions are need to treat this increasing number of patients as many public health care systems are already stressed due to lack of resources. Better value-based solutions are needed to avoid rationing of traditional open spine surgery [3, 4]. The traditional image-based clinical decision-making now seems outdated and does not work well with the personalized spine care approach required to make endoscopic spine care focused on treating validated pain generators work [5 - 9]. Instead, the authors' endoscopic interventional spine surgery approach has focused limiting treatment to the lumbar level to which the patients' subjective weakness, and intermittent claudication limiting walking endurance and other physical activities can be traced back to [10]. These diagnostic and pain management strategies often lead to a unilateral or single-level foraminal stenotic process as a frequent source of pain [11, 12].

The "inside-out" technique was the first transforaminal technique proposed for lumbar endoscopy. It was based on the available technology at the time [13, 14]. Kambin supported this treatment of lumbar decompression as "arthroscopic microdiscectomy" or abbreviated as "AMD." Kambin initially believed that avoiding going into the epidural space avoided the surgical scarring inherent from the translaminar approach for herniated lumbar discs. He later tried to develop an operating endoscope, and not very functional, even by including an "oval" cannula. The operating endoscope was too delicate and did not allow levering around bony anatomy. Yeung quickly modified Kambin's technique and used Kambin's arthroscopic micro-discectomy concept of visualizing intradiscal patho-anatomy such as annular tears, intradiscal visualization of annular defects, inflammatory conditions inside the disc correlating intradiscal with extradiscal and foraminal patho-anatomy. In 1998, Yeung *et al.* was the key opinion leader in the United States who first proposed the wide-spread use of spinal endoscopy based on his "inside-out" technique. The Yeung Endoscopic Spine System YESS™ was commercialized and accompanied by a wide array of specialized endoscopic decompression tools [15 - 22]. In the late 1990ies, the "outside-in" technique came about because other surgeons, including Thomas Hoogland's [23 - 25], became interested in addressing pathology in the epidural space outside the intervertebral disc as previously shown by Leu and Hauser [26 - 28]. These surgeons recognized that stenosis in the lateral canal and foramen needed to be addressed in conjunction with endoscopic herniated disc surgery as many patients suffered from both conditions [29 - 31]. The first author began with the "outside-in" transforaminal endoscopic decompression technique [29 - 31]. As endoscopic visualization of painful pathology improved with advances in endoscopic design and illumination technology, combining treatment of intradiscal pathology with the "outside-in" technique complementing the "inside out" technique allowed a gradual evolution of surgical protocols into a hybrid procedure for transforaminal lumbar decompression targeting the pain generator. Gradually highly skilled MIS surgeons included open and endoscopic decompression of the cervical, thoracic, and lumbar spine. Yeung also studied and stratified his indication every five years, taking more technically tricky cases at the request of his growing patient population requesting individualized options. Yeung accepted more endoscopically difficult cases based on his surgical successes that did not "burn any bridges" for a subsequent procedure if the endoscopic procedure failed.

In time and as a result of detailed statistical analysis of their respective clinical outcomes, both authors of this chapter merged their "outside-in" [32] approach with the "inside-out" [33] technique and vice versa, effectively hybridizing the two methods. In a joint analysis of their clinical outcome data, they realized that direct visualization of pain generators might be located in the posterior annulus directly underneath the dural sac. Their endoscopic treatment is just as important as treating such conditions in the epidural space [33 - 35]. Neither one of the two techniques alone afford the surgeon the ability to endoscopically treat all relevant pain generators in a symptomatic lumbar spinal motion segment. The "outside-in" has limitations since the working cannula is placed posterolaterally to the dural sac and above the intervertebral disc. The inside-out technique is limited because the working cannula sits underneath the dural sac, and painful pathology outside the intervertebral disc is not visualized and, hence, not treated. To overcome these shortcomings, the authors decided to hybridize these two approaches. In this chapter, the authors present an illustrative case series of 411 patients of the more advanced spinal conditions where many if most fellowship-trained spine surgeons prefer to depend on what they learned in their training. By employing a hybridization of these two transforaminal techniques, they found it to be more efficacious and cost-effective in cases of end-stage degenerative vacuum disc disease that are usually treated by fusion procedures. To make their case, the authors illustrate the individual technical steps and demonstrate how improved clinical outcomes could be achieved more reliably with these hybridized endoscopic spine surgery techniques [33].

TECHNIQUE DESCRIPTION

The surgical case example used to demonstrate the steps of the hybridized inside-out and outside-in technique is of a 63-year old female patient with symptomatic left-sided foraminal and lateral recess stenosis at the L4/5 level. The hybridized method consists of initial outside-in decompression with an opening foraminoplasty. The initial foraminoplasty is performed to clear the lateral aspect of the facet joint of soft tissue, control bleeding, and to controllably and under direct visualization safely place the working cannula into the triangular safe zone of the neuroforamen. Once the working cannula is placed and the neural exiting nerve root is safely retracted, the working cannula may be introduced into the intervertebral disc space employing the "inside-out" technique. Typically, the endoscopic working cannula sits between the endplates at the end of the case.

1. Preoperative Planing

• A complete preoperative diagnostic work-up includes plain film radiographs and magnetic resonance imaging (Fig. 1). Imaging studies should be reviewed for evidence of deformity, instability, and anatomical abnormalities that could be problematic when attempting to access the neuroforamen at the symptomatic level. Additional concerns that may be of relevance in the access planning relate to transitional anatomy. It should be taken into account for the planning of the attack angles and surgical approaches.

2. Patient Positioning

• The patient should be placed on the Wilson frame in the prone position so that the OR setup is ergonomic for the operating surgeon. All the tubing and cabling for the endoscopic decompression should be secured to the patient to not interfere with the free handling of the spinal endoscope. Preferably, the drapes are watertight, and the video tower and fluoroscopy unit should be opposite from the surgeon.

3. Access Planning and Marking

• In the posterior-anterior fluoroscopy plane (PA), the midline should be drawn along with the spinous processes. The authors prefer to mark the iliac wings by drawing lines outlining their location. A horizontal line connecting the iliac crests typically should run across the L4/5 level. If not, transitional anatomy, advanced vertical collapse, or deformity due to degenerative disc disease should be considered and accounted for during the access planning. The attack angles and distances should be measured on each patient as outlined below. The typical distance from the midline at the L4/5 level is approximately 10 to 12 cm. However, these numbers are not dogmatic and should be measured.

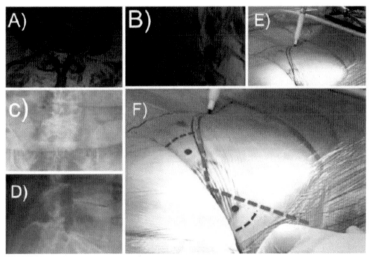

Fig. (1). Axial (**A**) and sagittal (**B**) and posterior-anterior (PA; **C**) and lateral (LAT; **D**) views of lumbar the spine of the same 63-year old female patient who suffered from the left sciatica-type leg- and back pain with decreased walking endurance due to claudication stemming from the left-sided foraminal and lateral recess stenosis at the L4/5 level. The patient underwent transforaminal endoscopic transforaminal outside-in followed by inside-out decompression. Access planning involves outlining the iliac crest and the midline (**E**). The most suitable access point can be estimated by drawing out trajectories on the PA and LAT fluoroscopy images (red dashed line). The skin incision is best placed where the two lines intersect (red dashed lines). The angles formed by these PA and LAT access trajectory lines form equal complementary angles (purple dashed lines and angle dot) with the horizontal line drawn across the surgical level (**F**).

• In the lateral projection (LAT), point the marker instrument's tip at the posterior annulus of the surgical neuroforamen. Align the marker instrument to be in line with the intervertebral disc. Draw a line on the patients' flank.

• Next, draw a similar line in the posteroanterior (PA) plane at your preferred attack angle by placing the pointing instrument's tip at the lateral aspect of the inferior pedicle of the surgical level. The ideal access point is where the PA and LAT lines intersect. Typically, these angles of the PA and LAT line with the horizontal line across the surgical level in the PA plane should form complementary angles (Fig. **2**).

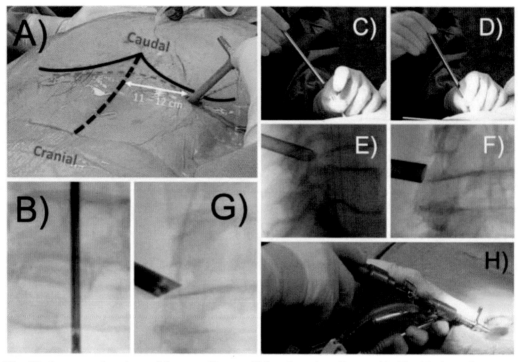

Fig. (2). Intraoperative views of the same 63-year old female patient discussed in Fig. (**1**) shown in a prone position (**A**) with PA (**B**) fluoroscopy image. A straight line is drawn connecting the lumbar spinous processes. The ilium is drawn out on the approach side to help to place the access cannula. The determined most suitable access point is to make a skin incision and access the neuroforamen with serial dilators (**C**) for placement of the working cannula (**D**). The initial working cannula placement is checked on PA (**E**) and LAT (**F**) fluoroscopy views. The initial foraminoplasty is performed with a 4 mm power drill (**G, H**) to reach the lateral recess and to obtain a good seal with the working cannula within the foramen.

4. Local Anesthesia & Monitored Anesthesia Care (MAC) Sedation

• The surgical area should be anesthetized by injecting the skin entry point with 3-5 cc of 0.5% long-lasting 0.5% bupivacaine (Marcain®) with epinephrine to the extent of the duration of postoperative relief from incisional pain.

• Next, an 18G 6-inch spinal needle should be advanced onto the surgical facet joint's lateral aspect, where additional local anesthesia should be injected by applying 2-4 cc of the same local anesthetic.

• The spinal needle should then be advanced into the surgical neuroforamen, where less than one cc of local anesthetic may be injected for additional pain control during the transforaminal decompression surgery. The surgeon should always aspirate before injecting any medication into the neuroforamen to avoid intravenous injection.

5. Placement of the Working Cannula

• The surgeon is ready to advance an 18 G 6-inch spinal needle into the neuroforamen at this juncture. It should be positioned against the inferior pedicle.

• Once the obturator is removed from the spinal needle, a guidewire measuring 300-mm in length can be introduced into the neuroforamen. The spinal needle can be pulled over the guidewire, which is now in place for the dilators.

• The commercially available dilators over which the working cannular is introduced may have a variable number of dilators which will fit snugly over each other. Most endoscopic spine systems have three dilators. Others have as many as five or just two. The guidewire's position should be monitored on the intraoperative fluoroscopy images as the dilators are advanced to ensure that the guidewire is not bent or dislodge, thus avoiding moving the dilators in no other area than the neuroforamen. This team of authors prefers working cannulas, some custom designed by the YESS™ system, and some with a 45-60 degree bevel, which may be placed flush against the facet joint's lateral aspect. This technique should provide a tight seal to minimize leakage of irrigation fluid into the surrounding tissue. Upon completion of these steps, the progress of the endoscopic instruments' decompression and the position may be monitored with the fluoroscopy unit positioned in the PA plane (Fig. **2**).

6. Initial Foraminoplasty

• First, the authors perform an initial foraminoplasty. A safe starting point is at the lateral aspect of the inferior pedicle. The decompression should start there. The power drill should then be moved posteriorly and superiorly in a sweeping motion to detach multifidus fibers and finally enter the facet joint complex and resect the superior articular process's tup.

• Visualizing the facet joint space is a safe way to get to the lateral recess and the triangular safe zone. At this juncture, epidural fat and foraminal ligaments may be encountered. The latter may cause tethering of the exiting nerve roots, for which reason they may have to be transected. The inferior pedicle's limited resection and drilling down any osteophytes from the ring apophysis impinging the traversing nerve root may be required to complete the decompression (Fig. **2**).

• Additional endoscopic instruments the authors of this chapter found useful during the traversing and exiting nerve root decompression, include Kerrison rongeurs and chisels. They may be effectively used in increasing the width of the lateral recess. Final inspection of the neuroforamen should be performed to ascertain the exiting and traversing nerve root. Their respective dorsal root ganglion is decompressed and float around freely in the epidural space before considering entering the intervertebral disc space.

OUTSIDE-IN PORTION

7. Pain Generators in the Epidural Space

• After initial foraminoplasty, the beveled working cannula should be advanced into the neuroforamen up to the lateral recess. The working cannula should be rotated clockwise and counterclockwise to inspect all areas of the neuroforamen and beyond.

• To visualize any painful pathology, the surgeon should attempt a 360-degree view of the neuroforamen (Fig. **2**).

• Intraoperative anesthetic injections and provocative and analgesic chromo discography may prove useful in the sedated yet awake patient to confirm whether any appearing abnormal tissue is painful.

8. Target the Center of the Disc Space

• The intervertebral disc space is best accessed by advancing a guidewire into its center, as verified by the PA and LAT fluoroscopic views. Dilators may be used over the guidewire. A nitinol guidewire may come in handy to avoid any kinking and advancement of the guidewire through the often structurally incompetent anterior annulus. The guidewire could cause vascular or bowel injury.

• Again, several sequential dilators or a single dilator matching the working cannula's inner diameter - in the authors' preferred system Ø 8.9 mm - may be used to advance the working cannula inside the intervertebral disc. Finally, intradiscal inspection and removal of abnormal disc tissue are feasible (Fig. **3**).

INSIDE-OUT PORTION

9. Discectomy

• Once the endoscopic working cannula is inside the intervertebral disc, removing any devitalized, delaminated, fissured, or abnormal appearing discal tissue should be performed (Fig. **4**).

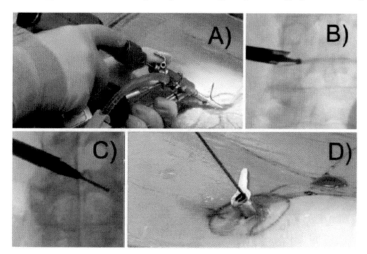

Fig. (3). The initial foraminoplasty with a low-speed (400 RPM), high-torque single-shafted, non-sheathed drill for rapid removal of bony- and soft tissue without causing a "white-out" effect from floating debris or excessive bleeding due to the suction-vortex impact of the drill shaft spinning inside the oval working channel of the spinal endoscope. The hand-held power drill is used to perform most of the foraminoplasty, including a small pediculectomy of the inferior pedicle and removal of common osteophytes of the ring-apophysis typically located below the traversing nerve root (A). Once the tip of the 4-mm round orbital drill bit has reached the lateral recess, the decompression of the traversing nerve root is typically complete. Drilling out the inferior portion of the neuroforamen by removing parts of the superior pedicle wall from lateral to medial also increases neuroforaminal volume (B).

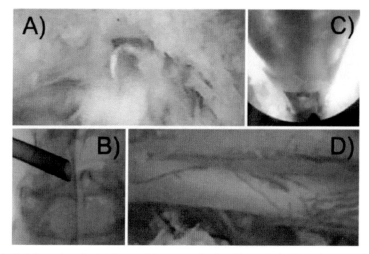

Fig. (4). After initial foraminoplasty, the working cannula should reach the lateral recess. At this point, the lateral recess's width is increased by egg-shelling out the superior articular process (SAP), which after initial decompression shows the traversing nerve root (A). After resection of the SAP tip from anterior to posterior, the roof of the lateral recess is effectively raised. A partial pediculectomy may be performed as well to achieve complete decompression. Then, the working cannula is advanced into the vacuum disc (B) to complete the discectomy with pituitary rongeurs (C), decompressing the undersurface of the dural sac until epidural fat is surrounding the free-floating nerve roots and the dural sac is seen (D).

• Yeung utilizes a flexible cannula initially designed by Endius™ to decompress the contra-lateral foramen *via* uniportal transforaminal discectomy to reduce the risk of recurrent intradiscal herniations.

• The endplates and the posterior annulus should be carefully inspected for entrapped loose disc tissue, annular tears, inflammatory granulomas, or scar tissue, particularly if the surgeon identifies them as painful during the operation. Again the use of diagnostic injection mentioned above may come in handy.

10. Intradiscal Assessment of Painful Pathology

• Beginning with the posterior annulus inspection, this team of authors prefers to perform a systematic examination of the intervertebral disc space. Removing a large central disc herniation may be effectively carried out from within the intervertebral disc space by pulling it in toto or piecemeal from the dural sac into the center for the interspace. Creating an annular window may prove useful during this portion of the operation (Fig. **3**).

• The authors of this chapter employ this standardized choreography of the endoscopic transforaminal lumbar decompression surgery by combing elements of the "outside-in" and the "inside-out" technique. This hybridized protocol allows the surgeon to visualize the posterior annulus and the inferior and superior endplate from one lateral recess to another.

CLINICAL SERIES

Clinical outcomes with the hybridized "outside-in" and "inside-out" procedures were analyzed in consecutive case series of 411 patients with an average age of 54.84 ± 16.32 years. The study included 192 (46.7%) females and 219 (53.3%) males. The average follow-up was 43.2 ± 26.53 months. In most patients, the indication for surgery was herniated disc (135;32.8%). An additional 13 patients (3.2%) had low-grade spondylolisthesis without translational motion on dynamic extension/flexion views. Another 101 patients (24.6%) suffered from spinal stenosis related symptoms affecting the foramen and lateral recess. A combination of herniated disc and stenosis was responsible for the sciatica-type back and leg symptoms in the remaining 162 (39.4%) patients. The surgical level in decreasing order was as follows: L4/5 (201/411; 48.9%), followed by L5/S1 (113/411; 27.5%) and L3/4 (36/411; 8.8%). Most endoscopic surgeries were unilateral (385/411; 93.7%) and single-level surgeries (361/411; 87.83%). For more detailed clinical outcome analysis, the disc herniations were subclassified as central in 167 (40.6%) patients, paracentral in 124 (30.2%) patients, or extraforaminal posterolateral in the remaining 120 (29.2%) of patients. VAS and ODI were used as the primary outcome measure [36 - 43]. Their analysis showed significant reductions. The ODI and VAS reductions were 37.6 ± 16.98 and 5.49 ± 2.06, respectively. They were statistically significant (p 0.0001). The analysis of the modified Macnab criteria [44, 45] showed that 134 (32.6%) patients had Excellent, 228 (55.5%) patients had Good, 40 (9.7%) patients had Fair, and the remaining 9 (2.2%) patients had poor outcomes. Vacuum end-stage degenerative vacuum disc disease was found in 411 patients, 304 (74%), and the remaining 107 (26%) patients. There was a statistically significantly higher proportion (p < 0.0001) of patients with Excellent and Good Macnab outcomes and the presence of a structurally defunct vacuum disc. Patients with vacuum disc had Excellent and Good 37.5% and 50% of the time, *versus* patients without vacuum discs, which had Excellent and Good 18.7% and 71.%, respectively.

DISCUSSION

Transforaminal endoscopy is typically performed by choosing one of the two popularized techniques – either the outside-in or the inside-out technique. Initially, the inside-out technique was developed by its proponents based on the technology available at the time. There were limits to the image quality and size of the working channel of the contemporary 1990ies endoscopes that were not entirely conducive to their epidural application focusing on foraminoplasty. Proponents of the outside-in approach were able to make the transition from working inside the disc to working outside the disc space because of technological advances mainly with spinal endoscopes and in part because of the more sophisticated decompression tools that were developed at the request of surgeon leaders who were more interested in a foraminoplasty. However, one of the most frequently unrecognized advantages of the inside-out technique is its simplicity and direct visualization of painful pathology inside the disc. As trivial as it may appear in retrospect today, proponents of the insight-out method recognized early on in the late 1980ies that all degenerative- or injury-related processes affecting the health of the lumbar intervertebral disc depends on the integrity of the intradiscal structures and that pain may arise from within the disc. In other words, those key opinion leaders (KOLs) in favor of inside out recognized that all trouble starts inside the disc, and working outside the disc in the epidural space with the transforaminal approach made little sense to them. This seemingly trivial discussion on which method to favor has long moved on from describing it as a dogma-like philosophy and has attained a foundation in sophisticated clinical outcome research that highlighted the impact of the directly visualized endoscopic work on clinical outcomes when using either approach. More appropriately, this discussion between inside-out and outside-in should, in fact, be changed to working inside the disc to visualize in treat pain generators within the nucleus or annulus and work outside the disc to address pain generators that are only accessible from the epidural space because that is where these pain generators can be found. Therefore, the idea of hybridizing these two common techniques seems like a natural continuation of the thought process on endoscopically visualized pain generators. Because of this deduction, the authors of this chapter have combined these two techniques in one in the same surgery as dictated by the directly visualized pathology and the required treatments to address them. The dogmatic way of describing the approach technique is, in the authors' opinion, truly outdated and no longer appropriate as superior clinical outcomes have been found if the two techniques are combined during the same operation. Hence, the concept of a hybridized outside-in and inside-out technique crystallized [33, 34].

Improved clinical outcomes were serendipitously noted by both authors of this chapter independently. The senior author has been performing transforaminal inside-out lumbar endoscopy for decades. In time, his technique needed to evolve from treating spinal stenosis, particularly in the foramen and in the lateral recess. Therefore, he began to decompress the lateral recess by taking down osteophytes through a small annular window with a side-firing laser and later with custom trephines, essentially carrying out the same procedure as the first author with the endpoint being the same but with the individual steps being carried out in a different order. The first author slowly adopted the inside-out technique after years of outside-in decompression because he noted better results with the endoscopic treatment of intradiscal pain generators when he serendipitously found vacuum disc in his patients. The analysis of individual 5-year clinical outcomes and a combined analysis comparing the two treatments between the two authors' patient groups revealed improved long-term outcomes with lower reoperation rates forming the basis for the proposed hybridization of these two techniques during the same operation. Consequently, the authors started combining the two techniques sometimes in different order of steps but eventually arriving at the same end-result – a combined "outside-in" and "inside-out" endoscopic decompression procedure to treat pain generators in the epidural space as well as inside the disease intervertebral disc.

To the novice surgeon deciding on entering the field of spinal endoscopy and seemingly has to choose between the two techniques, the fundamental difference between them is often not immediately evident [35]. The apparent difference is the initial location of the working cannula. For example, when a surgeon employs the "inside-out" method, the posterior annulus under the dural sac may be directly visualized [15]. This portion of the posterior annulus cannot be visualized with the "outside-in" method since the working cannula's tip sits directly posterolateral to the dural sac in the neuroforamen. The two fundamental differences in cannula position determine what the surgeon can initially see, evaluate, and treat endoscopically. Intraoperative confirmation of suspected pain generators may be done in the awake yet sedated patient where provocative or analgesic testing with disco- and epidurography may aid in their correct identification. The most commonly visualized painful epidural conditions may range from (1) inflamed disc; (2) inflamed nerve; (3) hypervascular scar; (4) hypertrophied superior articular process (SAP) and ligamentum flavum; (5) tender capsule; (6) impacting facet margin; (7) superior foraminal facet osteophyte; (8) superior foraminal ligament impingement; to (9) a hidden shoulder osteophyte, (10) autonomic nerve, (11) synovial cysts and (12) furcal nerves, or conjoined nerves. Intradiscal pain generators include medial annular tears and unstable disc fragments delaminated from the endplates, and devitalized detached disc tissue [16].

In the authors' opinion, the ability to turn the working cannula's opening towards the posterior annulus to visualize the posterior annulus is likely the most misunderstood aspect of the "inside-out" technique. The annular window technique, which at times may involve an annular resection, allows the surgeon to decompress the neural elements by removing offending pathology adequately. Such pathology may include bony osteophytes indenting the dural sac from below or pain generators residing within the annulus itself. An additional benefit of the inside-out technique is that all aspects of the posterior annulus from one side to the other from the approach side can be assessed without putting the neural elements at risk. The inside-out technique has few limitations to treat painful conditions in the epidural space by way of the annular window. This direct view underneath the dural sac is unique to the "inside-out" technique. Combing the "outside-in" and "inside-out" extends the surgeon the opportunity to treat all pain generators within the symptomatic lumbar motion segment. In the elderly, advanced degenerative vacuum disc disease often is found during routine lumbar transforaminal endoscopy. Up to 73% of patients over age 45 were found to have a vacuum disc that is often collapsed without structural integrity [46 - 50]. The "inside-out" look inside a vacuum disc ultimately was proven to produce more reliable long-term clinical improvements with fewer revision surgeries. In younger patients, the authors are concerned with propagating progressive vertical disc collapse with the "inside-out" technique. For this reason, they routinely start the transforaminal decompression with the "outside-in" technique and only enter the intervertebral disc space if there is a lack of structural integrity to improve outcomes.

CONCLUSION

The traditional "outside-in" and "inside-out" concepts depend on the execution of different initial steps. The inside-out technique requires to place the cannula inside the intervertebral disc first. The outside-in technique places it in the neuroforamen or at the lateral aspect of the facet joint complex. It often requires an initial foraminoplasty regardless of whether there is boney foraminal stenosis. This hybridization of the "outside-in" and the "inside-out" technique presented by the authors is intended to solve more complex problems such as severe central and lateral canal stenosis. The concept of staged management [53] advocated for by the authors and employment of the hybridization protocols leads to improved clinical outcomes and higher patients' satisfaction [16, 19, 51 - 56].

CONSENT FOR PUBLICATION

Not applicable.

CONFLICT OF INTEREST

The authors declare no conflict of interest, financial or otherwise.

ACKNOWLEDGEMENT

Declared none.

REFERENCES

[1]   Lewandrowski KU, Soriano-Sánchez JA, Zhang X, *et al.* Regional variations in acceptance, and utilization of minimally invasive spinal surgery techniques among spine surgeons: results of a global survey. J Spine Surg 2020; 6(S1) (Suppl. 1): S260-74.
[http://dx.doi.org/10.21037/jss.2019.09.31] [PMID: 32195433]

[2]   Lewandrowski KU, Soriano-Sánchez JA, Zhang X, *et al.* Surgeon motivation, and obstacles to the implementation of minimally invasive spinal surgery techniques. J Spine Surg 2020; 6(S1) (Suppl. 1): S249-59.
[http://dx.doi.org/10.21037/jss.2019.08.02] [PMID: 32195432]

[3]   Lewandrowski KU, Ransom NA. Five-year clinical outcomes with endoscopic transforaminal outside-in foraminoplasty techniques for symptomatic degenerative conditions of the lumbar spine. J Spine Surg 2020; 6(S1) (Suppl. 1): S54-65.
[http://dx.doi.org/10.21037/jss.2019.07.03] [PMID: 32195416]

[4]   Yeung A, Roberts A, Zhu L, Qi L, Zhang J, Lewandrowski KU. Treatment of Soft Tissue and Bony Spinal Stenosis by a Visualized Endoscopic Transforaminal Technique Under Local Anesthesia. Neurospine 2019; 16(1): 52-62.
[http://dx.doi.org/10.14245/ns.1938038.019] [PMID: 30943707]

[5]   Lewandrowski KU, Dowling A, de Carvalho P, *et al.* Indication And Contraindication Of Endoscopic Transforaminal Lumbar Decompression. World Neurosurg 2020.
[PMID: 32201296]

[6]   Lewandrowski KU. The strategies behind "inside-out" and "outside-in" endoscopy of the lumbar spine: treating the pain generator. J Spine Surg 2020; 6(S1) (Suppl. 1): S35-9.
[http://dx.doi.org/10.21037/jss.2019.06.06] [PMID: 32195412]

[7]   Dowling Á, Lewandrowski KU, da Silva FHP, Parra JAA, Portillo DM, Giménez YCP. Patient selection protocols for endoscopic transforaminal, interlaminar, and translaminar decompression of lumbar spinal stenosis. J Spine Surg 2020; 6(S1) (Suppl. 1): S120-32.
[http://dx.doi.org/10.21037/jss.2019.11.07] [PMID: 32195421]

[8]   Wasinpongwanich K, Pongpirul K, Lwin KMM, Kesornsak W, Kuansongtham V, Ruetten S. Full-

Endoscopic Interlaminar Lumbar Discectomy: Retrospective Review of Clinical Results and Complications in 545 International Patients. World Neurosurg 2019; 132: e922-8.
[http://dx.doi.org/10.1016/j.wneu.2019.07.101] [PMID: 31326641]

[9]   Wang Y, Yan Y, Yang J, *et al.* Outcomes of percutaneous endoscopic trans-articular discectomy for huge central or paracentral lumbar disc herniation. Int Orthop 2019; 43(4): 939-45.
[http://dx.doi.org/10.1007/s00264-018-4210-6] [PMID: 30374637]

[10]   Yeung A, Lewandrowski KU. Early and staged endoscopic management of common pain generators in the spine. J Spine Surg 2020; 6(S1) (Suppl. 1): S1-5.
[http://dx.doi.org/10.21037/jss.2019.09.03] [PMID: 32195407]

[11]   Xin Z, Huang P, Zheng G, *et al.* Using a percutaneous spinal endoscopy unilateral posterior interlaminar approach to perform bilateral decompression for patients with lumbar lateral recess stenosis. Asian J Surg 2019.
[PMID: 31594687]

[12]   Park JH, Bae CW, Jeon SR, Rhim SC, Kim CJ, Roh SW. Clinical and radiological outcomes of unilateral facetectomy and interbody fusion using expandable cages for lumbosacral foraminal stenosis. J Korean Neurosurg Soc 2010; 48(6): 496-500.
[http://dx.doi.org/10.3340/jkns.2010.48.6.496] [PMID: 21430975]

[13]   Yeung AT. The evolution of percutaneous spinal endoscopy and discectomy: state of the art. Mt Sinai J Med 2000; 67(4): 327-32.
[PMID: 11021785]

[14]   Yeung AT. Minimally Invasive Disc Surgery with the Yeung Endoscopic Spine System (YESS). Surg Technol Int 1999; 8: 267-77.
[PMID: 12451541]

[15]   Gore S, Yeung A. The "inside out" transforaminal technique to treat lumbar spinal pain in an awake and aware patient under local anesthesia: results and a review of the literature. Int J Spine Surg 2014; 8: 8.
[http://dx.doi.org/10.14444/1028] [PMID: 25694940]

[16]   Yeung AT, Gore S. *In-vivo* Endoscopic Visualization of Patho-anatomy in Symptomatic Degenerative Conditions of the Lumbar Spine II: Intradiscal, Foraminal, and Central Canal Decompression. Surg Technol Int 2011; 21: 299-319.
[PMID: 22505004]

[17]   Yeung AT, Yeung CA. Minimally invasive techniques for the management of lumbar disc herniation. Orthop Clin North Am 2007; 38(3): 363-72.
[http://dx.doi.org/10.1016/j.ocl.2007.04.005] [PMID: 17629984]

[18]   Yeung AT. The Evolution and Advancement of Endoscopic Foraminal Surgery: One Surgeon's Experience Incorporating Adjunctive Techologies. SAS J 2007; 1(3): 108-17.
[http://dx.doi.org/10.1016/S1935-9810(07)70055-5] [PMID: 25802587]

[19]   Yeung AT, Yeung CA. *In-vivo* endoscopic visualization of patho-anatomy in painful degenerative conditions of the lumbar spine. Surg Technol Int 2006; 15: 243-56.
[PMID: 17029183]

[20]   Tsou PM, Alan Yeung C, Yeung AT. Posterolateral transforaminal selective endoscopic discectomy and thermal annuloplasty for chronic lumbar discogenic pain: a minimal access visualized intradiscal surgical procedure. Spine J 2004; 4(5): 564-73.
[http://dx.doi.org/10.1016/j.spinee.2004.01.014] [PMID: 15363430]

[21]   Yeung AT, Yeung CA. Advances in endoscopic disc and spine surgery: foraminal approach. Surg Technol Int 2003; 11: 255-63.
[PMID: 12931309]

[22]   Yeung AT, Tsou PM. Posterolateral endoscopic excision for lumbar disc herniation: Surgical

technique, outcome, and complications in 307 consecutive cases. Spine 2002; 27(7): 722-31. [http://dx.doi.org/10.1097/00007632-200204010-00009] [PMID: 11923665]

[23] Hoogland T, Scheckenbach C. [Percutaneous lumbar nucleotomy with low-dose chymopapain, an ambulatory procedure]. Z Orthop Ihre Grenzgeb 1995; 133(2): 106-13. [http://dx.doi.org/10.1055/s-2008-1039420] [PMID: 7754655]

[24] Hoogland T, Scheckenbach C. Low-dose chemonucleolysis combined with percutaneous nucleotomy in herniated cervical disks. J Spinal Disord 1995; 8(3): 228-32. [http://dx.doi.org/10.1097/00002517-199506000-00009] [PMID: 7670215]

[25] Hoogland T. Percutaneous endoscopic discectomy. J Neurosurg 1993; 79(6): 967-8. [PMID: 8246070]

[26] HJ L. R H. Die perkutan posterolaterale Foraminoskopie: Prinzip, Technik und Erfahrungen seit 1991. Arthroskopie 1996; 26-31.

[27] Leu H, Schreiber A. [Endoscopy of the spine: minimally invasive therapy]. Orthopade 1992; 21(4): 267-72. [Endoscopy of the spine: minimally invasive therapy]. [PMID: 1408118]

[28] Leu H, Schreiber A. [Percutaneous nucleotomy with disk endoscopy--a minimally invasive therapy in non-sequestrated intervertebral disk hernia]. Schweiz Rundsch Med Prax 1991; 80(14): 364-8. [Percutaneous nucleotomy with disk endoscopy--a minimally invasive therapy in non-sequestrated intervertebral disk hernia]. [PMID: 2034933]

[29] Hoogland T, van den Brekel-Dijkstra K, Schubert M, Miklitz B. Endoscopic transforaminal discectomy for recurrent lumbar disc herniation: a prospective, cohort evaluation of 262 consecutive cases. Spine 2008; 33(9): 973-8. [http://dx.doi.org/10.1097/BRS.0b013e31816c8ade] [PMID: 18427318]

[30] Hoogland T, Schubert M, Miklitz B, Ramirez A. Transforaminal posterolateral endoscopic discectomy with or without the combination of a low-dose chymopapain: a prospective randomized study in 280 consecutive cases. Spine 2006; 31(24): E890-7. [http://dx.doi.org/10.1097/01.brs.0000245955.22358.3a] [PMID: 17108817]

[31] Schubert M, Hoogland T. Endoscopic transforaminal nucleotomy with foraminoplasty for lumbar disk herniation. Oper Orthop Traumatol 2005; 17(6): 641-61. [http://dx.doi.org/10.1007/s00064-005-1156-9] [PMID: 16369758]

[32] Lewandrowski KU. "Outside-in" technique, clinical results, and indications with transforaminal lumbar endoscopic surgery: a retrospective study on 220 patients on applied radiographic classification of foraminal spinal stenosis. Int J Spine Surg 2014; 8: 8. [http://dx.doi.org/10.14444/1026] [PMID: 25694915]

[33] Yeung A, Lewandrowski KU. Five-year clinical outcomes with endoscopic transforaminal foraminoplasty for symptomatic degenerative conditions of the lumbar spine: a comparative study of *inside-out* versus *outside-in* techniques. J Spine Surg 2020; 6(S1) (Suppl. 1): S66-83. [http://dx.doi.org/10.21037/jss.2019.06.08] [PMID: 32195417]

[34] Lewandrowski K-U, Ransom NA. Five-year clinical outcomes with endoscopic transforaminal outside-in foraminoplasty techniques for symptomatic degenerative conditions of the lumbar spine. J Spine Surg 2020; 6(S1) (Suppl. 1): S54-65. [http://dx.doi.org/10.21037/jss.2019.07.03] [PMID: 32195416]

[35] Lewandrowski K-U. The strategies behind "inside-out" and "outside-in" endoscopy of the lumbar spine: treating the pain generator. J Spine Surg 2020; 6(S1) (Suppl. 1): S35-9. [http://dx.doi.org/10.21037/jss.2019.06.06] [PMID: 32195412]

[36] Tandon R, Kiyawat V, Kumar N. Clinical Correlation between Muscle Damage and Oswestry Disability Index Score after Open Lumbar Surgery: Does Open Surgery Reduces Functional Ability?

Asian Spine J 2018; 12(3): 518-23.
[http://dx.doi.org/10.4184/asj.2018.12.3.518] [PMID: 29879780]

[37]   van Hooff ML, Mannion AF, Staub LP, Ostelo RW, Fairbank JC. Determination of the Oswestry Disability Index score equivalent to a "satisfactory symptom state" in patients undergoing surgery for degenerative disorders of the lumbar spine-a Spine Tango registry-based study. Spine J 2016; 16(10): 1221-30.
[http://dx.doi.org/10.1016/j.spinee.2016.06.010] [PMID: 27343730]

[38]   Asher AL, Chotai S, Devin CJ, *et al.* Inadequacy of 3-month Oswestry Disability Index outcome for assessing individual longer-term patient experience after lumbar spine surgery. J Neurosurg Spine 2016; 25(2): 170-80.
[http://dx.doi.org/10.3171/2015.11.SPINE15872] [PMID: 26989974]

[39]   van Hooff ML, Spruit M, Fairbank JC, van Limbeek J, Jacobs WC. The Oswestry Disability Index (version 2.1a): validation of a Dutch language version. Spine 2015; 40(2): E83-90.
[http://dx.doi.org/10.1097/BRS.0000000000000683] [PMID: 25575092]

[40]   Gum JL, Glassman SD, Carreon LY. Clinically important deterioration in patients undergoing lumbar spine surgery: a choice of evaluation methods using the Oswestry Disability Index, 36-Item Short Form Health Survey, and pain scales: clinical article. J Neurosurg Spine 2013; 19(5): 564-8.
[http://dx.doi.org/10.3171/2013.8.SPINE12804] [PMID: 24010900]

[41]   Fairbank JC, Pynsent PB. The Oswestry Disability Index. Spine (Phila Pa 1976) 2000; 25(22): 2940-52. discussion 52.
[http://dx.doi.org/10.1097/00007632-200011150-00017] [PMID: 11074683]

[42]   Fairbank J. Use of Oswestry Disability Index (ODI). Spine (Phila Pa 1976) 1995; 20(13): 1535-7.
[http://dx.doi.org/10.1097/00007632-199507000-00020] [PMID: 8623078]

[43]   Reed CC, Wolf WA, Cotton CC, Dellon ES. A visual analogue scale and a Likert scale are simple and responsive tools for assessing dysphagia in eosinophilic oesophagitis. Aliment Pharmacol Ther 2017; 45(11): 1443-8.
[http://dx.doi.org/10.1111/apt.14061] [PMID: 28370355]

[44]   Macnab I. The surgery of lumbar disc degeneration. Surg Annu 1976; 8: 447-80.
[PMID: 936011]

[45]   Macnab I. Negative disc exploration. An analysis of the causes of nerve-root involvement in sixty-eight patients. J Bone Joint Surg Am 1971; 53(5): 891-903.
[http://dx.doi.org/10.2106/00004623-197153050-00004] [PMID: 4326746]

[46]   Latif AB. [Vacuum phenomenon in the intervertebral disc]. Magy Traumatol Orthop Helyreallito Seb 1991; 34(4): 297-300. [Vacuum phenomenon in the intervertebral disc].
[PMID: 1685543]

[47]   Schweitzer ME, el-Noueam KI. Vacuum disc: frequency of high signal intensity on T2-weighted MR images. Skeletal Radiol 1998; 27(2): 83-6.
[http://dx.doi.org/10.1007/s002560050342] [PMID: 9526773]

[48]   Pak KI, Hoffman DC, Herzog RJ, Lutz GE. Percutaneous intradiscal aspiration of a lumbar vacuum disc herniation: a case report. HSS J 2011; 7(1): 89-93.
[http://dx.doi.org/10.1007/s11420-010-9168-x] [PMID: 22294964]

[49]   Lewandrowski KU, León JFR, Yeung A. Use of "Inside-Out" Technique for Direct Visualization of a Vacuum Vertically Unstable Intervertebral Disc During Routine Lumbar Endoscopic Transforaminal Decompression-A Correlative Study of Clinical Outcomes and the Prognostic Value of Lumbar Radiographs. Int J Spine Surg 2019; 13(5): 399-414.
[http://dx.doi.org/10.14444/6055] [PMID: 31741829]

[50]   Lewandrowski K-U, Zhang X, Ramírez León JF, de Carvalho PST, Hellinger S, Yeung A. Lumbar vacuum disc, vertical instability, standalone endoscopic interbody fusion, and other treatments: an

opinion based survey among minimally invasive spinal surgeons. J Spine Surg 2020; 6(S1) (Suppl. 1): S165-78.
[http://dx.doi.org/10.21037/jss.2019.11.02] [PMID: 32195425]

[51]   Kim HS, Adsul N, Kapoor A, *et al.* A Mobile Outside-in Technique of Transforaminal Lumbar Endoscopy for Lumbar Disc Herniations. J Vis Exp 2018; (138):
[http://dx.doi.org/10.3791/57999] [PMID: 30148483]

[52]   Yeung A, Lewandrowski K-U. Early and staged endoscopic management of common pain generators in the spine. J Spine Surg 2020; 6(S1) (Suppl. 1): S1-5.
[http://dx.doi.org/10.21037/jss.2019.09.03] [PMID: 32195407]

[53]   Bini W, Yeung AT, Calatayud V, Chaaban A, Seferlis T. The role of provocative discography in minimally invasive selective endoscopic discectomy. Neurocirugia (Astur) 2002; 13(1): 27-31.
[http://dx.doi.org/10.1016/S1130-1473(02)70646-5] [PMID: 11939090]

[54]   Lewandrowski KU. Successful outcome after outpatient transforaminal decompression for lumbar foraminal and lateral recess stenosis: The positive predictive value of diagnostic epidural steroid injection. Clin Neurol Neurosurg 2018; 173: 38-45.
[http://dx.doi.org/10.1016/j.clineuro.2018.07.015] [PMID: 30075346]

[55]   Chang MC, Lee DG. Outcome of Transforaminal Epidural Steroid Injection According to the Severity of Lumbar Foraminal Spinal Stenosis. Pain Physician 2018; 21(1): 67-72.
[http://dx.doi.org/10.36076/ppj.1.2018.67] [PMID: 29357335]

[56]   MacVicar J, King W, Landers MH, Bogduk N. The effectiveness of lumbar transforaminal injection of steroids: a comprehensive review with systematic analysis of the published data. Pain Med 2013; 14(1): 14-28.
[http://dx.doi.org/10.1111/j.1526-4637.2012.01508.x] [PMID: 23110347]

CHAPTER 7

Full Endoscopic Interlaminar Contra-Lateral Lumbar Foraminotomy

Harshavardhan Dilip Raorane[1], Hyeun-Sung Kim[1,*] and Il-Tae Jang[1]

[1] *Department of Neurosurgery, Nanoori Hospital, Gangnam, Seoul, South Korea*

Abstract: Foraminal stenosis is often underestimated due to difficulties in approaching the region surgically. The evolution of the transforaminal approach allowed safe surgical exploration of foraminal pathology under direct vision. Postoperative Dysesthesia (POD) due to irritation of the dorsal root ganglion (DRG) of lumbar nerve roots at the surgical level is a common sequela associated with the transforaminal approach. Minimal dorsal root ganglion (DRG) retraction is critical to prevent POD. Full endoscopic interlaminar contra-lateral lumbar foraminotomy consists of a sublaminar approach or translaminar approach. It is followed by contralateral foraminotomy and extraforaminal decompression. The contralateral approach's principle is to create a safe path to the contralateral foramen, preserving the ipsilateral anatomy. It allows simultaneous lateral recess, contra-lateral foramen, and extraforaminal decompression along the nerve root with minimal nerve root manipulation in the foramen. However, the learning curve for the technique is steep compared to the transforaminal technique.

Keywords: Dorsal root ganglion, Foraminal stenosis, Postoperative dysesthesia, Transforaminal approach.

INTRODUCTION

Lumbar foraminal stenosis (LFS) is defined as a spinal nerve root's entrapment into the narrowed intervertebral foramen caused by degenerative disease. The incidence of LFS has proportionally risen, accounting for approximately 8-11% of degenerative lumbar diseases requiring surgical treatment [1]. However, it's often underestimated due to difficulties to surgically approach the region. Conventionally, there are two types of surgeries defined for foraminal stenosis. The first is total facetectomy with lumbar interbody fusion, and the second is open micro-foraminotomy as defined by Wiltse and Spencer [2]. However, lumbar

---

* **Corresponding author Hyeun-Sung Kim:** Nanoori hospital, Nonhyeon-dong, Gangnam-gu, Seoul, South Korea; Tel: +82-10-2440-2631; E-mail: neurospinekim@gmail.com

Kai-Uwe Lewandrowski, Jorge Felipe Ramírez León, Anthony Yeung, Hyeun-Sung Kim, Xifeng Zhang, Gun Choi, Stefan Hellinger and Álvaro Dowling (Eds.)

interbody fusion has its own drawbacks such as pseudoarthrosis, implant failure, and adjacent segment disease.

Though micro-foraminotomy is considered the gold standard procedure, it was associated with poor visualization and incomplete decompression. The success rate has been reported between 58-80% [3, 4].

Endoscopic spine surgery has evolved in the last few decades [5]. The introduction of the transforaminal approach by Young *et al.* [6] allowed safe surgical removal of disc material and exploration of foraminal anatomy under direct vision. It helped us understand that causes for the foraminal stenosis are extrinsic compressive pathology and intrinsic pathologies. We have described the technique of full endoscopic interlaminar contra-lateral lumbar foraminotomy for the foraminal decompression. Simultaneous lateral recess, contra-lateral foramen, and extraforaminal decompression along the course of the nerve root can be carried out through a single approach [7].

SURGICAL ANATOMY

Lee *et al.* [8] defined the intervertebral foramen into 3 zones: Subarticular (entry zone), Foraminal (mid zone) and Extraforaminal (exit zone). The intervertebral foramen is an inverted teardrop-shaped structure bounded anteriorly by the posterior wall of the segmental vertebra body and intervertebral disc, superiorly and inferiorly by the pedicles of cephalad and corresponding caudal vertebra, and posteriorly by the facet joint. The neuroforaminal content consists of the spinal nerve roots, dorsal root ganglion of the exiting nerve root, the radicular artery and vein, lymphatics, and the intervertebral- and foraminal ligaments [9]. The foraminal ligaments are comprised of the transforaminal ligaments – namely the superior, middle and inferior transforaminal ligaments, and the radial ligaments – and the extraforaminal ligaments – the superior- and inferior corpotranverse ligaments, and intertransverse ligaments. Hence causes of foraminal stenosis are not only compressive pathologies from outside but also intrinsic inflammatory pathologies.

SURGICAL INDICATIONS

Depending on the pathology, causes of foraminal stenosis can be divided into:

a. Extrinsic pathology
   ○ Foraminal disc herniation
   ○ Extra-foraminal disc herniation
   ○ Double crush syndrome

- Degenerative disc disease with lateral wedging
- Ligamentum flavum hypertrophy
- Superior articular process overriding
- Decreased foraminal height
- Osteophytes/Syndesmophytes
- Facet arthropathy/hypertrophy
- Facet cyst
- Post-traumatic
- Post-surgical (failed back syndrome)

b. Intrinsic pathology
- Foraminal adhesion or fibrosis either due to inflammatory, infective or post-surgical scar tissue formation
- Transforaminal ligament due to hypertrophy, fibrosis or calcification

CONTRAINDICATIONS

There are a few contraindications to the full endoscopic interlaminar contra-lateral lumbar foraminotomy worth mentioning:

- Gross segmental instability evident on dynamic radiographs (> 4mm of translation or > 10^0 angular opening)
- Grade 2 or more spondylolisthesis according to Meyerding's criteria
- Bilateral foraminal stenosis (more suitable for fusion)
- Severe degenerative scoliosis
- Infection
- Malignancy

SURGICAL TECHNIQUE

Preoperative Planning

We routinely perform plain radiograph AP, lateral, oblique, and dynamic views of the lumbar spine. The plain radiographs are evaluated for the alignment of the spine for the presence of degenerative scoliosis. Dynamic views are assessed for segmental instability. For surgical planning, the AP view is evaluated for the width of cranial, caudal laminae, and the extent of the interlaminar window, which is reduced in most spinal canal stenosis cases. The height and width of the foramen are evaluated for safe bony decompression.

Ligamentum flavum's sublaminar and subarticular extent, along with thickness, is evaluated in MRI. CT scan assessed in axial cut for the size, shape, and orientation of facets (Facet tropism). It gives an idea about the safe range of the medial facet resection without causing iatrogenic instability. 3D reconstructed CT scan image gives a detailed 3-dimensional view of the interlaminar window narrowed by deviated spinous process and hypertrophied bony spurs. The cross-section area of the canal and dura is measured pre-operatively for the severity of stenosis and post-operatively for decompression adequacy.

Anaesthesia

The procedure is preferably performed under General anesthesia. It allows the patient's comfortable positioning over the frame and facilitates a comprehensive exploration of the spinal canal. It also can be performed under epidural anesthesia with sedation. We routinely use Ropivacaine (0.75%) mixed with an equivalent amount of radiocontrast dye for epidural anesthesia. About 10 to 15ml of epidural anesthetics are used and can be extended according to the number of spinal levels. It can be supplemented with sedation (Midazolam 0.05mg/kg).

Patient Preparation & Position

The patient is placed in a prone position over a radiolucent table with Wilson's frame. The surgeon stands on the opposite side of the pathology. A single dose of antibiotics is administered in the preoperative period. The entire procedure is performed under constant saline irrigation. We prefer to use an arthro-pump with a pressure set at 30-40 mm Hg. The irrigation fluid pressure should be adjusted according to the clarity of surgical fluid. A single dose of antibiotics is administered before the procedure (Fig. **1**).

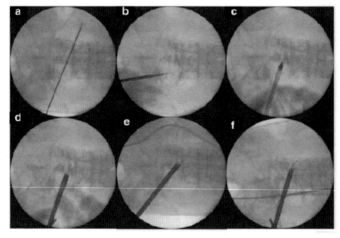

Fig. (1). (a) Intraoperative fluoroscopic view demonstrating. **(b)** An oblique line is drawn from the medial border of the ipsilateral facet to the contralateral foramen. **(c & d)** Skin incision. **(e)** Docking of obturator and working cannula at spinolaminar junction. **(f)** Contralateral sublaminar approach. Exploration of contralateral foraminal and extraforaminal region.

Surface Marking & Docking

An oblique line is drawn from the ipsilateral facet's medial border to the contralateral foramen under image intensifier guidance. About 1cm skin incision is taken at 1-1.5cm lateral to midline intersecting the oblique line. Skin incision location depends upon the approach (sublaminar or translaminar) and pathology (foraminal or extraforaminal). Multilevel stenosis can be decompressed through separate incisions.

The guidewire and serial dilators are passed through the skin incision, and the beveled working cannula is docked on the target point. Depending upon the approach, two target points are selected Point A: The spinolaminar junction of cranial vertebra on the ipsilateral side and point B: The deepest point of the caudal lamina. Finally, the endoscope is inserted into the working cannula. We routinely use an endoscope of a 30° viewing angle, 7.3 mm outer diameters, or equivalent, the working length of 171 mm.

Contralateral Approach

The contralateral approach's principle is to create a safe path to the contralateral foramen, preserving the ipsilateral anatomy. The sublaminar approach begins with drilling a base of the spinous process of the cranial vertebra from the midline to get access to the contralateral side. The midline of the spine is marked with a defect between ipsilateral and contralateral LF covered with epidural fat. The surgeons may encounter bleeding due to the constant presence of vessels around the defect. The interspinous ligament is another landmark that represents the midline of the spine. It can be differentiated from LF by its glistening white appearance compared to dull yellow LF. A working space is created for the instruments between the contralateral LF and cranial lamina. This technique's advantage is that vital neural structures are protected by a tough deep layer of LF throughout the procedure.

The drilling is performed in the sequence from the spinous process base, followed by the inferior margin of cranial lamina until we reach the SAP. It is continued until the free margins of deep LF and epidural fat begin to appear. The contralateral deep layer of LF is released from its superior and inferior attachments with a tissue dissector. It is then resected 'en bloc' with the help of endoscopic forceps. Once the deep LF is resected, contralateral traversing and exiting nerve root can be seen. The translaminar approach is preferred in patients with contralateral lateral recess stenosis marked by a trefoil shaped canal on the axial cut of MRI/CT scan. It involves contralateral complete laminectomy (Fig.

2).

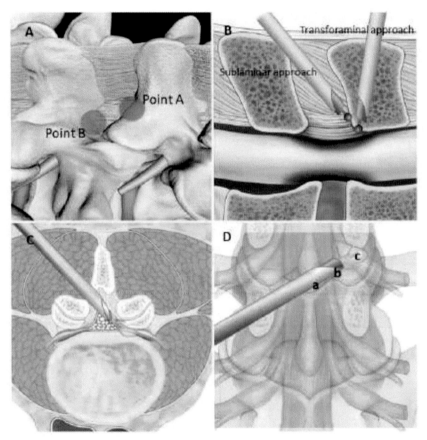

Fig. (2). A: docking sites. Point A in red: spinolaminar junction. Point B in green: Deepest point of caudal lamina B: Sublaminar and Translaminar Approach C. Axial view of the direction of scope to contralateral foramen D. systematic sequence of drilling; point a: spinolaminar junction to reach the contralateral side point b: ventral lower half of cephalad lamina attachment of LF point c: contralateral foraminal discectomy.

Foraminal & Extraforaminal Decompression

Foraminotomy can be performed by circumferentially enlarging the foraminal boundaries. The hypertrophied SAP or subluxated SAP tip on a dorsal side can be removed with an endoscopic drill and Kerrison rongeur. The osteophytes or syndesmophytes on a ventral side can be removed with a bone cutter and forceps. The working cannula and endoscope are gradually advanced into an enlarged foramen to visualize the foraminal pathology. The foraminal and extraforaminal decompression is done according to the location of the respective pathology. For example, hypertrophied bony facet is trimmed with an endoscopic burr and a punch. A hypertrophied foraminal ligament, a foraminal extruded disc fragment, or a loose osteophytes can be removed with endoscopic punch and forceps. The soft tissue debris or adhesions can be cleared with the help of a radiofrequency. Care must be taken to perform soft tissue dissection along the course of inflamed exiting nerve root without mobilizing it to minimize the postoperative dysesthesia for irritation of the dorsal root ganglion (DRG) – typically of the exiting nerve root. First, a discectomy is performed to create a ventral working space to approach the ventral osteophytes or syndesmophytes. The foraminal bleeding is meticulously coagulated with a radiofrequency to prevent further adhesions and fibrosis. An epidural drain is kept to avoid post-operative hematoma collection.

Final Check

The adequacy of decompression is checked with a flexible probe under endoscopic as well as fluoroscopic vision. The characteristic signs of an adequate foraminal decompression are mobility of exiting nerve root; colour changes of anaemic nerve root into pinkish red view and free pulsation of nerve root. The End-point is the "Beak Point" of the far lateral area the exiting root starts to curve downward. It represents the contour of the caudal and most lateral part of the upper vertebral body, after drilling out the syndesmophytes under the exiting nerve root. The extent of decompression can be cross-checked under fluoroscopic vision (Fig. **3**).

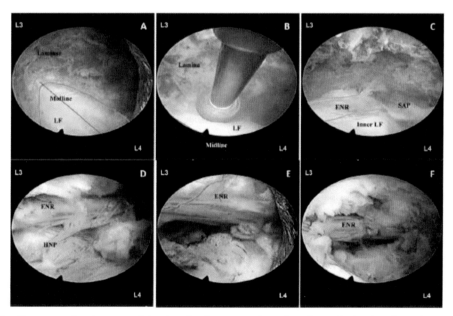

Fig. (3). Intraoperative images of the interlaminar contralateral endoscopic lumbar foraminotomy and discectomy. A: Docking and drilling of spinolaminar junction (Blue line) to create the midline sublaminar corridor (red line). B: Contralateral sublaminar approach C: Entrance of contralateral foramen. An imaginary tract of exiting nerve root (ENR) (green dotted line). D: contralateral herniated nucleus pulposus (HNP) and compressed contralateral L4 exiting nerve root in the foramen E: Exiting nerve root after discectomy. F: the entire course of exiting nerve root from the axillar part to the far-out part.

Postoperative Protocol

MRI and CT scan is performed as a routine on day 1 to check the adequacy of decompression. The epidural suction drain is removed on day 2. The patient is allowed to mobilize from postoperative day one as per tolerated. We encourage the patients to use bracing in the postoperative period to minimize the chances of micro-instability.

CLINCIAL SERIES

A total of 50 patients underwent interlaminar contralateral endoscopic lumbar foraminotomy and discectomy (ICELF) with a mean age of 64 years. The mean follow-up duration was 11 months. One patient operated at L2-3, six at L3-4, 22 at L4-5, and 21 at L5-S1 level. The clinical outcome was evaluated in the form of the visual analog score (VAS) of back and leg, Oswestry disability index (ODI), and Macnab's criteria. There was a statistical significant improvement in VAS score with mean value and range of pre-operative, one week, three months and final follow up are 7.42±0.99, 3.2±0.76, 2.54±0.99, and 2.16±0.98, respectively. The ODI score improved significantly from 73.4±7.33, 31.8±6.86, 28±6.83 and 25.2±6.34 in pre-operative, one week, three months, and final follow up. MacNab's criteria showed 12 (24%) Excellent, 35 (70%) Good, and 3 (6%) Fair outcomes in the ICELF and 23 (46%) Excellent, 19 (38%) Good, and 8 (16%) Fair outcomes in the TELD. Postoperative dysesthesia occurred less frequently in the ICELF (n=7) than the TELD (n=13). The POD incidence showed in the ICELF (7 out of 50, 14%) and the TELD (13 out of 50, 26%). We experienced incidental durotomy in 3 patients managed with the fibrin patch intra-operatively. There were no delayed postoperative complications such as recurrence or iatrogenic instability noted in our study.

COMPLICATIONS AND AVOIDANCE

Intraoperative Bleeding

Bleeding is encountered in several places in the contralateral approach. The midline defect between LF, axilla of exiting nerve root, and extraforaminal area are due to the segmental artery's anastomosing branches. Placing the working cannula close to the bone can prevent the obscuration of view by the bleeding. It can be controlled with a radiofrequency coagulator or laser. Some surgeons use hemostatic agents introduced through the working channel.

Dural Tear & Nerve Injury

The creation of sufficient working space between the lamina and ligamentum flavum for endoscopic instruments gives access to the contralateral side. The deep layer of ligamentum flavum acts as a protective barrier between the working space and vitals structures inside the spinal canal. The working cannula is placed firmly against the ventral surface of the lamina and facet to minimise the pressure over the underlying dura (Fig. **4**).

- Direct manipulation of an ischemic exiting nerve root inside the stenotic foramen is avoided to prevent transient dysesthesia or neuropraxia. The discectomy is performed first to create a ventral working space to approach the ventral osteophytes or syndesmophytes.
- In some patients with reduced foraminal height, pedicles of the caudal vertebra can be drilled along with SAP to minimize the neural manipulation by working cannula inside the foramen.
- The sharp instruments or laser is pointed away from the nerve root to avoid injury.
- In case of intraoperative dural tear, we prefer to repair a dural tear with layers of gel foam and fibrin patch. The fibrin patch is inserted between 2 layers of gel foam to cover the dural tear. We had not experienced any delayed sequela of the dural tear with this technique [10].

Incomplete Decompression

- The extent of decompression is cross-checked under fluoroscopy at every step of the surgery (*i.e.*, Contralateral recess, foramen, and extraforaminal region)
- Many authors have reported that mobilization of the nerve root and clinical results can be improved by removing the foraminal ligaments.

Recurrence

- The chances of recurrence can be avoided by the 'annular sealing technique' for foraminal disc herniation.
- The dissection in the foramen is kept minimal to avoid post-operative adhesion.

Iatrogenic Instability

- The iatrogenic instability is usually the result of an excessive bony removal in the region of pars or excessive ventral facetectomy.

Infection

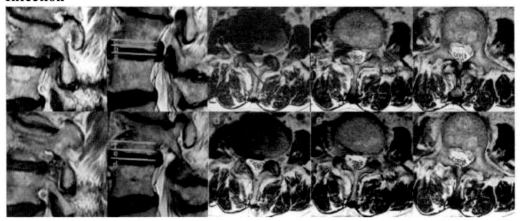

Fig. (4). Representative case – 71-year-old female patient with symptomatic L4-5 right foraminal to extraforaminal stenosis treated with full endoscopic interlaminar contralateral foraminotomy. Long red arrow showing the path of contralateral approach; short red arrow showing extruded disc fragment.

DISCUSSION

Macnab *et al.* [11, 12] originally described the "hidden zone" – a common site of foraminal stenosis between the traversing and exiting nerve root. In this region, foraminal stenosis is often underestimated. Hence, treatment is usually not directed at this area. However, direct visualization of this hidden zone has become feasible because of endoscopic spine surgery evolution. In the last few decades, this "hidden zone of Macnab" has become the focus of treatment and investigation. Knight *et al.* [3] introduced the percutaneous transforaminal laser foraminoplasty for the foraminal soft tissue decompression. Hoogland and Schubert [4] used serial reamers and trephines to enlarge the narrowed foramen. Both the procedures have specific limitations, for example, the laser foraminoplasty may effectively ablate soft tissue of the herniated disc or the hypertrophied ligamentum flavum. The later procedure is relatively blind and may be associated with significant bone resection. Ahn *et al.* [5] described the endoscopic lumbar foraminotomy for the foraminal decompression under direct endoscopic vision to produce good clinical results. Although the transforaminal approach provides excellent visualization of foraminal pathology, safe docking into narrowed stenotic foramen may be challenging. It may prevent the proper intraforaminal positioning of a working cannula and may irritate the exiting nerve root.

A contralateral approach can do adequate lateral recess and foraminal decompression with maximum preservation of the facet joint. Preservation of the facet joint and paraspinal muscles maintains the integrity of the motion segments. The contralateral approach allows the gradual advancement of the endoscope from the wide subarticular part of the foramen into the narrowed foraminal and extraforaminal area under direct vision. The entire course of the nerve root can be easily explored for compressive as well as inflammatory pathology. Multiple pathologies (such as double crush and triple crush syndrome) can be addressed through a single approach [7, 13].

As we have not experienced any significant pitfalls for the technique, it is applicable only for the patients with the unilateral symptoms. In patients with bilateral foraminal stenosis, interbody fusion is to be considered. As we approach the foramen from the spinal canal, local anesthesia is not preferred for this technique. Hence anesthesia-related complications are inevitable. The learning curve for the technique is steep compared to the transforaminal technique. However, surgical skills can be mastered over some time with adequate mentorship.

CONCLUSION

The contralateral technique provides adequate circumferential decompression of the foramen under direct vision. Multiple foraminal pathologies can be tackled through a single approach. Preservation of ipsilateral anatomy with contralateral facet improves the stability of the motion segment. It provides safe and minimally invasive options for foraminal decompression.

CONSENT FOR PUBLICATION

Not applicable.

CONFLICT OF INTEREST

The authors declare no conflict of interest, financial or otherwise.

ACKNOWLEDGEMENT

Declared none.

REFERENCES

[1]   Jenis LG, An HS. Spine update. Lumbar foraminal stenosis. Spine (Phila Pa 1976) 2000; 25(3): 389-94.
[http://dx.doi.org/10.1097/00007632-200002010-00022] [PMID: 10703115]

[2]   Wiltse LL, Spencer CW. New uses and refinements of the paraspinal approach to the lumbar spine. Spine 1988; 13(6): 696-706.
[http://dx.doi.org/10.1097/00007632-198813060-00019] [PMID: 3175760]

[3]   Donaldson WF III, Star MJ, Thorne RP. Surgical treatment for the far lateral herniated lumbar disc. Spine 1993; 18(10): 1263-7.
[http://dx.doi.org/10.1097/00007632-199308000-00003] [PMID: 8211356]

[4]   Kunogi J, Hasue M. Diagnosis and operative treatment of intraforaminal and extraforaminal nerve root compression. Spine 1991; 16(11): 1312-20.
[http://dx.doi.org/10.1097/00007632-199111000-00012] [PMID: 1750006]

[5]   Kim H, Kim M, Kim H, Oh SW, Adsul NM. Evolution of Spinal Endoscopic Surgery 2019; 16(1): 6-14.

[6]   Gore S, Yeung A. The "inside out" transforaminal technique to treat lumbar spinal pain in an awake and aware patient under local anesthesia: results and a review of the literature. Int J Spine Surg 2014; 8: 28.
[http://dx.doi.org/10.14444/1028] [PMID: 25694940]

[7]   Wu PH, Kim HS, Jang IT. How I do it? Uniportal full endoscopic contralateral approach for lumbar foraminal stenosis with double crush syndrome. Acta Neurochir (Wien) 2020.

[8]   Lee CK, Rauschning W, Glenn W. Lateral lumbar spinal canal stenosis: classification, pathologic anatomy and surgical decompression. Spine 1988; 13(3): 313-20.
[http://dx.doi.org/10.1097/00007632-198803000-00015] [PMID: 3388117]

[9]   Uchikado H, Nishimura Y, Hattori G, Ohara Y. Micro-anatomical structures of the lumbar intervertebral foramen for full-endoscopic spine surgery: review of the literatures. J Spine Surg 2020; 6(2): 405-14.
[http://dx.doi.org/10.21037/jss.2019.10.07] [PMID: 32656378]

[10]   Kim HS, Raorane HD, Wu PH, Heo DH, Sharma SB, Jang IT. Incidental Durotomy During Endoscopic Stenosis Lumbar Decompression: Incidence, Classification, and Proposed Management Strategies. World Neurosurg 2020; 139: e13-22.
[http://dx.doi.org/10.1016/j.wneu.2020.01.242] [PMID: 32059965]

[11]   Kim H-S, Sharma S, Wu P, Raorane H, Adsul N, Singh R, *et al.* Complications and limitations of endoscopic spine surgery and percutaneous instrumentation. Indian Spine J. 2020.
[http://dx.doi.org/10.4103/isj.isj_27_19]

[12]   Macnab I. Negative disc exploration. An analysis of the causes of nerve-root involvement in sixty-eight patients. J Bone Joint Surg Am 1971; 53(5): 891-903.
[http://dx.doi.org/10.2106/00004623-197153050-00004] [PMID: 4326746]

[13]   Kim HS, Paudel B, Jang JS, *et al.* Percutaneous Full Endoscopic Bilateral Lumbar Decompression of Spinal Stenosis Through Uniportal-Contralateral Approach: Techniques and Preliminary Results. World Neurosurg 2017; 103: 201-9.
[http://dx.doi.org/10.1016/j.wneu.2017.03.130] [PMID: 28389410]

CHAPTER 8

Mobile Outside In, SCOT (Suprapedicular Circumferential Opening Technique) Approach for Highly Inferior Migrated HNP

Nitin Maruti Adsul[1,2], **Hyeun Sung Kim**[1,*] and **Il-Tae Jang**[1]

[1] *Department of Neurosurgery, Nanoori Gangnam Hospital, Seoul, South Korea*

[2] *Sir Ganga Ram Hospital, Ortho-Spine Surgery, New Delhi, India*

Abstract: Downward migrated lumbar disc herniation can present a challenge to any spine surgeon. Open spine surgery requires an aggressive decompression of the posterior bony elements, which ultimately may lead to postlaminectomy syndrome and instability – both of which have been associated with higher reoperation rates. The interlaminar endoscopic approach is a reasonable alternative to open translaminar surgery but still carries the risk of dural tear and does not afford the ability for an intradiscal discectomy. The authors offer a modification of the outside-in transforaminal approach - the suprapedicular circumferential opening technique (SCOT) to gain better access to downward- and far-migrated extruded lumbar disc herniations.

Keywords: Downward migrated lumbar herniated disc, Suprapedicular decompression, Transforaminal approach.

INTRODUCTION

Lumbar disc herniations (LDH) are increasingly treated with the transforaminal endoscopic lumbar discectomy (TELD) procedure. Besides minor tissue damage, fewer problems with iatrogenic instability, epidural scarring, and retraction of the neural tissue are also notable advantages [1 - 6]. One of the more challenging clinical scenarios are downward migrated disc herniations alongside and below the traversing nerve root. Access to these high-grade interiorly migrated disc herniations may be obstructed by the pedicle and osteophytes of the ring apophysis [1 - 6]. Unless all fragments are removed in their entirety, the operation may fail [1, 4, 5]. Technological advances have made it possible for the experienced spinal endoscopist to go after these downward-migrated extruded

* **Corresponding author Hyeun Sung Kim:** Department of Neurosurgery, Nanoori Gangnam Hospital, Seoul, South Korea; Tel: +82-10-2440-2631; E-mail: neurospinekim@gmail.com

Kai-Uwe Lewandrowski, Jorge Felipe Ramírez León, Anthony Yeung, Hyeun-Sung Kim, Xifeng Zhang, Gun Choi, Stefan Hellinger and Álvaro Dowling (Eds.)

disc herniations, which many perhaps earlier would have considered an indication for open surgery [6 - 8]. In this chapter, the authors describe their transforaminal suprapedicular circumferential opening technique (SCOT) intended to master the challenges of endoscopically removing high-grade inferiorly migrated lumbar disc herniations.

RATIONALE FOR SCOT

One might ask why the transforaminal and not the interlaminar approach is used for these inferior migrated disc herniations, causing painful compression syndromes of the traversing nerve root? However, the transforaminal approach has several advantages that the authors of this chapter ask the reader to consider [9, 10]. These obvious advantages include a much lower risk of a dural tear. Typically, the dural sac is displaced posteriorly by these bulky disc herniations creating a surgical compartment where the surgeon can work safely *via* the transforaminal approach without much nerve root retraction. The contrary is the case with the interlaminar approach. The endoscopic spine surgeon will encounter the posterior displaced compressed dural sac if the interlaminar approach is chosen.

Another advantage of the transforaminal approach lies in its minimal disruption of the lumbar motion segment and the preservation of its anatomical structures. There is no need to remove bone from the overhanging rostral lamina, such as during the interlaminar approach. Conceivably, this could destabilize the motion segment and prompt more surgery later on. Another consideration is that such laminotomy to establish the interlaminar access to the disc herniation is time-consuming, making this technique less suitable for an outpatient surgery center where rapid turn-overs and early discharge are crucial to making such a clinical decision operation work. Besides, the transforaminal approach can easily be carried out at all lumbar levels, where the interlaminar approach may have some limitations above the L5/S1 level since the interlaminar windows are much smaller or may not exist because of anatomical variations or vertical collapse due to progressive degenerative disease in the aging spine.

Another shortcoming of the interlaminar approach is that the endoscopic visualization is limited to the epidural space. An intradiscal exploration is challenging, if not impossible, from the intradiscal approach. On the other hand, the transforaminal approach allows the surgeon to work in the epidural space and the intradiscal compartment by advancing the working cannula into the interspace. Any unstable intradiscal tissue that could lead to recurrent postoperative disc extrusions could be preemptively removed during the intradiscal portion of the transforaminal decompression procedure. The transforaminal approach is also more conducive to performing decompression surgery under local anesthesia than the interlaminar approach, which patients do not tolerate unless it is done under general anesthesia.

SURGICAL STEPS

As described in many other chapters in this Bentham series on spinal endoscopy, the patient should undergo the transforaminal SCOT procedure in the prone position on a radiolucent Wilson frame. Under local anesthesia, the authors establish a transforaminal endoscopic access portal under fluoroscopic control. The authors' preference is to inject the skin entry point with 1% lidocaine followed by injection of another 7–10 cc 1% lidocaine into the neuroforaminal area and 2-3 cc of 1.6% lidocaine with epinephrine 3–5 minutes after the first injection [5, 10 - 12]. The planning and placement of the skin entry point and the access trajectory to the surgical neuroforamen have also been described by many able authors in this Bentham series. The spinal access needle should be aimed at the most distal and caudal portion of the disc space. The authors recommend performing a discogram in the center-section of the surgical disc space to visualize any extruded disc fragments and their relationship to the disc tissue within the interspace using 6 ml of iohexol dye mixed with 1 ml indigo carmine. Neither of these substances is neurotoxic. The insertion of sequential dilators over a guidewire follows the THESYS technique popularized by Hoogland *et al.*, which culminates in the docking of a beveled working cannula into the neuroforamen. The authors use the endoscopic spine surgery system provided by JoimaxGmbH, Raumfabrik 33A, Amalienbadstraße, Karlsruhe, Germany.

Initially, the authors employ the inside-out technique to complete the intradiscal decompression. Then, the working cannula is retracted and directed caudally within the epidural space at the suprapedicular notch employing outside-in maneuvers [8]. A radiofrequency probe (Elliquence, New York, USA) and pituitary forceps are used to clear the pedicle of any soft tissue. The core steps of the SCOT procedure are executed by first drilling the central part of the superior articular process using a power drill (Primado 2, NSK, Tochigi, Japan). Then, the suprapedicular notch is further drilled out. Finally, the ring apophysis of the caudal vertebral body is drilled down directly underneath the traversing nerve root to increase the neuroforaminal volume to pursue the inferiorly migrated disc herniation further. The indigo carmine-stained extruded disc tissue is typically easily discernable during the video-endoscopic examination of the epidural space below the traversing nerve root (Figs. **1** and **2**). A semirigid flexible probe that can be curved by squeezing its handle can be used as an alternative to rigid probe and forceps should it be challenging to extirpate the extruded disc in its entirety. After all, extruded disc herniations are highly inflammatory. Bleeding may occur due to the engorgement of previously compressed epidural veins that could be severed when adherent to the extruded disc tissue. The endoscopic spine surgeon should be prepared to deal with adhesions and scar tissue, possibly preventing removing all of the extruded disc tissue. The radiofrequency probe is the tool of choice to handle such bleeding problems. Alternatively, retracting the endoscope for a few minutes to let a clot form may sometimes be all it takes to control bleeding. The authors recommend reviewing a postoperative MRI 4~24 hours after SCOT to confirm the removal of the migrated disc fragment.

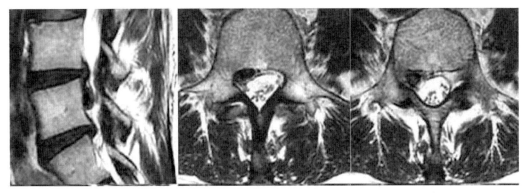

Fig. (1A). a) Preoperative MRI showing high grade inferior migration at L4-5 level.

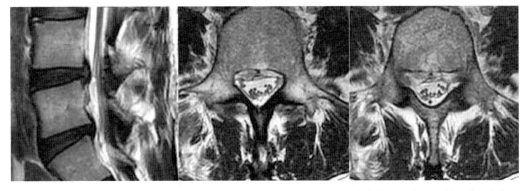

Fig. (1B). b) Postoperative MRI showing complete removal of high grade inferiorly migrated herniated disc.

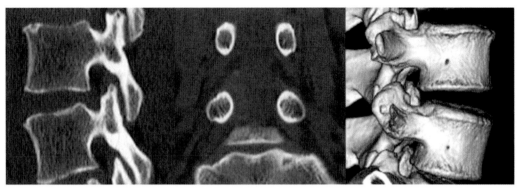

Fig. (2A). a) Preoperative CT.

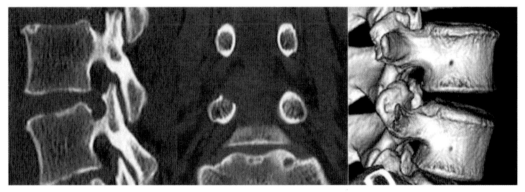

Fig. (2B). Postoperative showing widened neuroforamen without structural damage (Highlighted red area was drilled during the procedure).

DISCUSSION

Nowadays, the advancement of endoscopic technology allows the skilled endoscopic spine surgeon to decompress highly migrated sequestrated discs fragments to be removed [1 - 3]. Traditionally, clinical outcomes with these types of disc herniation are less favorable [4 - 6]. The reliability of recent endoscopic spine surgery techniques is now on par with traditional microsurgical decompression [3 - 7]. Attempting to treat more complex problems posed, for example, by high-grade inferiorly migrated disc herniations is now within reach of the well-trained endoscopic spine surgeon [6, 8, 9]. Removing the anatomic barrier posed by the pedicle with the SCOT procedure is one such step forward made possible with the advent of power drills and flexible graspers. Inadequate decompression leaving remnants of the extruded disc herniations behind has been reported by Lee *et al.* as one of the main reasons for failed endoscopic discectomy failure and a high revision surgery rate. The latter may additionally be impacted by the size of and location of the herniation [4].

There are few technical details worth discussing regarding the SCOT technique. Most notably, the skin entry point is more cranial, and the trajectory is much more aimed towards the caudal pedicle when compared to traditional endoscopic surgical approaches, where the working cannula is lined up more parallel to the disc space. Ultimately, the initial docking point for the working cannula is at the junction between the lower vertebral body and the superior articular process (SAP). For the initial foraminoplasty, portions of the SAP may be removed partially removed with reamers. In contrast to the original TESSYS outside-in technique, parts of the superior margin of the caudal pedicle and lower vertebral body just below the traversing nerve root are removed during the foraminoplasty. Therefore, the ideal entry point for the SCOT suprapedicular approach is the upper margin of the inferior vertebral pedicle. In patients with spondylosis, more of the upper margin of the caudal vertebral may have to be removed to increase the neuroforaminal volume [9 - 11].

The motivation for developing the SCOT technique was derived from the frustrating experience of the previous transforaminal methods, which had limited ability to deal with high-grade inferiorly migrated discs. The SCOT technique circumvents this problem by removing a high-grade inferior migrated disc through the narrow foraminal space above the caudal vertebra's pedicle. This new technique has the advantage of a prone procedure done under local anesthesia with minimal tissue disruption and postoperative complications, as discussed above, such as dural tears [8, 12]. The access angles are much steeper to warrant access to these downward- and far-migrated discs, whose removal can be quite tricky at times. When measured in the coronal and sagittal plane, the steep, nearly vertical access angles are intended to facilitate the decompression below the traversing root. Adequate decompression may result in bleeding. Achieving hemostasis is typically not problematic. Placement of a hemovac drainage system is a consideration; however, the authors leave that decision at the discretion of the attending spine surgeon. Conversion to open surgery is rarely needed.

CONCLUSION

The SCOT technique represents a modern modification of the transforaminal approach. It consists of steeper access angles to reach far- and downward migrated lumbar herniated disc herniations. Clinical outcomes are typically more favorable with the SCOT- than with the standard transforaminal outside-in technique while delivering lower recurrence and reoperation rates.

CONSENT FOR PUBLICATION

Not applicable.

CONFLICT OF INTEREST

The authors declare no conflict of interest, financial or otherwise.

ACKNOWLEDGEMENTS

Declared none.

REFERENCES

[1]   Lee S, Kim S-K, Lee S-H, *et al.* Percutaneous endoscopic lumbar discectomy for migrated disc herniation: classification of disc migration and surgical approaches. Eur Spine J 2007; 16(3): 431-7.
        [http://dx.doi.org/10.1007/s00586-006-0219-4] [PMID: 16972067]

[2]   Jang J-S, An S-H, Lee S-H. Transforaminal percutaneous endoscopic discectomy in the treatment of foraminal and extraforaminal lumbar disc herniations. J Spinal Disord Tech 2006; 19(5): 338-43.
        [http://dx.doi.org/10.1097/01.bsd.0000204500.14719.2e] [PMID: 16826005]

[3]   Tsou PM, Yeung AT. Transforaminal endoscopic decompression for radiculopathy secondary to intracanal noncontained lumbar disc herniations: outcome and technique. Spine J 2002; 2(1): 41-8.
        [http://dx.doi.org/10.1016/S1529-9430(01)00153-X] [PMID: 14588287]

[4]   Schubert M, Hoogland T. Endoscopic transforaminal nucleotomy with foraminoplasty for lumbar disk herniation. Oper Orthop Traumatol 2005; 17(6): 641-61.
        [http://dx.doi.org/10.1007/s00064-005-1156-9] [PMID: 16369758]

[5]   Lee S-H, Kang BU, Ahn Y, *et al.* Operative failure of percutaneous endoscopic lumbar discectomy: a radiologic analysis of 55 cases. Spine 2006; 31(10): E285-90.
        [http://dx.doi.org/10.1097/01. brs.0000216446.13205.7a] [PMID: 16648734]

[6]   Kim CH, Chung CK, Woo JW. Surgical outcome of percutaneous endoscopic interlaminar lumbar discectomy for highly migrated disk herniation. Clin Spine Surg 2016; 29(5): E259-66.
        [http://dx.doi.org/10.1097/BSD.0b013e31827649ea] [PMID: 23073149]

[7]   Yeung AT, Yeung CA. Advances in endoscopic disc and spine surgery: foraminal approach. Surg Technol Int 2003; 11: 255-63.
        [PMID: 12931309]

[8]   Ahn Y. Transforaminal percutaneous endoscopic lumbar discectomy: technical tips to prevent complications. Expert Rev Med Devices 2012; 9(4): 361-6.
        [http://dx.doi.org/10.1586/erd.12.23] [PMID: 22905840]

[9]   Kim HS, Ju CI, Kim SW, Kim JG. Endoscopic transforaminal suprapedicular approach in high grade inferior migrated lumbar disc herniation. J Korean Neurosurg Soc 2009; 45(2): 67-73.
        [http://dx.doi.org/10.3340/jkns.2009.45.2.67] [PMID: 19274114]

[10]   Lee C-W, Yoon K-J, Ha S-S, Kang J-K. Foraminoplastic superior vertebral notch approach with reamers in percutaneous endoscopic lumbar discectomy: technical note and clinical outcome in limited indications of percutaneous endoscopic lumbar discectomy. J Korean Neurosurg Soc 2016; 59(2): 172-81.
        [http://dx.doi.org/10.3340/jkns.2016.59.2.172] [PMID: 26962427]

[11]   Iprenburg M. Transforaminal endoscopic surgery in lumbar disc herniation in an economic crisis-the TESSYS method. US Musculoskeletal Rev 2008; 3: 47-9.

[12]   Ahn Y, Jang I-T, Kim W-K. Transforaminal percutaneous endoscopic lumbar discectomy for very high-grade migrated disc herniation. Clin Neurol Neurosurg 2016; 147: 11-7.
        [http://dx.doi.org/10.1016/j.clineuro.2016.05.016] [PMID: 27239898]

CHAPTER 9

Over-The-Top *versus* Transforaminal Lumbar Endoscopic Techniques

Álvaro Dowling[1,2] and Kai-Uwe Lewandrowski[3,4,5,*]

[1] *Endoscopic Spine Clinic, Santiago, Chile*

[2] *Department of Orthopaedic Surgery, USP, Ribeirão Preto, Brazil*

[3] *Center for Advanced Spine Care of Southern Arizona and Surgical Institute of Tucson, Tucson, AZ, USA*

[4] *Department of Orthopaedic Surgery, UNIRIO, Rio de Janeiro, Brazil*

[5] *Department of Orthoapedic Surgery, Fundación Universitaria Sanitas, Bogotá, D.C., Colombia, USA*

Abstract: A systematic review of contemporary lumbar endoscopic decompression techniques shows that the lion's share of lumbar endoscopic decompressions is done *via* the transforaminal and interlaminar approach. Many modifications and diverse applications for the more complex clinical applications have been described. Clinical outcomes in well-trained, experienced hands suggest that these modified endoscopic procedures are genuine advances. However, from the point of view of the community-based or academic traditionally trained spine surgeon adoption of these complex endoscopic procedures may still seem either impractical or out of reach when these endoscopic procedures are considered for each individual patient. The surgeon will have to figure out how to implement these procedures into their routine clinical operations by replacing the well-tried, time-proven and reliable open or other forms of minimally invasive spine surgeries. Recognizing a surgical technique's clinical advantages over another is one thing, but transforming one's practice is much more complex and depends not only on one's training or comfort level, but in most cases, the actual experience for each surgeon that will evolve due to the feedback from their patients. In patients who have experienced both the transforaminal and translaminar endoscopic approach, each surgeon will likely use the approach that gives the safest, most cost-effective, as well as the approach chosen by the surgeon for each anatomically based and guided approach. Many additional factors could potentially impede endoscopic spine surgery implementation, most of which will evolve, as the surgeon circle around the anatomic limitations of each approach. The availability or lack of equipment, trained staff, and support system also plays a role.

***** **Corresponding author Kai-Uwe Lewandrowski:** Center for Advanced Spine Care of Southern Arizona and Surgical Institute of Tucson, Tucson, AZ, USA, Department of Orthopaedic Surgery, UNIRIO, Rio de Janeiro, Brazil and Department of Orthoapedic Surgery, Fundación Universitaria Sanitas, Bogotá, D.C., Colombia, USA; Tel: +1 520 204-1495; Fax: +1 623 218-1215; E-mail: business@tucsonspine.com

The institutionalized spine surgeons may encounter additional hurdles since endoscopic spine surgery's disparate nature may disrupt well-established revenue cycles, making its implementation difficult. The surgeon's institutions may have to shoulder the burden of capital equipment purchases while facing lower reimbursement. To aid the prospective endoscopic spine surgeons in overcoming these implementation hurdles, the authors aimed to provide a systematic step-by-step comparison of the lumbar endoscopic over-the-top *versus* the transforaminal decompression techniques to illustrate their various technical aspects and clinical indications to aid the reader in selecting a "preferred" endoscopic technique.

Keywords: Endoscopy, Lumbar endoscopic surgery, Over the top technique, Transforaminal approach.

INTRODUCTION

Endoscopic procedures demonstrate equivalent clinical outcomes compared to the traditional open microsurgery with minor tissue trauma. Additionally, shorter hospital stays, lower costs of post-operative care may result in lower direct and indirect costs and earlier return to work due to rapid rehabilitation. The increase in the number of elderly patients and the need for an early return to work has increased the demand for developing the percutaneous endoscopic decompression and fusion techniques in the lumbar spine. In the last two decades, the technical evolution has been outstanding because of better optics design, improvements in surgical instruments and surgical approaches. The paradigm of percutaneous endoscopic spine surgery is shifting. Many original research articles and reviews relevant to this special issue confirm optimal endoscopic spinal surgery results.

The history of endoscopic lumbar spine surgery shows that its protagonists reached significant millstones by employing disruptive techniques and protocols that were disparaging to traditional and translaminar minimally invasive surgical technology. These newer endoscopic protocols came to prominence due to the need for safe, and more cost-effective minimally invasive techniques that are also associated with fewer dural leaks and iatrogenic instability or disabling back pain due to failed back surgery. In 1939, JG Love was the first to publish a description of the interlaminar approach. His original report indicated high patient satisfaction and nerve root compression signs had a significant improvement. The reduction of collateral damage was the driving force for the pioneers of microsurgery [1].

In 1977, Caspar [2] and Yasargil [3] independently described a microsurgical interlaminar approach. Microsurgery was shown to improve the short-term clinical outcome of lumbar discectomy significantly, mainly by reducing iatrogenic collateral damage. Postoperative pain was much better controlled with this surgical approach techniques. The intraoperative blood loss and infection risk were recognized to be lower, and hospital stays were shorter. Various factors than short-term results predict long-term clinical outcomes due to the nature of the progressive underlying degenerative lumbar spine disease [4]. Historically, current modern endoscopic techniques are centered around Yeung and Hoogland. Both endoscopic surgeon's operative techniques only differed on their approaches to the same patho-anatomy. Others have since contributed in the past few years. In the authors' opinion, recent modern concepts contributed to the current adoption of minimally invasive and endoscopic spinal surgery techniques by traditionally trained open and endoscopic spine surgeons.

In a more comprehensive historical review, in 1964, Lyman Smith published a paper about the enzymatic dissolution of the lumbar nucleus pulposus [5, 6]. The long-term outcomes were good and complications were rare and chemonucleolysis seemed to become a viable alternative to surgical discectomy [7, 8]. Parviz Kambin, a Philadelphian surgeon, further developed the posterolateral approach in 1980 [9 - 12]. He described a safe corridor to the lumbar disc between the exiting nerve root and the superior facet in his pioneering works. This safe zone was later universally accepted as Kambin's Triangle. Later, Suezawa, Schreiber, and Leu improved upon Kambin's percutaneous technique by visualizing the procedure with an endoscope. They called this modification of Kambin's original technique discoscopy [13 - 15]. In the 90s, Anthony Yeung [16, 17] and Hal Matthews [18, 19] described a more lateral access route. Their transforaminal approach aimed at far lateral disc herniations and more medially located pathologies. These surgical procedures were now possible because the surgical access corridor was aimed more parallel at the annulus's posterior rim. Anthony Yeung advanced the intradiscal therapies concepts *via* the transforaminal approach by describing visualized endoscopic treatments of validated pain generators. Based on these advances, he developed the YESS™ endoscopic spine system, which turned out to be versatile for both the transforaminal and interlaminar approach techniques [17, 20]. Sebastian Ruetten chiefly popularized the latter [21 - 25]. While several chapters in this Bentham book series recognize these individual contributing surgeons, in this chapter, the authors describe the most commonly employed contemporary lumbar endoscopic approaches and their associated techniques.

TRANSFORAMINAL APPROCHES

The transforaminal approach has significantly evolved in the last few decades. From the first attempts in 1963 with Smith injecting chymopapain into the disk to the very early origins with Hijikata [13] in 1975 with percutaneous nucleotomy and nonspecific disc depressurization in the 80s [9, 10, 26 - 28]. The "previsualization era," as defined by Kim *et al.* [29], reached its peak with the description of the triangular safe zone by Kambin in 1991 [30 - 32] and later with the maximum cannula diameter allowed in the triangular safe zone in the cadaveric study by Mirkovic and Schwartz [33]. The "postvisualization era" [29] arrived in the 90s with transforaminal endoscopic microdiscectomy described by Matthews [18] and endoscopic assisted surgery described by Foley [34, 35] and Destandau [36].

In 1999, Yeung presented the YESS system [17], and later in 2000, he described the original "inside-out" transforaminal technique with emphasis on a standardized methodology [16]. Around the same time, the "outside-in" approach was first described by Hoogland and Knight and allegedly permitted the resection of a broader range of disc herniations through a foraminoplasty [37 - 39]. Knight's emphasis was for foraminoplasty using a laser. Later, in 2006, the interlaminar approach was described by Ruetten [25], focusing on the troublesome L5-S1 herniated disc. Choi *et al.* introduced the use of an endoscopic drill for the foraminoplasty, allowing the surgeon to reach further migrated fragments through the transforaminal approach [40].

INSIDE-OUT TECHNIQUE

The original standardized inside-out technique for transforaminal endoscopic surgery was described by Yeung *et al.* [41, 42]. The inside-out approach and methodology focus on targeting the pain generators in the foramen and treat pain by visualizing inflammation and compression of nerves [43 - 46]. The technique is always performed under local anesthesia allowing the patient to feel pain when manipulating the inflamed root and guide the surgeon through the procedure by provocative methods like evocative chromo-discography [47]. The inside-out technique aims to dock the working cannula inside the disc space allowing the surgeon to remove degenerative fragmented disc material, pursuing indirect decompression of epidural space, and perform intradiscal thermal modulation of annular tears [41 - 44, 47]. If needed, the endoscope is withdrawn from the disc space to inspect the foramen and remove extruded fragments after foraminoplasty [45]. Probing ventral and dorsal to the traversing nerve and the exiting nerve's axilla confirms adequate removal of all mechanical lesions. Accepted indications include the following:

1. Annular tears with discogenic lumbar pain as determined by evocative discography,
2. All disc herniations and protrusions accessible through the foramen, whether contained, extruded, or sequestered,
3. Failed back syndrome from foraminal fibrosis, recurrent HNP, and subarticular lateral recess stenosis,

4. Mild and soft tissue central spinal stenosis,
5. Foraminal and extraforaminal stenosis,
6. Discitis,
7. Juxtafacet and pedunculated cysts.

There are some contraindications and limitations to the inside-out approach. Some authors argue that the inside-out technique is not ideal for extra discal pathologies like migrated disc herniations or central protruded disc with severe canal compromise. It may be more destructive as it requires removing more normal tissue to achieve decompression [25]. Other authors affirm that in badly degenerated discs or older disc prolapses, the sequestered material often loses its continuity, making the retrograde sequester resection from intradiscal technically limited [48].

OUTSIDE-IN TECHNIQUE

The outside-in approach was first described and popularized by Dr. Hoagland [37 - 39, 49 - 51], the "Thomas endoscopic spine surgery system" (THESSYS), as a modification of the inside-out technique. It is based on serial dilation of the foramen using dilators, trephines, or cannulated reamers [50]. With this technique, a progressive foraminoplasty allows the surgeon to access the more diminutive intervertebral foramen at the lower levels and degenerative stenotic foramen. This procedure's main advantage is that it can be applied for a broader range of pathologies like extruded, sequestrated, migrated, and calcified disc when the intended retrograde sequester resection from intradiscal is often technically limited [48, 52]. Nevertheless, blind fluoroscopically guided facetectomy can jeopardize the neurovascular and ligamentous structures in the foramen [45] or result in post-operative pain and segmental instability due to over-enthusiastic reaming. Further modifications of the original technique, such as introducing an endoscopic drill by Choi, have made the procedure safer [53, 54]. In 2005, Ruetten introduced another modification, the "extreme lateral access." The objective was to direct the endoscope through a far lateral approach that permitted to reach the spinal canal tangentially to better address disc prolapses sequestered within the spinal canal [48]. In addition to the indications of inside-out technique, the outside-in approach can better address:

1. Severe central protruded disc with high canal compromise,
2. Sequestrated disc with low grade superior and inferior migration,
3. Recurred disc,
4. Calcified disc,
5. Lateral recess and foraminal stenosis.

The well-recognized contraindications and limitations related to sequestrated disc with high-grade migration require to remove significant bone with the outside-in technique. This can significantly elevate the chance of neural tissue damage (DRG) [55 - 57], instability, and even fracture in osteoporotic bone [58, 59].

FROM INTERLAMINAR TO OVER-THE-TOP TECHNIQUES

In 2005, Ruetten first reported the full-endoscopic interlaminar technique (FED-IL) with successful outcomes reported with the endoscopic treatment of lumbar stenosis [23, 52, 60 - 65]. Choi *et al.* reported variations of the interlaminar technique [66]. He recommended that the targeting spinal needle be inserted under fluoroscopy guidance, passing through LF into the lateral recess and the intervertebral disc. Serial dilators were passed over the guidewire into the intervertebral disc to insert a round working cannula [66]. Kim and Chung modified the original Ruetten technique by advancing the dilators through an 8-millimeter small incision to the ligamentum flavum followed by a short cut through it under the direct endoscopic vision to enter the epidural space [67]. The large working cannula was used to retract and maintain a roomy opening in the ligamentum flavum to allow access to the epidural space. Hwang *et al.* described a contralateral approach to remove sequestrated or migrated herniations [68]. With Hwang's technique, the endoscope passes over the dura by undercutting the spinous process visualizing the contralateral nerve route and disc fragment. Gun Choi described the intermittent method. The puncture needle was inserted through a one-centimeter incision lateral to the posterior median line. Advanced use of the standard loss-of-resistance techniques employed by pain management physicians during interlaminar epidural steroid injections allowed safe access to the epidural space. An epidurogram was created by injecting lignocaine, outlining the nerve root and dural sac, thus confirming that the needle reached the epidural space safely [40]. Specifically intended for the L5/S1 segment, the needle was then advanced into the disc from where serial dilation and working cannula placement may commence [40]. The epidural fat and nerve root, and dural sac may be retracted with an upward rotation of the working cannula [69]. Song *et al.* compared intermittent techniques with a full-endoscopic approach [69]. They found that the herniated disc's intermittent method was effective and economically more advantageous due to shorter surgery times and lower hospitalization costs when compared to traditional translaminar lumbar decompression [69]. The over-the-top technique has evolved as a bilateral variation of the interlaminar approach to the lumbar herniated disc.

UNILATERAL AND BILATERAL ENDOSCOPIC OVER THE TOP TECHNIQUES

Transitioning to the over-the-top decompression technique may be easier for the traditionally trained spine surgeon since it resembles the traditional translaminar surgeries carried out with an endoscope instead through a midline or paraspinal incision with and without a minimally invasive retractor. The videoendoscopic visualization of the familiar posterior lumbar anatomy may be easier than learning the transforaminal anatomy. The evaluation of the amount of decompression is debatable but deemed sufficient when there is an apparent increase of the dura's pulsations or a clear view of a pulsating nerve root. High-grade three-dimensional anatomical knowledge of the facet joints, ligaments, the nerves is mandatory. However, you need to plan the anatomical goals to release the neural structure and pain generator efficiently when you need a decompression. In the last decade, the Authors developed the over-the-top technique for the transforaminal approach. It consists of a well-executed preoperative anatomical planning and parametric analysis of the angular orientation of the facets joint, the laminae, and the intervertebral disc in the sagittal plane to maximize the endoscopic decompression in the lateral recess by maneuvering over the top of the dural sac from the into the lateral recesses. Special consideration should be given to the preoperative planning at the L5/S1 level.

After insertion of the working cannula, a transforaminal endoscopic diagnostic inspection of the neuroforamen should be performed to look for unexpected pain generators, and other anatomical abnormalities. Using a combination of various tools such as drills, Kerrison, trephines, chisels, the direct posterior interlaminar decompression is completed from the rostral pedicle to the caudal pedicle to reach both lateral recesses and the entry zone to both neuroforaminae (Fig. **1**). The goal of this over-the-top endoscopic decompression is decompression of the dural sac and the bilateral recesses. It, therefore, is particularly suitable for endoscopic removal of central bony and soft tissue stenosis. To accomplish this, it is imperative to start the midline decompression and understand the endoscopically visualized anatomy in context with the imaging provided by the preoperative MRT and CT scan.

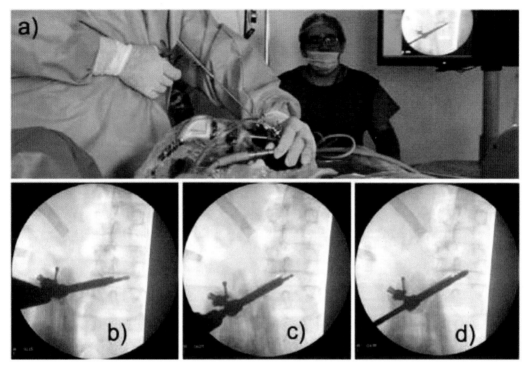

Fig. (1). Intraoperative fluoroscopic images obtained during the over-the-top contralateral decompression showing use an endoscopic Kerrison (a, b), a high-speed drill (c), and a trephine (d).

High-speed drills are often necessary to initially gain access to the central spinal canal. Incidental durotomies are of concern. This team of authors recommends that spine surgeons familiarize themselves with the proper use of high-speed endoscopic drills in training labs or other forms of endoscopic spine surgery where the dural sac is at lower risk of being injured. Some high-speed drill sets provide a protector sleeve or retractor blade that should be strategically placed during this portion of the decompression to protect the dural sac. After the surgeon deems the endoscopic decompression complete, one should always take fluoroscopic images in both planes with a probe touching the pedicles or placed in the foramina to be certain that no portion of the painful pathology was missed. Lastly, a comprehensive endoscopic view with complete side-to-side dural sac decompression should be obtained.

OVER-THE-TOP LUMBAR DECOMPRESSION FOR CENTRAL CHANNAL STENOSIS

The aging population in most countries will increasingly require treatment of lumbar spinal canal stenosis [70 - 73]. In the elderly, many spines are choosing the endoscopic lumbar decompression procedures because of multiples advantages such as less blood loss, lower complication- and infection rates, less postoperative pain, and earlier return to their usual activities and work. Multiple the Spine Outcome Research Trial (SPORT) studies showed that surgical decompression of lumbar spinal stenosis offers a substantially more significant improvement in pain and function than non-operative treatment over four- and eight-year follow up [74 - 79]. Without attempting to engage in an exhaustive discussion of the indications, pros, and cons of instrumented lumbar fusion surgery, the authors of this chapter are stipulating that most surgeons would agree that the addition of instrumentation for fusion during a decompression surgery adds significantly higher perioperative morbidity, complication- and reoperation rates [80 - 85]. On this flip side of this argument stands the lengthy learning curve with endoscopic spine surgery. Each surgeon should review surgical candidates deemed appropriate for the endoscopic over-the-top or transforaminal procedure on a case-by-case basis to maximize clinical benefit and achieve consistent clinical outcomes [86].

OVER THE TOP SURGICAL TECHNIQUE

The patient is placed in the prone position. The surgery is performed under local anesthesia with sedation utilizing monitored anesthesia protocols (MAC). Alternatively, surgeons may choose to perform these surgeries under general anesthesia. These choices are typically made in the context of skill level, available support, and training by the anesthesia- and surgical support teams. First, the midline and the rostral lamina's inferior border are marked at the surgical level in the posterior-anterior plane (PA). In the lateral (LAT) place, the surgeon should draw a line parallel to the intervertebral space, thus, indicating the endoscopic attack angle required to access the interlaminar area.

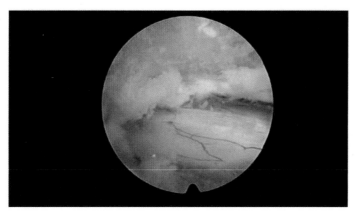

Fig. (2). View of the dural sac during the initial decompression with the over-the-top technique.

The incision is preferably placed slightly in the cranial aspect of the interlaminar window facilitating widening of the interlaminar window rostrally by resecting portions of the upper lamina with the high-speed burr. For safe access to the central canal, the endoscope is placed at the transitional junction between the ligamentum flavum and the facet joint. Decompression starts with the upper lamina and part of the inferior articular process in an L's shape before starting partial resection of the inferior lamina (Fig. **2**). These maneuvers are all done with the intent of widening the interlaminar window. In patients with a very thick ligament flavum, a more comprehensive decompression of the superior lamina may require detaching it from its rostral attachment area to the upper lamina's undersurface before attempting to peel the yellow ligament back. These procedural variations are essential to avoid dural tears. At this juncture, all portions of the accessible ligamentum flavum should be removed endoscopically until the midline. Both lateral recesses are visualized, including the axillary takeoff of the exiting nerve roots. A combination of Kerrison rongeurs, burs, trephines, and chisels are used to accomplish this. Surgeons will choose these types of instruments often according to their personal preference and factors dictated by the compressive pathology's anatomy. The need for complete decompression cannot be overstressed to avoid the need for revision decompression surgery in patients with failure to cure (Fig. **3**).

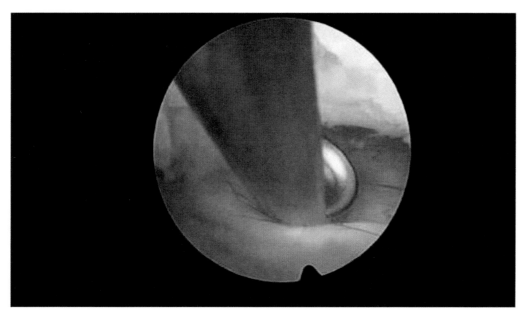

Fig. (3). Panoramic view during the over-the-top endoscopic decompression showing the Kerrison instrument in the contralateral recess.

As with any endoscopic spine surgery, training and mentorship programs should be effectively used by the aspiring endoscopic spine surgeon before attempting to perform the technically demanding over-the-top and transforaminal decompression procedure independently. Concerning the decompression's rostral-to-caudal extent, the authors recommend decompressing each recess and from rostral pedicle to caudal pedicle and verifying this under fluoroscopic control intraoperatively. Similarly, should the foraminal decompression adequacy be checked in both the PA and LAT plane fluoroscopically by passing a probe out through the foramen. Simplified wound closure can be accomplished with a single suture horizontal mattress stitch. Patients are fully mobilized immediately after surgery without a brace and we discharge them two to three hours after surgery. Typically, the first postoperative visit is scheduled within a week from the operation. Patients are advised to move around normally and that bedrest is not advised.

PATIENT SELECTION PROTOCOLS FOR LUMBAR SPINE DECOMPRESSION

The question now becomes which patient to select for which type of lumbar endoscopic decompression? What are the best criteria for the transforaminal *versus* the interlaminar approach and its over-the-top variation. A formal definition of these patient selection criteria is albeit from the literature, and very few articles were published on this subject. The authors have done so concerning the transforaminal and interlaminar approach. Beyond the apparent limitations of available equipment resources, surgeon's skill level, and general support staff, the authors present a work flow chart for selecting patients for the best endoscopic lumbar decompression procedure based on the merits of the type location of the patient's painful pathology.

Although the authors are not bent on using image-based criteria to define the painful pathology, they have developed an image-based algorithm to choose patients for the most appropriate endoscopic approach and decompression technique to maximize clinical improvements. This algorithm identifies four types of lumbar spinal stenosis. It stratifies patients according to the location, type, and extent of bony and soft tissue stenosis to suggest a preferred endoscopic approach (Fig. **4**). Additional anatomical factors regarding the symptomatic compressive pathology restricting access to it at the surgical level are considered. Employing this patient selection algorithm, the authors [87] analyzed clinical outcomes over a five-year follow-up period. Visual Analogue Scale (VAS) [88] and modified Macnab criteria [89] were used as the primary clinical outcome measures.

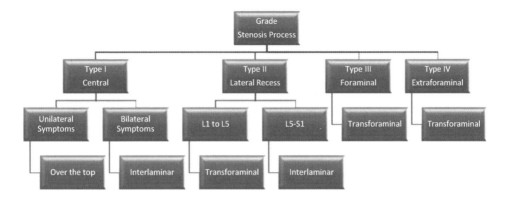

Fig. (4). Algorithm employed in the grading spinal stenosis by location of the compressive pathology: type I-Central canal stenosis, type II – lateral recess stenosis, type III – foraminal stenosis, and type IV – extraforaminal stenosis. The endoscopy approach was chosen on the basis of this protocol.

CLINICAL SERIES

The authors' clinical study to validate the patient selection algorithm for the best endoscopic stenosis decompression approach and technique included 249 patients [87]. The study ran from 2013 to 2018 and included 137 (55%) men and 112 (45%) women with an average age of 56.03±16.8 years with an average follow-up of 38.27±27.9 months. These patients had endoscopic decompression for symptomatic bony and soft tissue spinal stenosis. The primary clinical outcome measures were the Oswestry Disability Index (ODI) [90 - 92], Visual Analogue Scale (VAS) [88], and modified Macnab criteria [89]. This study's results were published in a special focus issue in the Journal of Spine Surgery [87]. The authors would recommend this chapter's readers to look for further information on this study in the provided reference. Briefly, the authors found the following frequency distribution of common spinal stenosis scenarios. Stratifying patients by the predominant anatomic location of the compression pathology, type I stenosis in the central spinal canal was seen in nearly half the study patients (121/249; 48.6%). Exclusive lateral recess stenosis (Type II) was observed in only 15 of 249 patients (6%). Foraminal stenosis (Type III) was the second-largest group of patients (104/249; 41.8%). Extraforaminal stenosis was the least common clinical finding, with 9/249 patients having this constellation of compressive pathology (3.6%). The transforaminal technique was used in 137 of the 249 study patients (55.0%) with type II to IV stenosis. The interlaminar method was employed in 78 of the 249 study patients (31.3%). The combination of these two techniques was applied in 12 of the 249 patients (4.8%). Type I central stenosis lesions were treated with an interlaminar approach in 8 of the 249 patients (3.2%). Clinical outcomes were Excellent (47;18.9%) and Good

(178;71.5%) in the vast majority of patients. Fair (18; 7.2%) and Poor (6;2.4%) outcome results occurred in a few patients. These findings suggest that the clinical application of this stenosis patient selection algorithm is useful for patient selection. This clinical series shows that this decision algorithm's application is suitable in selecting patients for the interlaminar approach and endoscopic decompression technique and its over-the-top variant. These findings were corroborated by the VAS analysis, where the paired two-tailed t-testing showed statistically significant average VAS reductions of 5.46±2.1 (P<0.0001). The ODI reductions were with 37.1±16.9 points, similarly significant (P<0.0001).

DISCUSSION

The over-the-top bilateral recess and foraminal decompression may have favorable clinical outcomes, particularly if patients with central stenosis are stratified for the procedure. Patient selection protocol focusing on determining the best endoscopic approach to asymptomatic stenotic processes in the lumbar spine is needed to maximize clinical outcomes with the endoscopic decompression procedure. The formalized preoperative decision-making algorithm discussed by the authors is suitable for selecting patients for the over-the-top procedure appropriately. Besides patient selection, the surgeon's skill level determines clinical outcomes with the chosen endoscopic decompression procedure. The choice of a preferred approach should be based on the preoperatively identified and validated pain generator. Its extent and location should be considered carefully with attention to detail in working up the painful pathoanatomy. At L5/S1, several anatomical limitations may restrict the utility of the transforaminal approach. Again, the over-the-top variation of the interlaminar approach may be the best solution in these particular scenarios.

CONCLUSION

Selecting the best approach may facilitate achieving the goals of this surgery. The over-the-top technique is a variation of the unilateral interlaminar approach, emphasizing bilateral lateral recess decompression and decompression of the central spinal canal. In skilled hands, clinical outcomes are favorable. Employing a patient stratification algorithm may aid in appropriate patient selection. Surgeon skill level is the most relevant factor in determining patient outcomes with the endoscopic procedure. Adequate training and mentorship alongside an experienced endoscopic spine surgeon is the most effective way to master the over-the-top endoscopic decompression procedure's steep learning curve. It should be considered an alternative to the transforaminal techniques whenever the patients' painful pathology is mainly located in the lateral recesses or central canal.

The over-the-top decompression should be considered at the L5/S1 level unless the patient has extraforaminal painful compressive pathology.

CONSENT FOR PUBLICATION

Not applicable.

CONFLICT OF INTEREST

The authors declare no conflict of interest, financial or otherwise.

ACKNOWLEDGEMENTS

Declared none.

REFERENCES

[1]   Love JG. Removal of the protruded interlaminar discs without laminectomy. Mayo Clin Proc 1939; 14.

[2]   Caspar W. A new surgical procedure for lumbar disc herniation causing less tissue damage through a microsurgical approach. Berlin, Heidelberg, Germany: Springer 1977; p. 7.
        [http://dx.doi.org/10.1007/978-3-642-66578-3_15]

[3]   Lumbar Disc Adult Hydrocephalus GYM. Advances in Neurosurgery. Berlin, Heidelberg, Germany: Springer 1977; pp. 81-1.

[4]   Lewis PJ, Weir BK, Broad RW, Grace MG. Long-term prospective study of lumbosacral discectomy. J Neurosurg 1987; 67(1): 49-53.
        [http://dx.doi.org/10.3171/jns.1987.67.1.0049] [PMID: 3598671]

[5]   Smith L. Enzyme Dissolution of the Nucleus Pulposus in Humans. JAMA 1964; 187(187): 137-40.
        [http://dx.doi.org/10.1001/jama.1964.03060150061016] [PMID: 14066733]

[6]   The classic. Enzyme dissolution of the nucleus pulposus in humans. By Lyman W. Smith. 1964. Clin Orthop Relat Res 1986; (206): 4-9.
        [PMID: 3519036]

[7]   Flanagan N, Smith L. Clinical studies of chemonucleolysis patients with ten- to twenty-year follow-up evaluation. Clin Orthop Relat Res 1986; 206(&NA;): 15-7.
        [http://dx.doi.org/10.1097/00003086-198605000-00004] [PMID: 3708968]

[8]   Mansfield F, Polivy K, Boyd R, Huddleston J. Long-term results of chymopapain injections. Clin Orthop Relat Res 1986; (206): 67-9.
        [PMID: 3708994]

[9]   Kambin P, Sampson S. Posterolateral percutaneous suction-excision of herniated lumbar intervertebral discs. Report of interim results. Clin Orthop Relat Res 1986; (207): 37-43.
        [PMID: 3720102]

[10]   Kambin P, Brager MD. Percutaneous posterolateral discectomy. Anatomy and mechanism. Clin Orthop Relat Res 1987; (223): 145-54.
        [PMID: 3652568]

[11]   Kambin P. Percutaneous lumbar diskectomy JAMA 1989; 262: 1776.

[12]   Kambin P, Schaffer JL. Percutaneous lumbar discectomy. Review of 100 patients and current practice. Clin Orthop Relat Res 1989; 238: 24-34.

[http://dx.doi.org/10.1097/00003086-198901000-00004] [PMID: 2910608]

[13] Schreiber A, Suezawa Y, Leu H. Does percutaneous nucleotomy with discoscopy replace conventional discectomy? Eight years of experience and results in treatment of herniated lumbar disc. Clin Orthop Relat Res 1989; 238: 35-42.
[http://dx.doi.org/10.1097/00003086-198901000-00005] [PMID: 2910617]

[14] Leu H, Schreiber A. [Percutaneous nucleotomy with disk endoscopy--a minimally invasive therapy in non-sequestrated intervertebral disk hernia]. Schweiz Rundsch Med Prax 1991; 80(14): 364-8. [Percutaneous nucleotomy with disk endoscopy--a minimally invasive therapy in non-sequestrated intervertebral disk hernia].
[PMID: 2034933]

[15] Leu H, Schreiber A. [Endoscopy of the spine: minimally invasive therapy]. Orthopade 1992; 21(4): 267-72. [Endoscopy of the spine: minimally invasive therapy].
[PMID: 1408118]

[16] Yeung AT. The evolution of percutaneous spinal endoscopy and discectomy: state of the art. Mt Sinai J Med 2000; 67(4): 327-32.
[PMID: 11021785]

[17] Yeung AT. Minimally Invasive Disc Surgery with the Yeung Endoscopic Spine System (YESS). Surg Technol Int 1999; 8(8): 267-77.
[PMID: 12451541]

[18] Mathews HH. Transforaminal endoscopic microdiscectomy. Neurosurg Clin N Am 1996; 7(1): 59-63.
[http://dx.doi.org/10.1016/S1042-3680(18)30405-4] [PMID: 8835146]

[19] Mathews ES, Scrivani SJ. Percutaneous stereotactic radiofrequency thermal rhizotomy for the treatment of trigeminal neuralgia. Mt Sinai J Med 2000; 67(4): 288-99.
[PMID: 11021779]

[20] Yeung A, Kotheeranurak V. Transforaminal Endoscopic Decompression of the Lumbar Spine for Stable Isthmic Spondylolisthesis as the Least Invasive Surgical Treatment Using the YESS Surgery Technique. Int J Spine Surg 2018; 12(3): 408-14.
[http://dx.doi.org/10.14444/5048] [PMID: 30276099]

[21] Ruetten S, Komp M, Merk H, Godolias G. Recurrent lumbar disc herniation after conventional discectomy: a prospective, randomized study comparing full-endoscopic interlaminar and transforaminal *versus* microsurgical revision. J Spinal Disord Tech 2009; 22(2): 122-9.
[http://dx.doi.org/10.1097/BSD.0b013e318175ddb4] [PMID: 19342934]

[22] Ruetten S, Komp M, Merk H, Godolias G. Surgical treatment for lumbar lateral recess stenosis with the full-endoscopic interlaminar approach *versus* conventional microsurgical technique: a prospective, randomized, controlled study. J Neurosurg Spine 2009; 10(5): 476-85.
[http://dx.doi.org/10.3171/2008.7.17634] [PMID: 19442011]

[23] Ruetten S, Komp M, Merk H, Godolias G. Full-endoscopic interlaminar and transforaminal lumbar discectomy *versus* conventional microsurgical technique: a prospective, randomized, controlled study. Spine 2008; 33(9): 931-9.
[http://dx.doi.org/10.1097/BRS.0b013e31816c8af7] [PMID: 18427312]

[24] Ruetten S, Komp M, Merk H, Godolias G. Use of newly developed instruments and endoscopes: full-endoscopic resection of lumbar disc herniations *via* the interlaminar and lateral transforaminal approach. J Neurosurg Spine 2007; 6(6): 521-30.
[http://dx.doi.org/10.3171/spi.2007.6.6.2] [PMID: 17561740]

[25] Ruetten S, Komp M, Godolias G. A New full-endoscopic technique for the interlaminar operation of lumbar disc herniations using 6-mm endoscopes: prospective 2-year results of 331 patients. Minim Invasive Neurosurg 2006; 49(2): 80-7.
[http://dx.doi.org/10.1055/s-2006-932172] [PMID: 16708336]

[26] Onik G, Helms CA, Ginsberg L, Hoaglund FT, Morris J. Percutaneous lumbar diskectomy using a new aspiration probe: porcine and cadaver model. Radiology 1985; 155(1): 251-2.
[http://dx.doi.org/10.1148/radiology.155.1.3975407] [PMID: 3975407]

[27] Onik GM, Kambin P, Chang MK. Minimally invasive disc surgery. Nucleotomy *versus* fragmentectomy. Spine 1997; 22(7): 827-8.
[http://dx.doi.org/10.1097/00007632-199704010-00024] [PMID: 9106327]

[28] Kambin P, Nixon JE, Chait A, Schaffer JL. Annular protrusion: pathophysiology and roentgenographic appearance. Spine 1988; 13(6): 671-5.
[http://dx.doi.org/10.1097/00007632-198813060-00013] [PMID: 2972071]

[29] Kim HS, Raorane HD, Wu PH, Yi YJ, Jang IT. Evolution of endoscopic transforaminal lumbar approach for degenerative lumbar disease. J Spine Surg 2020; 6(2): 424-37.
[http://dx.doi.org/10.21037/jss.2019.11.05] [PMID: 32656380]

[30] Kambin P. Arthroscopic microdiskectomy. Mt Sinai J Med 1991; 58(2): 159-64.
[PMID: 1857361]

[31] Kambin P, Schaffer JL. A multicenter analysis of percutaneous discectomy. Spine 1991; 16(7): 854-5.
[http://dx.doi.org/10.1097/00007632-199107000-00031] [PMID: 1925764]

[32] Schaffer JL, Kambin P. Percutaneous posterolateral lumbar discectomy and decompression with a 6.9-millimeter cannula. Analysis of operative failures and complications. J Bone Joint Surg Am 1991; 73(6): 822-31.
[http://dx.doi.org/10.2106/00004623-199173060-00005] [PMID: 1830052]

[33] Mirkovic SR, Schwartz DG, Glazier KD. Anatomic considerations in lumbar posterolateral percutaneous procedures. Spine 1995; 20(18): 1965-71.
[http://dx.doi.org/10.1097/00007632-199509150-00001] [PMID: 8578369]

[34] Foley KT, Smith MM, Rampersaud YR. Microendoscopic approach to far-lateral lumbar disc herniation Neurosurg Focus 1999; 7: e5.
[http://dx.doi.org/10.3171/foc.1999.7.6.6]

[35] Perez-Cruet MJ, Foley KT, Isaacs RE, *et al.* Microendoscopic lumbar discectomy: technical note. Neurosurgery 2002; 51(5) (Suppl.): S129-36.
[PMID: 12234440]

[36] Destandau J. A special device for endoscopic surgery of lumbar disc herniation. Neurol Res 1999; 21(1): 39-42.
[http://dx.doi.org/10.1080/01616412.1999.11740889] [PMID: 10048052]

[37] Hoogland T, Scheckenbach C. [Percutaneous lumbar nucleotomy with low-dose chymopapain, an ambulatory procedure]. Z Orthop Ihre Grenzgeb 1995; 133(2): 106-13.
[http://dx.doi.org/10.1055/s-2008-1039420] [PMID: 7754655]

[38] Hoogland T, Scheckenbach C. Low-dose chemonucleolysis combined with percutaneous nucleotomy in herniated cervical disks. J Spinal Disord 1995; 8(3): 228-32.
[http://dx.doi.org/10.1097/00002517-199506000-00009] [PMID: 7670215]

[39] Hoogland T. Percutaneous endoscopic discectomy. J Neurosurg 1993; 79(6): 967-8.
[PMID: 8246070]

[40] Choi G, Lee SH, Raiturker PP, Lee S, Chae YS. Percutaneous endoscopic interlaminar discectomy for intracanalicular disc herniations at L5-S1 using a rigid working channel endoscope. Neurosurgery 2006; 58(1) (Suppl.): ONS59-68.
[http://dx.doi.org/10.1227/01.NEU.0000362000.35742.3D] [PMID: 16479630]

[41] Yeung AT, Yeung CA. *In-vivo* endoscopic visualization of patho-anatomy in painful degenerative conditions of the lumbar spine. Surg Technol Int 2006; 15(15): 243-56.
[PMID: 17029183]

[42] Yeung AT. The Evolution and Advancement of Endoscopic Foraminal Surgery: One Surgeon's Experience Incorporating Adjunctive Techologies. SAS J 2007; 1(3): 108-17.
[http://dx.doi.org/10.1016/S1935-9810(07)70055-5] [PMID: 25802587]

[43] Tsou PM, Alan Yeung C, Yeung AT. Posterolateral transforaminal selective endoscopic discectomy and thermal annuloplasty for chronic lumbar discogenic pain: a minimal access visualized intradiscal surgical procedure. Spine J 2004; 4(5): 564-73.
[http://dx.doi.org/10.1016/j.spinee.2004.01.014] [PMID: 15363430]

[44] Yeung AT, Gore S. *In-vivo* Endoscopic Visualization of Patho-anatomy in Symptomatic Degenerative Conditions of the Lumbar Spine II: Intradiscal, Foraminal, and Central Canal Decompression. Surg Technol Int 2011; 21(21): 299-319.
[PMID: 22505004]

[45] Gore S, Yeung A. The "inside out" transforaminal technique to treat lumbar spinal pain in an awake and aware patient under local anesthesia: results and a review of the literature. Int J Spine Surg 2014; 8
[http://dx.doi.org/10.14444/1028]

[46] Yeung A, Lewandrowski KU. Early and staged endoscopic management of common pain generators in the spine. J Spine Surg 2020; 6(6) (Suppl. 1): S1-5.
[http://dx.doi.org/10.21037/jss.2019.09.03] [PMID: 32195407]

[47] Yeung AT, Yeung CA. Advances in endoscopic disc and spine surgery: foraminal approach. Surg Technol Int 2003; 11(11): 255-63.
[PMID: 12931309]

[48] Ruetten S, Komp M, Godolias G. An extreme lateral access for the surgery of lumbar disc herniations inside the spinal canal using the full-endoscopic uniportal transforaminal approach-technique and prospective results of 463 patients. Spine 2005; 30(22): 2570-8.
[http://dx.doi.org/10.1097/01.brs.0000186327.21435.cc] [PMID: 16284597]

[49] Hoogland T, van den Brekel-Dijkstra K, Schubert M, Miklitz B. Endoscopic transforaminal discectomy for recurrent lumbar disc herniation: a prospective, cohort evaluation of 262 consecutive cases. Spine 2008; 33(9): 973-8.
[http://dx.doi.org/10.1097/BRS.0b013e31816c8ade] [PMID: 18427318]

[50] Schubert M, Hoogland T. Endoscopic transforaminal nucleotomy with foraminoplasty for lumbar disk herniation. Oper Orthop Traumatol 2005; 17(6): 641-61.
[http://dx.doi.org/10.1007/s00064-005-1156-9] [PMID: 16369758]

[51] Hoogland T, Schubert M, Miklitz B, Ramirez A. Transforaminal posterolateral endoscopic discectomy with or without the combination of a low-dose chymopapain: a prospective randomized study in 280 consecutive cases. Spine 2006; 31(24): E890-7.
[http://dx.doi.org/10.1097/01.brs.0000245955.22358.3a] [PMID: 17108817]

[52] Ruetten S, Komp M, Merk H, Godolias G. Full-endoscopic cervical posterior foraminotomy for the operation of lateral disc herniations using 5.9-mm endoscopes: a prospective, randomized, controlled study. Spine 2008; 33(9): 940-8.
[http://dx.doi.org/10.1097/BRS.0b013e31816c8b67] [PMID: 18427313]

[53] Lee S, Kim SK, Lee SH, *et al.* Percutaneous endoscopic lumbar discectomy for migrated disc herniation: classification of disc migration and surgical approaches. Eur Spine J 2007; 16(3): 431-7.
[http://dx.doi.org/10.1007/s00586-006-0219-4] [PMID: 16972067]

[54] Choi G, Prada N, Modi HN, Vasavada NB, Kim JS, Lee SH. Percutaneous endoscopic lumbar herniectomy for high-grade down-migrated L4-L5 disc through an L5-S1 interlaminar approach: a technical note. Minim Invasive Neurosurg 2010; 53(3): 147-52.
[http://dx.doi.org/10.1055/s-0030-1254145] [PMID: 20809458]

[55] de Carvalho PST, Ramos MRF, da Silva Meireles AC, *et al.* Feasibility of Using Intraoperative Neuromonitoring in the Prophylaxis of Dysesthesia in Transforaminal Endoscopic Discectomies of the

Lumbar Spine Brain Sci 2020.
[http://dx.doi.org/10.3390/brainsci10080522]

[56]   Cho JY, Lee SH, Lee HY. Prevention of development of postoperative dysesthesia in transforaminal percutaneous endoscopic lumbar discectomy for intracanalicular lumbar disc herniation: floating retraction technique. Minim Invasive Neurosurg 2011; 54(5-6): 214-8.
[http://dx.doi.org/10.1055/s-0031-1287774] [PMID: 22287030]

[57]   Lewandrowski KU, Dowling A, Calderaro AL, *et al.* Dysesthesia due to irritation of the dorsal root ganglion following lumbar transforaminal endoscopy: Analysis of frequency and contributing factors. Clin Neurol Neurosurg 2020; 197: 106073.
[http://dx.doi.org/10.1016/j.clineuro.2020.106073]

[58]   Lu H, Zhao F, Cao J, *et al.* Zhongguo Xiu Fu Chong Jian Wai Ke Za Zhi 2013; 2012(26): 1420-4. [Spinal canal decompression with microendoscopic disectomy and pillar vertebral space insertion for thoracolumbar neglected fracture].

[59]   Ishimoto Y, Yamada H, Curtis E, *et al.* Spinal Endoscopy for Delayed-Onset Lumbar Radiculopathy Resulting from Foraminal Stenosis after Osteoporotic Vertebral Fracture: A Case Report of a New Surgical Strategy Case Rep Orthop 2018; 2018: 1593021.
[http://dx.doi.org/10.1155/2018/1593021]

[60]   Ruetten S, Komp M, Merk H, Godolias G. Full-endoscopic anterior decompression *versus* conventional anterior decompression and fusion in cervical disc herniations. Int Orthop 2009; 33(6): 1677-82.
[http://dx.doi.org/10.1007/s00264-008-0684-y] [PMID: 19015851]

[61]   Wasinpongwanich K, Pongpirul K, Lwin KMM, Kesornsak W, Kuansongtham V, Ruetten S. Full-Endoscopic Interlaminar Lumbar Discectomy: Retrospective Review of Clinical Results and Complications in 545 International Patients. World Neurosurg 2019; 132: e922-8.
[http://dx.doi.org/10.1016/j.wneu.2019.07.101] [PMID: 31326641]

[62]   Markovic M, Zivkovic N, Spaic M, *et al.* Full-endoscopic interlaminar operations in lumbar compressive lesions surgery: prospective study of 350 patients. "Endos" study. J Neurosurg Sci 2016; •••: 2016.
[PMID: 27362665]

[63]   Ruetten S. Full-endoscopic Operations of the Spine in Disk Herniations and Spinal Stenosis. Surg Technol Int 2011; 21(21): 284-98.
[PMID: 22505003]

[64]   Ruetten S, Hahn P, Oezdemir S, *et al.* Full-endoscopic Uniportal Odontoidectomy and Decompression of the Anterior Cervicomedullary Junction Using the Retropharyngeal Approach. Spine 2018; 43(15): E911-8.
[http://dx.doi.org/10.1097/BRS.0000000000002561] [PMID: 29438218]

[65]   Ruetten S, Hahn P, Oezdemir S, Baraliakos X, Godolias G, Komp M. Full-endoscopic uniportal retropharyngeal odontoidectomy for anterior craniocervical infection. Minim Invasive Ther Allied Technol 2019; 28(3): 178-85.
[http://dx.doi.org/10.1080/13645706.2018.1498357] [PMID: 30179052]

[66]   Lee CH, Choi M, Ryu DS, *et al.* Efficacy and Safety of Full-endoscopic Decompression *via* Interlaminar Approach for Central or Lateral Recess Spinal Stenosis of the Lumbar Spine: A Meta-analysis. Spine 2018; 43(24): 1756-64.
[http://dx.doi.org/10.1097/BRS.0000000000002708] [PMID: 29794584]

[67]   Kim CH, Chung CK, Jahng TA, Yang HJ, Son YJ. Surgical outcome of percutaneous endoscopic interlaminar lumbar diskectomy for recurrent disk herniation after open diskectomy. J Spinal Disord Tech 2012; 25(5): E125-33.
[http://dx.doi.org/10.1097/BSD.0b013e31825bd111] [PMID: 22744610]

[68]   Hwang JH, Park WM, Park CW. Contralateral Interlaminar Keyhole Percutaneous Endoscopic

Lumbar Surgery in Patients with Unilateral Radiculopathy. World Neurosurg 2017; 101(101): 33-41.
[http://dx.doi.org/10.1016/j.wneu.2017.01.079] [PMID: 28153626]

[69]   Song H, Hu W, Liu Z, *et al.* Percutaneous endoscopic interlaminar discectomy of L5-S1 disc herniation: a comparison between intermittent endoscopy technique and full endoscopy technique. J Orthop Surg Res 2017; 12: 162.
[http://dx.doi.org/10.1186/s13018-017-0662-4]

[70]   Palliyil NS, Shah S, Rai RR, Dalvie S, Monteiro J. Age - Does it really count? A study of the Perioperative Morbidity and Long-Term Outcome in Patients Above 70 Years of Age Undergoing Spine surgery for Lumbar Degenerative Disorders. Rev Bras Ortop 2020; 55(3): 298-303.
[http://dx.doi.org/10.1055/s-0039-1700833] [PMID: 32616974]

[71]   Costa F, Alves OL, Anania CD, *et al.* Decompressive Surgery for Lumbar Spinal Stenosis: WFNS Spine Committee Recommendations. World Neurosurg X 2020; 7: 100076.
[http://dx.doi.org/10.1016/j.wnsx.2020.100076]

[72]   Ponkilainen VT, Huttunen TT, Neva MH, *et al.* National trends in lumbar spine decompression and fusion surgery in Finland, 1997-2018. Acta Orthop 2020; 2020: 1-5.
[http://dx.doi.org/10.1080/17453674.2020.1839244] [PMID: 33106074]

[73]   Amitkumar M, Singh PK, Singh KJ, *et al.* Surgical Outcome in Spinal Operation in Patients Aged 70 Years and Above. Neurol India 2020; 68(1): 45-51.
[http://dx.doi.org/10.4103/0028-3886.279672] [PMID: 32129242]

[74]   Pearson AM, Blood EA, Frymoyer JW, *et al.* SPORT lumbar intervertebral disk herniation and back pain: does treatment, location, or morphology matter? Spine 2008; 33(4): 428-35.
[http://dx.doi.org/10.1097/BRS.0b013e31816469de] [PMID: 18277876]

[75]   Weinstein JN, Tosteson AN, Tosteson TD, *et al.* The SPORT value compass: do the extra costs of undergoing spine surgery produce better health benefits? Med Care 2014; 52(12): 1055-63.
[http://dx.doi.org/10.1097/MLR.0000000000000250] [PMID: 25334052]

[76]   Weinstein JN, Lurie JD, Tosteson TD, *et al.* Surgical compared with nonoperative treatment for lumbar degenerative spondylolisthesis. four-year results in the Spine Patient Outcomes Research Trial (SPORT) randomized and observational cohorts. J Bone Joint Surg Am 2009; 91(6): 1295-304.
[http://dx.doi.org/10.2106/JBJS.H.00913] [PMID: 19487505]

[77]   Weinstein JN, Lurie JD, Tosteson TD, *et al.* Surgical *versus* nonoperative treatment for lumbar disc herniation: four-year results for the Spine Patient Outcomes Research Trial (SPORT). Spine 2008; 33(25): 2789-800.
[http://dx.doi.org/10.1097/BRS.0b013e31818ed8f4] [PMID: 19018250]

[78]   Weinstein JN, Lurie JD, Tosteson TD, *et al.* Surgical *vs* nonoperative treatment for lumbar disk herniation: the Spine Patient Outcomes Research Trial (SPORT) observational cohort. JAMA 2006; 296(20): 2451-9.
[http://dx.doi.org/10.1001/jama.296.20.2451] [PMID: 17119141]

[79]   Pearson A, Lurie J, Tosteson T, Zhao W, Abdu W, Weinstein JN. Who should have surgery for spinal stenosis? Treatment effect predictors in SPORT. Spine 2012; 37(21): 1791-802.
[http://dx.doi.org/10.1097/BRS.0b013e3182634b04] [PMID: 23018805]

[80]   McAfee PC, DeVine JG, Chaput CD, *et al.* The indications for interbody fusion cages in the treatment of spondylolisthesis: analysis of 120 cases. Spine 2005; 30(6) (Suppl.): S60-5.
[http://dx.doi.org/10.1097/01.brs.0000155578.62680.dd] [PMID: 15767888]

[81]   Rouben D, Casnellie M, Ferguson M. Long-term durability of minimal invasive posterior transforaminal lumbar interbody fusion: a clinical and radiographic follow-up. J Spinal Disord Tech 2011; 24(5): 288-96.
[http://dx.doi.org/10.1097/BSD.0b013e3181f9a60a] [PMID: 20975594]

[82]   Kim CW, Doerr TM, Luna IY, *et al.* Minimally Invasive Transforaminal Lumbar Interbody Fusion

Using Expandable Technology: A Clinical and Radiographic Analysis of 50 Patients. World Neurosurg 2016; 90(90): 228-35.
[http://dx.doi.org/10.1016/j.wneu.2016.02.075] [PMID: 26921700]

[83] Försth P, Ólafsson G, Carlsson T, *et al.* A Randomized, Controlled Trial of Fusion Surgery for Lumbar Spinal Stenosis. N Engl J Med 2016; 374(15): 1413-23.
[http://dx.doi.org/10.1056/NEJMoa1513721] [PMID: 27074066]

[84] Qiao G, Feng M, Wang X, *et al.* Revision for Endoscopic Diskectomy: Is Lateral Lumbar Interbody Fusion an Option? World Neurosurg 2020; 133(133): e26-30.
[http://dx.doi.org/10.1016/j.wneu.2019.07.226] [PMID: 31398523]

[85] O'Donnell JA, Anderson JT, Haas AR, *et al.* Treatment of Recurrent Lumbar Disc Herniation With or Without Fusion in Workers' Compensation Subjects. Spine 2017; 42(14): E864-70.
[http://dx.doi.org/10.1097/BRS.0000000000002057] [PMID: 28700387]

[86] Kim JE, Yoo HS, Choi DJ, Park EJ, Jee SM. Comparison of Minimal Invasive *Versus* Biportal Endoscopic Transforaminal Lumbar Interbody Fusion for Single-level Lumbar Disease. Clin Spine Surg 2021; 34(2): E64-71.
[http://dx.doi.org/10.1097/BSD.0000000000001024] [PMID: 33633061]

[87] Dowling Á, Lewandrowski KU, da Silva FHP, Parra JAA, Portillo DM, Giménez YCP. Patient selection protocols for endoscopic transforaminal, interlaminar, and translaminar decompression of lumbar spinal stenosis. J Spine Surg 2020; 6(6) (Suppl. 1): S120-32.
[http://dx.doi.org/10.21037/jss.2019.11.07] [PMID: 32195421]

[88] Reed CC, Wolf WA, Cotton CC, Dellon ES. A visual analogue scale and a Likert scale are simple and responsive tools for assessing dysphagia in eosinophilic oesophagitis. Aliment Pharmacol Ther 2017; 45(11): 1443-8.
[http://dx.doi.org/10.1111/apt.14061] [PMID: 28370355]

[89] Macnab I. Negative disc exploration. An analysis of the causes of nerve-root involvement in sixty-eight patients. J Bone Joint Surg Am 1971; 53(5): 891-903.
[http://dx.doi.org/10.2106/00004623-197153050-00004] [PMID: 4326746]

[90] van Hooff ML, Spruit M, Fairbank JC, van Limbeek J, Jacobs WC. The Oswestry Disability Index (version 2.1a): validation of a Dutch language version. Spine (Phila Pa 1976) 2015; 40(2): E83-90.
[http://dx.doi.org/10.1097/BRS.0000000000000683] [PMID: 25575092]

[91] Fairbank JC, Pynsent PB. The Oswestry Disability Index. Spine (Phila Pa 1976) 2000; 25(22): 2940-52.
[http://dx.doi.org/10.1097/00007632-200011150-00017] [PMID: 11074683]

[92] Fairbank J. Use of Oswestry Disability Index (ODI). Spine (Phila Pa 1976) 1995; 20(13): 1535-7.
[http://dx.doi.org/10.1097/00007632-199507000-00020] [PMID: 8623078]

CHAPTER 10

Endoscopic Treatment of Lumbar Facet Cysts

Stefan Hellinger[1,*] and **Kai-Uwe Lewandrowski**[2,3,4]

[1] *Department of Orthopedic and Spine Surgery, Arabellaklinik, Munich, Germany*

[2] *Center for Advanced Spine Care of Southern Arizona and Surgical Institute of Tucson, Tucson AZ, USA*

[3] *Associate Professor of Orthopaedic Surgery, Universidad Colsanitas, Bogota, Colombia, USA*

[4] *Visiting Professor, Department Orthopaedic Surgery, UNIRIO, Rio de Janeiro, Brazil*

Abstract: Cysts associated with degeneration of the lumbar facet joints are commonly encountered during routine lumbar endoscopy. They can be difficult to dissect and may heighten the risk of nerve root injury when they are fibrotically attached. Many of these cysts are extradural. Because of their highly inflammatory nature, they may be associated with radicular symptoms even without associated mechanical compression of the traversing or exiting nerve root of the symptomatic surgical level. These synovial cysts may be acutely painful. Their related symptoms may be difficult to distinguish from those caused by lumbar disc herniation or stenosis in the lateral spinal canal on clinical examination. The endoscopic spine surgeon is often forced to deal with them to complete the neural element decompression. What is less clear is what to do with patients with sizeable isolated facet joint based cysts without much other clinical pathology. The surgical indications and prognosticators of favorable clinical outcomes with endoscopic surgery are less well understood. Therefore, the authors performed a systematic analysis of their clinical series of patients they identified to have had synovial cysts either on preoperative advanced imaging studies or on those they found serendipitously during routine lumbar endoscopy. In total, 48 were identified in whom removal of the extradural cyst was performed during routine transforaminal and interlaminar endoscopy. The primary indication for surgery in these patients was painful foraminal and lateral recess stenosis. The patients were divided into 26 females and 22 males. The L4/5 level was the most frequent site of facet based cysts. It was found in 26 patients (72.2%). The second most common site was the L5/S1 level in 8 patients (22.2%), followed by two patients (5.6%) at the L3/4 level. A single patient had endoscopic decompression at the T9/10 level. Outcome analysis showed clinical improvements in all patients. According to the modified Macnab criteria, 19/48 (39.6%) patients had excellent outcomes. Good and fair results were achieved in 18/48 (37.5%) and 11/48 (22.9%) patients, respectively. The observed VAS leg pain score reductions were substantial and statistically significant ($p < 0.000$) from preoperative 8.06 ± 1.57 to postoperative 1.92 ± 1.49, and 1.77 ± 1.32 at final follow-up. One patient had a recurrent disc herniation, and another patient did not improve. Two patients

---

* **Corresponding author Stefan Hellinger:** Department of Orthopedic and Spine Surgery, Arabellaklinik, Munich, Germany; Tel: +4989264076; E-mail: hellinger@gmx.de

Kai-Uwe Lewandrowski, Jorge Felipe Ramírez León, Anthony Yeung, Hyeun-Sung Kim, Xifeng Zhang, Gun Choi, Stefan Hellinger and Álvaro Dowling (Eds.)

underwent fusion during the follow-up period. Patients with Fair outcomes had a statistically significant association (p < 0.001) with facet instability as suggested by axial T2-weighted MRI imaging findings of thickened ligamentum flavum, facet joint hypertrophy, and a bright white fluid-filled joint gap of > 2 mm. Endoscopic resection of extradural spinal cysts that nearly exclusively stem from degenerated lumbar facet joints in skilled hands is feasible. Instability was one of the prognosticators of Fair Macnab outcomes.

Keywords: Endoscopic decompression, Extradural cysts, Lumbar foraminal stenosis.

INTRODUCTION

Facet cysts are often encountered during routine lumbar endoscopy. These extradural cysts may cause raging sciatica-type back and leg pain since they are often highly inflammatory. Although they are less commonly problematic than a herniated disc or a stenotic process in the foramen or the lateral recess, the radiculopathy is often a result of inflammation of the dorsal root ganglion, tethering or scarring of the traversing or exiting nerve root. Therefore, symptoms may be seemingly out of proportion with the mechanical compression seen on the preoperative MRI scan [1 - 3]. One should consider synovial extradural cyst in the differential diagnosis, mainly if the patient's symptoms cannot be explained due to the absence of corresponding compressive pathology on the preoperative MRI scan. It is not uncommon to encounter a pain syndrome in the patient's presentation that on physical examination may be impossible to differentiate from those caused by lumbar disc herniation or stenosis in the lateral spinal canal. One of the patient's history elements that should elevate the surgeon's suspicion for the presence of a facet cyst is very painful radiculopathy without neurogenic claudication [4 - 9]. Therefore, a painful facet cyst diagnosis is based on a thorough history and physical examination and corroborating advanced magnetic resonance imaging (MRI), whose sensitivity has been reported as high as 90% compared to 70% of computed tomography (CT) scan [10 - 13].

ETIOLOGY

The etiology and natural history of cysts are unclear [13 - 15]. Acute trauma and repetitive micro-trauma are thought to have causative roles in the formation of cysts. Juxtafacet cysts occur most frequently at the L4-5, which is the most mobile lumbar segment. Cysts are positively associated with facet osteoarthritis, disc degeneration, and degenerative spondylolisthesis. Most cysts probably occur due to interaction between abnormal motion and progressive degenerative process at the facet joint. Lumbar juxtafacet cysts originate from degenerated facet joints or ligamentum flavum as part of a generalized segmental degenerative process.

Radicular symptoms can occur due to the exiting or traversing spinal nerve's irritation by the juxtafacet cyst, often in association with a protruding disc. When synovial cysts are seen, the presence of facet arthrosis may or may not be evident on X-ray or MRI but maybe visualized endoscopically. Some synovial cysts are located at the lateral recess and incidentally visualized by the spine endoscope. Lumbar juxtafacet cysts are extradural cysts of the spine originating from the degenerated facet joint (synovial cyst) or myxomatous degeneration of ligamentum flavum (ganglion cyst). Juxtafacet cysts with features of both synovial and ganglion cysts have been described. Calcification of cyst lining and hemosiderin deposits within the cyst has been seen histologically.

CLINICAL COURSE

Clinically, juxtafacet cysts can contribute to radicular as well as low back pain. Radicular pain occurs when the spinal nerve becomes inflamed due to chronic compression by the cyst. Although the cyst may be the significant compressive structure upon the nerve, significant contributions can come from co-existing annular tears, herniated disc, vertebral osteophyte, and foraminal stenosis. Radicular pain, radiculopathy (reflex, motor, and sensory changes), and neurogenic claudication patterns are dependent upon the size, shape, and location of the cyst to the spinal nerve. These findings are influenced by the fixed shape and size of the spinal canal within which the cyst and the nerve reside. Cysts can change in size, and this may explain clinical fluctuations. The juxtafacet cyst itself is generally not the cause of chronic low back pain. However, the cyst is usually associated with degenerated and hypermobile facets and disc, which can be the source(s) of pain. Excessive repetitive loading upon the facet/disc exceeding their mechanical strength and reparative ability result in capsular and annular strain/tears. Microscopic injury activates mediators of the inflammatory process and pain. The cyst is a marker of progressive motion segment deterioration involving the corresponding facet and the disc.

DIFFERENTIAL DIAGNOSIS

The differential diagnosis of facet cysts - which are also commonly called synovial or ganglion cysts [13] - consists of extradural arachnoid cysts [14, 15], perineural (Tarlov) cysts [16, 17], dermoid cysts [18, 19], neurofibroma with cystic degeneration [20]. Juxtafacet cysts are quite uncommon causes of radiculopathy, low back pain, and neurogenic claudication and are often associated with advanced spinal degenerative disease. Facet-based synovial cysts are by far the most common intraspinal cysts that are histologically distinct from the other types of cysts and have been deemed to be associated with instability of the degenerated lumbar spinal motion segment (Table 1).

Table 1. Comparison of etiology, clinical, and histological of synovial- *versus* ganglion cyst.

Feature	Synovial Cyst	Ganglion Cyst
MRI Appearance		
Histology	• Synovia of degenerated intervertebral facet joints	• Myxoid degeneration of the periarticular fibrous tissue
Fluid	• Clear fluid secreted by synovial cells	• Mucous fluid with collagenous capsule
Relationship to Joint	• Direct connection to the intervertebral joint space	• No connection to the joint space
Clinical Course	• Changing symptoms with changing size	• Increasing symptoms with increasing size

This deduction was made because facet cysts are most commonly found in the single-most mobile lumbar motion segment - L4/5 [13, 21, 22]. Patients often report acute episodes of sudden onset of severe pain. A chronic course is also common with long asymptomatic periods, with the overall clinical course being benign and at times self-limiting. Repeated flareups eventually prompt treatment.

NON-OPERATIVE CARE

The majority of facet cysts improve with supportive medical care and do not require surgical treatment. Initial nonoperative management of acute radicular pain in the absence of significant and progressive neurologic deficits can include rest, medications, physical therapy, facet injection, and selective spinal nerve injection. These synovial facet joint cysts may respond well to nonsteroidal anti-inflammatories (NSAIDs) and transforaminal epidural steroid injections (TESI). Opioids are usually not necessary, and if demanded by the patient, should only be prescribed for a short course. Patients should be told to maintain a light walking schedule, physical therapy (PT) with emphasis on core-strengthening exercises, and modification of their daily activities for at least six weeks to see the natural history of symptomatic lumbar synovial facet cysts playing out, which most of the time ends up in spontaneous resolution. If patients do not improve with these supportive care measures, should surgical treatment be considered once other possible causes for the patient's symptoms have been excluded? Surgical procedures are 1) image-guided percutaneous steroid injection and rupture procedures, and 2) laminectomy, facetectomy, and excision of the visualized cyst.

Specifically, instability-related pain, an infectious or undiagnosed inflammatory (rheumatoid arthritis, ankylosing spondylitis, or gout), or a tumorous process should be ruled out.

INTERVENTIONAL PROCEDURES

Image-guided percutaneous steroid injection into the cyst is a palliative procedure with short-term and inconsistent efficacy; its morbidity is low, but multiple injections are often required. Steroid injection/cyst rupture technique has been more effective than steroid injection alone, but the results are inferior to endoscopic surgical cyst excision. Injection techniques target only the cyst and do not address the frequently co-existing compressive lesions, including disc herniation, vertebral marginal osteophytes, hypertrophied facets), all of which can contribute to radiculopathy. Some authors have proposed a CT-guided needle aspiration or an injection into the affected facet joint complex and its associated cyst [23, 24]. Despite successful intraarticular needle placement confirmed on CT scan, symptom relief after needle aspiration of the facet cyst content is not reliable [24]. While patients may report immediate pain relief from the injection of a local anesthetic, the question of whether long-term pain relief can be attributed to the intra-articular aspiration remains controversial, particularly given that the overall clinical course is benign and symptoms resolve spontaneously [23]. In the chapter, the authors propose endoscopic treatment of lumbar facet cysts. They explain their surgical protocol in detail and analyze the clinical outcomes.

SURGICAL TREATMENT

Failed conservative care or rapid onset of the severe neurological deficit with severe pain [3, 8, 27, 28]. Open excision of juxtafacet cyst is highly effective in decompressing and removing the cyst. Open technique, however, is more destructive to soft-tissues (paraspinal muscles, ligaments, facet capsule) and bone (lamina, facet) structures not contributing to nerve impingement. Complications include dural tear, seroma, hematoma, deep infection, and acute/ late instability requiring immediate/delayed fusion is well documented. While open approaches may be effective, the transforaminal approach has less surgical morbidity.

ENDOSCOPIC MANAGEMENT

An alternative to injection and open procedures is decompression of the juxtafacet cysts utilizing an established endoscopic technique for the spine with mechanical, RF, and laser ablation. Endoscopic surgery has become a recognized minimally invasive standard for ablation, decompression, repair, release and shrinkage of a variety of abnormal structures in virtually all joints. Endoscopic decompression of intraarticular cysts in the shoulder, knee, and ankle have been reported.

Endoscopic assessment of joints is complementary with MRI and other imaging studies and at times can detect abnormalities undetected with these studies. Therapeutic endoscopic procedure can immediately follow diagnostic evaluation. The choice of endoscopic approach may be dictated by the size and localization of the synovial facet cyst and its relationship to the neural elements. Often, synovial cysts are multi-loculated and may repeatedly fill and leak onto the neural elements. A highly inflammatory cyst adherent to the neural elements should be expected at the time of surgery, thus increasing the risk of surgical dissection. Typically, they are encountered in the axilla between the exiting and traversing nerve root. Many cysts emanate from the tip of the superior articular process (SAP) and are close to the dorsal root ganglion (DRG) of the exiting nerve root. This area is also called the hidden zone of Macnab. It is in this area where sequelae and complications (incidental durotomy) with endoscopic surgery may occur. For example, postoperative dysesthesias and motor dysfunction may make the postoperative recovery harder even though they frequently resolve spontaneously with or without supportive care measures, such as a TESI, and medical management using gabapentin or pregabalin.

The juxtafacet cyst is located either in the lateral recess or medially to the facet's tip near the exiting nerve in the foramen. When the cyst wall is visualized, it is grabbed with endoscopic pituitary forceps and thermally ablated with a radiofrequency probe or laser. When the cyst is not visualized, the medial facet capsule is thermally ablated, proceeding from the base of the superior articular process at the foramen's caudal aspect sweeping cranially toward the rostral tip of the facet exiting nerve. The cyst is then punctured and the synovial-like wall removed through the access cannula. When the capsule is not directly accessible or when a hypertrophied facet encroaches upon the nerve, medial facet ablation is performed with a side-firing laser. Injection of Isovue-300 mixed with indigo carmine with a foraminal epidural injection contrast can help outline the cyst. Vertebral foraminal osteophytes in the foramen can also be trimmed with a laser. Adequate decompression is determined by relief of preoperative pain expressed by the awake patient and visualization of the now mobile and pulsating exiting and traversing nerve. The authors used the following two surgical techniques.

Transforaminal Approach

For the transforaminal decompression, the author's preference is to position the patient in the prone position. A lateral decubitus is an alternative position. Intraoperative determination of the best access angles to the surgical level seems easier to this team of authors in the posteroanterior (PA) fluoroscopic plane, where most of the surgery is carried out. After prepping and draping the patient in standard surgical fashion, the anatomic landmarks, including the midline, iliac crests, and a line parallel to the surgical disc space, can be marked directly on the patient/ In the lateral (LAT) fluoroscopic projection. A long pituitary rongeur can be used to determine the most appropriate access angle and distance in both planes from the skin to the disc's posterior aspect. The access planning and details of this method have been detailed in another chapter authored by the senior author on the hybridization of the "inside-out" and "outside-in" technique. To go into further details on the utilization of these two methods of the transforaminal approach would be beyond the scope of this book chapter. However, the authors recommend that the prospective endoscopic spine surgeon consider familiarizing him or herself with the indications of the transforaminal approach's methodological nuances.

Patients may undergo endoscopic surgery under local anesthesia and sedation employing monitored anesthesia care (MAC) protocols. Alternatively, general anesthesia can be considered mainly if the surgeon is highly confident and does not heavily rely on the patient's verbal communication during the surgeon. Overall, patient satisfaction with the surgery seems better when intraoperative pain is well controlled, and the wakeup was uneventful. There are separate book chapters in these three volumes of endoscopic spine text that the prospective surgeon could read on the application of modern enhanced recovery anesthesia protocols (ERAS)and the use of intraoperative neuromonitoring. Regardless, it is always a good idea to inject local anesthesia at the skin entry point and apply it to the entire surgical corridor before introducing the endoscopic dilators and working cannula. An intraoperative facet block and transforaminal injection of 0.5 to 1 cc of 1% bupivacaine may also go a long way in perioperative pain control and improve patient satisfaction while shortening the operation time. For the guidewire's initial placement, a 16 or 18 G long spine needle is advanced toward the target area. Serial dilators are introduced over said guidewire towards the foramen in a rotating motion. Finally, the working cannula is introduced over the dilators. These details of endoscopic access creation to the spine are well known to most surgeons and are described in great detail in numerous chapters by other contributing authors. After the introduction of the spinal endoscope, the authors prefer an initial foraminoplasty under direct visualization. They came to dislike blind reaming of the foramen with trephines or hand drills for this purpose as such maneuvers tend to destroy the local anatomy before the surgeon had an opportunity to assess it *via* direct visualization first. In doing so, the authors' position that the potential for nerve root injury is lower since tethered or furcal nerves and synovial cysts are readily identified without stirring up a lot of bleeding. During this initial foraminoplasty, power- shaves or burs in conjunction with Kerrison rongeurs, punches, and hooks may be used. These instruments are also useful during the lateral recess decompression. Depending on the surgeon's preference and skill level, a bipolar or a radiofrequency probe may useful to control bleeding and shrink soft tissue (Fig. **1**). It is not mandatory, though, to ablate. The synovial cyst is easily identified by following the SAP rostrally to its tip when entering the lumbar facet joint. This move is characteristically not too difficult since most of these degenerative facet joints are unstable and have a widened joint space. Adhesions of the synovial cyst material may pose some challenges to dissecting it off the neural elements. Radiofrequency may also be cautiously employed during this portion of the operation, and thermal damage to the dorsal root ganglion should definitively be avoided by burning it.

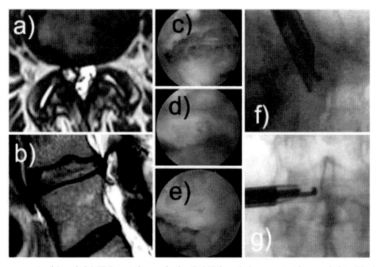

Fig. (1). Shown are: (a, b) axial MRI cut through the L4/5 level demonstrating a right-sided synovial facet cyst impinging on the traversing L5 nerve root, (c-e) the videoendoscopic view of the decompressed dural sac and traversing L5 nerve root at various stages of the decompression. The synovial facet cyst was adherent to the ligamentum flavum and the nerve root. The fluoroscopic images in the lateral (f) and the posteroanterior (g) projection show the use of a Kerrison rongeur during the transforaminal endoscopic lateral recess decompression and the resection of the tip of the superior articular process.

At this point, the surgeon has the option of advancing the working cannula into the intervertebral disc to perform an "inside-out" decompression under direct visualization of the interior of the intervertebral disc space. This part of the decompression takes place anteriorly below the dural sac and medially. However, most epidural synovial facet cysts arise in the lateral canal. The maneuvers out of the playbook of the "outside-in" technique are required to accomplish the decompression goals. Ultimately, the surgeon may decide to employ both methods as synovial facet cysts are typically associated with herniated disc and another associated spinal stenosis. Again, the axillary hidden zone of Macnab is a common site where most of the decompression work will be concentrated. The inside-out techniques may come in handy should one encounter excessive epidural fibrosis around the exiting nerve root. An annular window created below the dorsal root ganglion may be the only access to the undersurface of the exiting nerve root's dorsal root ganglion to tease off adhesions without undue retraction of the root and incidental dural tears. In some cases, it may be safer to perform a posterior annular resection in the axillary area and to leave some scar tissue on the neural elements rather than trying to dissect the interval between dura and cyst at all cost. This approach was performed in 79.2% (38/48) of the study patients.

Interlaminar Approach

At times, the interlaminar approach may be preferable to the transforaminal approach, mainly if the cyst is located in the lateral recess medial to the facet joint complex. Accessing the lateral spinal canal to address compressive pathology in that area has recently gained popularity mostly when found at the L5-S1 level. However, it is also feasible in other levels and in the author's series (see below) presented herein was chosen in 10 (20.8%) of the 48 patients. Performing a partial resection of the medial part of the facet joint - namely the inferior articular process (IAP) - is key to accessing juxtafacet cysts in this area. This part of the operation sometimes requires removing portions of the upper lamina and always of the ligmentum flavum and, thus, carries the risk of an incidental durotomy. High-speed burrs are a must to effectively carry out this part of the operation (Fig. **2**).

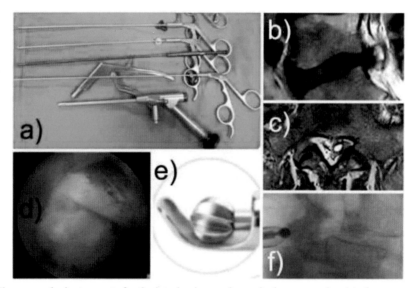

Fig. (2). Shown are the instruments for the interlaminar endoscopic decompression (a), the preoperative axial (b) and sagittal (c) MRI cuts through the L5/S1 level demonstrating a left-sided synovial facet cyst impinging on the traversing S1 nerve root, which was confirmed endoscopically *via* the interlaminar approach (d). The decompression of the facet joint and cyst removal hinges on the skillful application of a motorized drill bit (e).

As with the transforaminal approach, the authors of this chapter prefer the prone position for the interlaminar surgery employing similar landmarks but specifically outlining the interlaminar window using fluoroscopy to confirm the gateway's surgical level to the intervertebral disc space. Fluoroscopy is utilized to specifically outline the facet joints in the PA and lateral projections. The working cannula is inserted over sequential dilators positioning it at the medial aspect of the facet joint at its junction with the lamina. Different configurations of working cannulas are available, with some of them are useful as a nerve root retractor by turning the bevel of the working cannula towards the ligament flavum. The lamina's inferior lateral edge may be resected with Kerrisons or burs as needed.

First, the inferomedial portion of the facet joint should be removed. Remove the ligament flavum with a blunt dissector and subsequently with endoscopic rongeurs. Any adhesions of the cyst with the dura or the nerve roots should be carefully dissected. Removal in toto is rarely feasible, and piecemeal resection of the cyst may be more efficient. The hidden zone of Macnab in the axilla of the two nerve roots may be obscured. In cases of huge cysts, a combination of interlaminar and transforaminal full endoscopic decompression may be indicated to visualize the Macnab's axillary hidden zone better. The surgical area should be scrutinized with a nerve hook to be convinced that the neural elements are free of adhesions, tethering, and compression.

CLINICAL SERIES

This study of 48 patients included 26 females and 22 male patients with an average age of 60.58 years ranging from 30 to 91. All patients were diagnosed with unrelenting radiculopathy that did not improve with conservative care of a minimum of 12 weeks and had MRI evidence of a facet cyst with or without a concomitant herniated disc or lateral recess stenosis. Besides, patients' MRI scans and X-rays were evaluated for any evidence of instability, including an enlarged ligamentum flavum, a widened joint space of greater than 2 mm filled with white fluid on T2-weighted image sequences [25, 26]. Only patients without mobile spondylolisthesis were included. Patients' clinical improvements were assessed using the modified Macnab criteria at the final follow [27]. The mean follow-up was 55.46 months, ranging from 24 to 129 months. Twenty-six patients (72.2%) had cyst resection at L4/5, followed by the L5/S1 level in another 8 (22.2%). Two patients (5.6%) had surgery at the L3/4 level, and one patient at T9/10 (2.1%) (Table **2**).

Table 2. Level distribution of patients who underwent endoscopic resection of synovial facet cysts.

Level	Frequency	Percent	Valid Percent	Cumulative Percent
L3/4	6	12.5	12.5	12.5
L4/5	32	66.7	66.7	79.2
L5/S1	9	18.8	18.8	97.9
TH9/10	1	2.1	2.1	100.0
Total	48	100.0	100.0	-
Facet joint instability indicated by a widening of the joint space > 2 mm on axial MRI images				
-	**Frequency**	**Percent**	**Valid Percent**	**Cumulative Percent**
Joint < 2mm	28	58.3	58.3	58.3
Joint > 2mm	20	41.7	41.7	100.0
Total	48	100.0	100.0	-

Surgery was done *via* the transforaminal approach in 38 (79.2%) and the interlaminar approach in 10 (20.8%) patients, nine of which had surgery at the L5/S1 level. Intraoperatively, synovial cysts were often pedunculated, inflamed, red, suggesting intralesional bleeding with hemosiderin deposits (Fig. **3**).

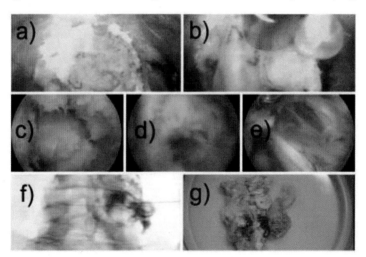

Fig. (3). Shown are various intraoperative endoscopic images of pedunculated inflamed synovial cysts (a, b) that can be removed with a rongeur. Cyst material can be quite adherent to the traversing nerve root (c-d). Intralesional injection of dye may show the cyst's multiloculated nature on intraoperative fluoroscopy images (f) and give the surgeon an idea of the size of the cystic lesion to remove it in its entirety (g). Images courtesy Dr. Anthony Yeung, Desert Institute of Spine Care, Phoenix Arizona, USA.

Six patients (12.5%) had dysesthesias postoperatively. Only one patient had a recurrent disc herniation (2.1%), and an additional patient failed to improve due to underlying chronic neuropathy previously unrecognized. Fusions with facet joint resection were necessary to control inferior surgical outcomes in two patients (4.2%). In these patients, the need for fusion was prompted by a recurrent disc herniation and in the other by the natural progression of the underlying disease. Twenty (41.7%) of the 48 study patients had red-flag signs of segmental instability on the routine T2-weighted axial MRI scans as suggested by widening the facet joint space to greater than 2 mm thickening of the ligamentum flavum (Table **2**). Clinical outcome assessment showed excellent Macnab outcomes in 39.6% (19/48) of patients and good in another 37.5% (18/48). The remaining 11 patients (22.9%) were graded to have fair Macnab outcomes (Table **3**). At final follow up, the average VAS score for leg pain reductions were statistically significant and reduced preoperative numbers of 8.06 ± 1.57 to 1.92 ± 1.49 immediately postoperatively, and 1.77 ± 1.32 at final follow-up.

Table 3. Macnab outcomes in patients who underwent endoscopic resection of synovial facet cysts.

-	-	**Frequency**	**Percent**	**Valid Percent**	**Cumulative Percent**
Valid	Excellent	19	39.6	39.6	39.6
-	Good	18	37.5	37.5	77.1
-	Fair	11	22.9	22.9	100.0
-	Total	48	100.0	100.0	-

Claudication symptoms stopped in all patients. Unfortunately, patients with Good (18/48) and Fair (11/48) Macnab outcomes bemoaned residual mechanical low back pain. Patients with Excellent Macnab outcomes did not. However, mechanical low back pain was successfully treated in all 29 patients nonoperatively by NSAIDs, activity modification, and physical therapy. There were no nerve root injuries or postoperative weakness. There was no statistically significant difference in outcome measures or complications in patients treated either with the transforaminal or interlaminar method. MRI findings suggestive of facet joint instability such as thickened ligamentum flavum and widening of the facet joint complex (Fig. **2a**) above 2 mm were recorded in 20 (41.7% of 48 patients). Fixed Grade I spondylolisthesis was found in 14 of these 20 patients. However, their preoperative dynamic extension/flexion views did not show any discernable motion.

Two patients showed 3 mm of anterolisthesis in flexion, reducing extension on preoperative dynamic lateral views. Such MRI instability markers were statistically significant in correlation with fair clinical Macnab outcomes (p < 0.001) (Table **4**).

Table 4. Crosstabulation of Macnab outcomes in patients who underwent endoscopic synovial cyst resection *versus* facet instability.

-		MRI Instability Criteria		-
Macnab	Outcome	Facet Joint Space < 2mm	Facet Joint Space > 2mm	Total
	Excellent	14	5	19
	Good	2	9	11
	Fair	12	6	18
Total	-	28	20	48
Pearson Chi-Square		9.652	2	.008
Likelihood Ratio		9.956	2	.007
N of Valid Cases		48	-	-
1 cells (16.7%) have expected count less than 5. The minimum expected count is 4.58.				

DISCUSSION

Endoscopic treatment of lumbar synovial facet cysts is a reasonable alternative to open spine surgery. The attraction with endoscopic surgery is its simplicity and the minimal collateral damage by the mere exposure-related postlaminectomy-syndrome and instability because of the minimal bony resection of the facet joint complex. The authors recommend an initial foraminoplasty to expose the facet cyst by decompressing the facet joint space at the superior articular process's rostral tip. The transforaminal approach can adequately address most facet cysts. However, in particular, the interlaminar approach and its over-the-top techniques may come in handy when there is central stenosis, or the cysts extend into the central canal, as was the case in 36 patients of this case series. However, the most significant upside to the endoscopic treatment of symptomatic lumbar facet cysts lies in its simplicity where many patients can be discharged to their home within one hour [29].

Facet cysts can be grossly classified as intraspinal cysts. Their etiology is not fully understood. The most common reason believed to be responsible for their formation is osteoarthritis and degenerative spondylolisthesis affecting the mechanical integrity of the facet joint complex. The resulting hypermobility, abnormal motion, and chronic trauma may contribute to forming these synovial cysts. What makes them symptomatic is even less well understood. Leaking synovial liquid followed by slime degeneration of the surrounding connective tissue onto the neural elements can be very painful. Postlaminectomy induced instability after previous decompression surgeries is also a commonly attributed factor, again following the notion that mechanical instability is at the heart of the problem [30]. As far as incidence, the contemporary literature suggests that there is a peak of intraspinal facet cysts incidence is up to 8.6% of patients within 3 to 12 months after microsurgery for a herniated disc or lateral canal stenosis [31]. Most patients experience spontaneous resolution of symptoms. In fact, up to 70% of cases resolve within 6 weeks, with half reported occurrences being asymptomatic [31, 32]. Some authors find post-laminectomy segmental and rotational instability with progression to spondylolisthesis and advanced disc degeneration as one of the most significant predictors of symptomatic facet cysts [33]. Myxoid degeneration and softening of collagen connecting tissue of the joint capsule, metaplasia of pluripotent mesenchymal cells, embryonal synovial tissue in the periarticular fibrous connective tissue growing through constant stimulus has been found to play a role on the cellular level. The proliferation of fibroblasts with increasing hyaluronic acid production due to irritation essentially presents a benign neoplastic source of newly formed tissue, which ultimately gets involved in developing nerve root compression. Regardless of etiology, synovial cysts are frequently misdiagnosed, and the patients' treating physicians frequently underestimate the severity of low back- and radicular leg pain they can cause. Tissue biopsy may be required to distinguish synovial from ganglion cysts definitively. History and physical examination or MRI scan may not suffice to establish the diagnosis. In rare cases, ganglion cysts were found even inside synovial cysts. Intralesional bleeding may render it impossible to arrive at an accurate histological classification of the cyst's content. Some may argue that the exact histopathological definition of the juxtafacet cyst is clinically irrelevant since the clinical presentation and their respective treatments are similar. Both types of cysts - synovial and ganglion cysts - have been classified as degenerative intraspinal cysts [34]. Others proposed the term periarticular cyst, joint cysts, synovial cysts, or juxtafacet cysts [11, 35]. The cyst may be filled with a clear, serous, or xanthochrome liquid containing substantial mucopolysaccharides [36, 37]. In comparison to synovial cysts, ganglion cysts stem from mucoid degeneration of periarticular connective tissue [10, 26, 33, 39 - 43].

When to intervene and when to wait? That is the question many surgeons will have to decide on, considering that most patients presenting synovial cysts are asymptomatic [36 - 38]. A recent positional MRI study included 852 asymptomatic volunteers who identified 50 patients with intraspinal juxtafacet cysts (5,87%) [42]. Another study determined that synovial facet cysts may become symptomatic in a short, time underlining that inflammation of the nerves may be one of the more significant factors determining their acuity. Most synovial joint cysts develop in the hand, elbow, hip, or knee. They are comparatively uncommon in the lumbar spine and even more rare in the thoracic and cervical regions [21].

Initially, most patients may respond fovorable to epidural corticosteroid injections or intraarticular injections of local anesthetic or steroids [24, 25]. Short-term bed rest, bracing, physical therapy, NSAIDs, and in rare cases, short term treatment with opioids should be tried before considering surgery. CT-guided needle aspiration can be considered for those patients who do not want surgery. However, they should be advised that cyst aspirations are not as effective and do not provide similar long-term relief, as observed with surgical decompression. Traditionally, microsurgical dissection *via* the hemilaminectomy approach is recommended. However, this translaminar operation dictates the removal of a significant portion of the facet joint's medial portion and the inferior portion of the adjacent lamina. Therefore, the endoscopic excision can be considered in patients refractory to conservative care with satisfactory clinical results. In the authors' experience, exposing both the exiting and traversing nerve roots carefully before attempting resection of the cyst in toto or piecemeal diminishes the risk of a dural tear. The application of this protocol produced no incidental durotomies in our patient population. The associated neovascularization and inflammatory cellular infiltration may be quite severe and lead to adhesions raising the degree of difficulty in accomplishing a complete neural decompression similar to that observed with herniated discs [44]. Application of a bipolar radiofrequency (RF) probe may help shrink the adherent and tethered cyst tissue.

Excision of the cysts is the cornerstone of surgical treatment [37, 38]. The authors of this chapter employed either the transforaminal or the interlaminar approach to remove the cysts endoscopically. The endoscopic approach is the preferred method by the authors since it minimizes trauma, postoperative scarring segmental instability. The latter may prompt spinal fusion [45]. That endoscopic resection of the cysts may suffice to successfully treat patients suffering from symptomatic synovial facet cysts, as evidenced by the authors' study results. Some 77.1% of patients had Excellent and Good Macnab outcomes. The VAS score reductions averaging 6.29 ± 1.9 corroborated the Macnab outcome analysis. The main reason for patients' rating of Good or Fair Macnab outcomes was mechanical back pain persistence. While mechanical instability of the surgically treated facet joint complex was the likely explanation for these persistent symptoms - proven by the statistically significant correlation between MRI instability criteria and advanced degeneration of the facet joints - most of these patients complaining of persistent low back pain were treated successfully with additional non-operative supportive care measures during the postoperative convalescence period. A more detailed analysis of these MRI instability markers seems warranted to determine whether they are useful prognosticators of clinical outcomes with the diseased facet joint's surgical treatment.

CONCLUSION

Hypertrophic synovitis resulting in pedunculated cysts may occur as an incidental para-articular mass without evidence on CT or MRI or as a benign intraspinal mass visualized on MRI. It may be underdiagnosed clinically when the clinician is focused only on the disc as the primary cause of sciatica. There is a demonstrated false negative rate on MRI. In degenerative lumbar discs, radicular symptoms may be multi-factorial, caused by annular tears, disc protrusion, facet synovitis, juxtafacet cysts, and osteophytosis tethering the spinal nerves. Synovial cysts may be found incidentally during endoscopic disc decompression. Even when incidental to disc herniation or annular tears, synovial cysts should be resected to avoid failed back surgery syndrome. When the foramen is visualized endoscopically, the radiofrequency ablation of juxta facet cysts may improve the surgical result. Endoscopic decompression of neural elements compromised by symptomatic lumbar facet cysts is an attractive alternative to open translaminar or microsurgical resection of this often highly inflammatory and painful pathology. Its most significant advantage is less exposure-related damage and lower postoperative instability rates. Direct endoscopic visualization of any facet cyst may help minimize the required joint-resection to diminish spinal fusion's need prompted by disease progression

CONSENT FOR PUBLICATION

Not applicable.

CONFLICT OF INTEREST

The authors declare no conflict of interest, financial or otherwise.

ACKNOWLEDGEMENT

Declared none.

REFERENCES

[1]   Yeung A, Yeung CA. Endoscopic Identification and Treating the Pain Generators in the Lumbar Spine that Escape Detection by Traditional Imaging Studies. J Spine 2017; 6(2): 369.
[http://dx.doi.org/10.4172/2165-7939.1000369]

[2]   Kouyialis AT, Boviatsis EJ, Korfias S, Sakas DE. Lumbar synovial cyst as a cause of low back pain and acute radiculopathy: a case report. South Med J 2005; 98(2): 223-5.
[http://dx.doi.org/10.1097/01.SMJ.0000129792.92433.B6] [PMID: 15759954]

[3]   Reddy P, Satyanarayana S, Nanda A. Synovial cyst of lumbar spine presenting as disc disease: a case report and review of literature. J La State Med Soc 2000; 152(11): 563-6.
[PMID: 11125509]

[4]   Howington JU, Connolly ES, Voorhies RM. Intraspinal synovial cysts: 10-year experience at the Ochsner Clinic. J Neurosurg 1999; 91(2) (Suppl.): 193-9.

[PMID: 10505504]

[5]   Kono K, Nakamura H, Inoue Y, Okamura T, Shakudo M, Yamada R. Intraspinal extradural cysts communicating with adjacent herniated disks: imaging characteristics and possible pathogenesis. AJNR Am J Neuroradiol 1999; 20(7): 1373-7.
[PMID: 10473000]

[6]   Trummer M, Flaschka G, Tillich M, Homann CN, Unger F, Eustacchio S. Diagnosis and surgical management of intraspinal synovial cysts: report of 19 cases. J Neurol Neurosurg Psychiatry 2001; 70(1): 74-7.
[http://dx.doi.org/10.1136/jnnp.70.1.74] [PMID: 11118251]

[7]   Kurz LT, Garfin SR, Unger AS, Thorne RP, Rothman RH. Intraspinal synovial cyst causing sciatica. J Bone Joint Surg Am 1985; 67(6): 865-71.
[http://dx.doi.org/10.2106/00004623-198567060-00006] [PMID: 4019534]

[8]   Baum JA, Hanley EN Jr. Intraspinal synovial cyst simulating spinal stenosis. A case report. Spine 1986; 11(5): 487-9.
[http://dx.doi.org/10.1097/00007632-198606000-00018] [PMID: 3750088]

[9]   Banning CS, Thorell WE, Leibrock LG. Patient outcome after resection of lumbar juxtafacet cysts. Spine 2001; 26(8): 969-72.
[http://dx.doi.org/10.1097/00007632-200104150-00024] [PMID: 11317123]

[10]   Hemminghytt S, Daniels DL, Williams AL, Haughton VM. Intraspinal synovial cysts: natural history and diagnosis by CT. Radiology 1982; 145(2): 375-6.
[http://dx.doi.org/10.1148/radiology.145.2.7134440] [PMID: 7134440]

[11]   Kao CC, Uihlein A, Bickel WH, Soule EH. Lumbar intraspinal extradural ganglion cyst. J Neurosurg 1968; 29(2): 168-72.
[http://dx.doi.org/10.3171/jns.1968.29.2.0168] [PMID: 5673315]

[12]   Jackson DE Jr, Atlas SW, Mani JR, Norman D. Intraspinal synovial cysts: MR imaging. Radiology 1989; 170(2): 527-30.
[http://dx.doi.org/10.1148/radiology.170.2.2911681] [PMID: 2911681]

[13]   Boviatsis E J, Stavrinou L C, Kouyialis A T, et al. 2008; Spinal synovial cysts: pathogenesis, diagnosis and surgical treatment in a series of seven cases and literature review. Eur Spine J 17(6): 831-837. 10.

[14]   Liu JK, Cole CD, Kan P, Schmidt MH. Spinal extradural arachnoid cysts: clinical, radiological, and surgical features. Neurosurg Focus 2007; 22(2): E6.
[http://dx.doi.org/10.3171/foc.2007.22.2.6] [PMID: 17608349]

[15]   Choi JY, Kim SH, Lee WS, Sung KH. Spinal extradural arachnoid cyst. Acta Neurochir (Wien) 2006; 148(5): 579-85.
[http://dx.doi.org/10.1007/s00701-006-0744-2] [PMID: 16505968]

[16]   Voyadzis JM, Bhargava P, Henderson FC. Tarlov cysts: a study of 10 cases with review of the literature. J Neurosurg 2001; 95(1) (Suppl.): 25-32.
[PMID: 11453427]

[17]   Mitra R, Kirpalani D, Wedemeyer M. 2008; Conservative management of perineural cysts. Spine 33(16): E565-8. 10.1097.
[http://dx.doi.org/10.1097/BRS.0b013e31817e2cc9]

[18]   Kanev PM, Park TS. Dermoids and dermal sinus tracts of the spine. Neurosurg Clin N Am 1995; 6(2): 359-66.
[http://dx.doi.org/10.1016/S1042-3680(18)30468-6] [PMID: 7620359]

[19]   Baker JK, Hanson GW. Cyst of the ligamentum flavum. Spine 1994; 19(9): 1092-4.
[http://dx.doi.org/10.1097/00007632-199405000-00019] [PMID: 8029749]

[20] Métellus P, Fuentes S, Dufour H, Do L, Figarella-Branger D, Grisoli F. An unusual presentation of a lumbar synovial cyst: case report. Spine 2002; 27(11): E278-80.
[http://dx.doi.org/10.1097/00007632-200206010-00021] [PMID: 12045529]

[21] Shah RV, Lutz GE. Lumbar intraspinal synovial cysts: conservative management and review of the world's literature. Spine J 2003; 3(6): 479-88.
[http://dx.doi.org/10.1016/S1529-9430(03)00148-7] [PMID: 14609693]

[22] Sabo RA, Tracy PT, Weinger JM. A series of 60 juxtafacet cysts: clinical presentation, the role of spinal instability, and treatment. J Neurosurg 1996; 85(4): 560-5.
[http://dx.doi.org/10.3171/jns.1996.85.4.0560] [PMID: 8814156]

[23] Sabers S R, Ross S R, Grogg B E, Lauder T D. 2005; Procedure-based nonsurgical management of lumbar zygapophyseal joint cyst-induced radicular pain Arch Phys Med Rehabil 86(9): 1767-71.
[http://dx.doi.org/10.1016/j.apmr.2004.11.051]

[24] Bjorkengren AG, Kurz LT, Resnick D, Sartoris DJ, Garfin SR Sr. Symptomatic intraspinal synovial cysts: opacification and treatment by percutaneous injection. AJR Am J Roentgenol 1987; 149(1): 105-7.
[http://dx.doi.org/10.2214/ajr.149.1.105] [PMID: 3495967]

[25] Snoddy MC, Sielatycki JA, Sivaganesan A, Engstrom SM, McGirt MJ, Devin CJ. Can facet joint fluid on MRI and dynamic instability be a predictor of improvement in back pain following lumbar fusion for degenerative spondylolisthesis? Eur Spine J 2016; 25(8): 2408-15.
[http://dx.doi.org/10.1007/s00586-016-4525-1] [PMID: 27106489]

[26] Khan AM, Girardi F, Park JH, Suh SW, Lee SH. Spinal lumbar synovial cysts. Diagnosis and management challenge. Eur Spine J 2006; 15(8): 1176-82.
[http://dx.doi.org/10.1007/s00586-005-0009-4] [PMID: 16440202]

[27] Lyons MK, Atkinson JL, Wharen RE, Deen HG, Zimmerman RS, Lemens SM. Surgical evaluation and management of lumbar synovial cysts: the Mayo Clinic experience. J Neurosurg 2000; 93(1) (Suppl.): 53-7.
[PMID: 10879758]

[28] Macnab I. Negative disc exploration. An analysis of the causes of nerve-root involvement in sixty-eight patients. J Bone Joint Surg Am 1971; 53(5): 891-903.
[http://dx.doi.org/10.2106/00004623-197153050-00004] [PMID: 4326746]

[29] Lewandrowski KU. Readmissions After Outpatient Transforaminal Decompression for Lumbar Foraminal and Lateral Recess Stenosis. Int J Spine Surg 2018; 12(3): 342-51.
[http://dx.doi.org/10.14444/5040] [PMID: 30276091]

[30] Oertel MF, Ryang Y-M, Gilsbach JM, Rohde V. Lumbar foraminal and far lateral juxtafacet cyst of intraspinal origin. Surg Neurol 2006; 66(2): 197-9.
[http://dx.doi.org/10.1016/j.surneu.2005.11.026] [PMID: 16876628]

[31] Sehati N, Khoo L, Holly L. Treatment of lumbar synovial cysts using minimally invasive surgical techniques, Neurosurg. Focus 2006; 20(3): E2 1-6.

[32] Yasuma T, Arai K, Yamauchi Y. The histology of lumbar intervertebral disc herniation. The significance of small blood vessels in the extruded tissue. Spine 1993; 18(13): 1761-5.
[http://dx.doi.org/10.1097/00007632-199310000-00008] [PMID: 7694378]

[33] Wildi LM, Kurrer MO, Benini A, Weishaupt D, Michel BA, Brühlmann P. Pseudocystic degeneration of the lumbar ligamentum flavum: a little known entity. J Spinal Disord Tech 2004; 17(5): 395-400.
[http://dx.doi.org/10.1097/01.bsd.0000109837.59382.0e] [PMID: 15385879]

[34] Shima Y, Rothman SL, Yasura K, Takahashi S. Degenerative intraspinal cyst of the cervical spine: case report and literature review. Spine 2002; 27(1): E18-22.
[http://dx.doi.org/10.1097/00007632-200201010-00029] [PMID: 11805654]

[35]   Kao CC, Winkler SS, Turner JH. Synovial cyst of spinal facet. Case report. J Neurosurg 1974; 41(3): 372-6.
[http://dx.doi.org/10.3171/jns.1974.41.3.0372] [PMID: 4416019]

[36]   Kjerulf TD, Terry DW Jr, Boubelik RJ. Lumbar synovial or ganglion cysts. Neurosurgery 1986; 19(3): 415-20.
[http://dx.doi.org/10.1227/00006123-198609000-00013] [PMID: 3489903]

[37]   Abdullah AF, Chambers RW, Daut DP. Lumbar nerve root compression by synovial cysts of the ligamentum flavum. Report of four cases. J Neurosurg 1984; 60(3): 617-20.
[http://dx.doi.org/10.3171/jns.1984.60.3.0617] [PMID: 6699708]

[38]   Khan AM, Synnot K, Cammisa FP, Girardi FP. Lumbar synovial cysts of the spine: an evaluation of surgical outcome. J Spinal Disord Tech 2005; 18(2): 127-31.
[http://dx.doi.org/10.1097/01.bsd.0000156830.68431.70] [PMID: 15800428]

[39]   Christophis P, Asamoto S, Kuchelmeister K, Schachenmayr W. "Juxtafacet cysts", a misleading name for cystic formations of mobile spine (CYFMOS). Eur Spine J 2007; 16(9): 1499-505.
[http://dx.doi.org/10.1007/s00586-006-0287-5] [PMID: 17203271]

[40]   Ikuta K, Tono O, Oga M. Prevalence and clinical features of intraspinal facet cysts after decompression surgery for lumbar spinal stenosis. J Neurosurg Spine 2009; 10(6): 617-22.
[http://dx.doi.org/10.3171/2009.2.SPINE08769] [PMID: 19558297]

[41]   Niggemann P, Kuchta J, Hoeffer J, Grosskurth D, Beyer H-K, Delank K-S. Juxtafacet cysts of the lumbar spine: a positional MRI study. Skeletal Radiol 2011.
[http://dx.doi.org/10.1007/s00256-011-1186-3] [PMID: 21560008]

[42]   Phuong LK, Atkinson JLD, Thielen KR. Far lateral extraforaminal lumbar synovial cyst: report of two cases. Neurosurgery 2002; 51(2): 505-7.
[http://dx.doi.org/10.1097/00006123-200208000-00038] [PMID: 12182792]

[43]   Salmon B L, Deprez M P, Stevenaert A E, Martin D H. The extraforaminal juxtafacet cyst as a rare cause of L5 radiculopathy: a case report. Spine 2003; 28(19): E405-7.
[http://dx.doi.org/10.1097/01.BRS.0000085101.37990.4C]

[44]   Pendeton P, Carl B, Pollay M. Spinal extradural bengin synovial or ganglion cyst: case report. Neurosurgery 1983; 13: 322-6.
[http://dx.doi.org/10.1227/00006123-198309000-00021] [PMID: 6621847]

[45]   Min , et al. Endoscopically managed synovial cyst of the lumbar spine. Korean Spine J 2006; 3: 242-5.

CHAPTER 11

Transforaminal Endoscopic Lumbar Foraminotomy TELF for Lumbar Stenosis in Patients Aged Over 80 Years

Jorge Felipe Ramírez León[1,2,*], **José Gabriel Rugeles Ortíz**[1,2], **Carolina Ramírez Martínez**[1,2], **Nicolás Prada Ramírez**[3] and **Gabriel Oswaldo Alonso Cuéllar**[4]

[1] *Clínica Reina Sofía, Bogotá, Colombia, USA*

[2] *Centro de Columna Cirugía Mínima Invasión Latinamerican Endoscopic Spine Surgeons LESS Invasiva Group Fundación Universitaria Sanitas. Bogotá, D.C., Colombia, USA*

[3] *Clínica Foscal, Bucaramanga, Colombia Latinamerican Endoscopic Spine Surgeons LESS Invasiva Group Universidad Autónoma de Bucaramanga, Bucaramanga, Colombia, USA*

[4] *Doctor in Veterinary Medicine. Director of Education and Research Latinamerican Endoscopic Spine Surgeons LESS Invasiva Group Bogotá, D.C., Colombia, USA*

Abstract: Neurogenic claudication due to a herniated disc, spinal stenosis, instability, or deformity is typical in the elderly. When conservative management fails, and the patient's disability prevents a healthy lifestyle, surgery is often recommended. There are multiple concerns with open spine surgery in the geriatric patient population, including medical comorbidities and fewer overall reserves to tolerate aggressive operations with high blood loss and long operating times. Endoscopic foraminal decompression has gained popularity and is now openly competing with open decompression and fusion operations by focusing the treatment on validated pain generators. Such simplified treatments often consist of targeted single-level and unilateral neuroforaminal decompressions. It is evident that appropriate patient selection and a diagnostic workup employing validated prognosticators of a favorable outcome are necessary to make such an endoscopic spinal surgery program work in the elderly. In this chapter, the authors describe their patient selection algorithms and preferred surgical techniques. In their experience, high patient satisfaction may be achieved when employing their clinical protocols.

Keywords: Geriatric patients, Neurogenic claudication, Spinal stenosis.

---

* **Corresponding author Jorge Felipe Ramírez León:** Orthopedic Surgeon, Minimally Invasive Spine Surgeon; Clínica Reina Sofía, Bogotá, Colombia, USA and Centro de Columna Cirugía Mínima Invasión Latinamerican Endoscopic Spine Surgeons LESS Invasiva Group Fundación Universitaria Sanitas. Bogotá, D.C., Colombia, USA; E-mail: jframirezl@yahoo.com

Kai-Uwe Lewandrowski, Jorge Felipe Ramírez León, Anthony Yeung, Hyeun-Sung Kim, Xifeng Zhang, Gun Choi, Stefan Hellinger and Álvaro Dowling (Eds.)

INTRODUCTION

Advances in medicine have dramatically increased average life expectancy. Some recent demographic studies expect that the 65 years of age and older population in the US will reach 20% by 2030 [1]. Similar data is expected in the UK (22%). In the rest of Europe and over the world, the number of persons aged 80 years will be 426 million in 2050, three times the 2019 data (143 million), this growing geriatric population create new challenges for the medical fields, including all the degenerative pain-related diseases that also have raised and now are quite prevalent in developing countries [2 - 5]. For instance, musculoskeletal pain's global prevalence in the elderly ranges from 65 to 85% [1] and is positively associated with reduced quality of life, depression, and adverse health effects [5]. Specifically, for low back pain LBP the prevalence is between 24 and 36%, being osteoarthrosis and lumbar stenosis, the most common pathologies (1). Studies found that chronic and severe LBP prevalence and incidence could increase up to three times in patients in their 80ies *versus* their 50ies [6 - 8].

LBP intensity and disability are more severe and is the primary cause for visiting a health care provider. Treating the older population can be challenging due to associated comorbidities, high risk of complications, elevated cost, poor outcomes, and functional disability. Therefore, many older patients are undertreated or receive no treatment for spinal stenosis at all. Although the first treatment option must be non-operative management, in some instances, the surgical treatment has proven to be a good option for relieving pain in older patients [4]. Recently, with the development of new technologies, endoscopic spine surgery has been an excellent and safe option to treat LBP and radiculopathy in older patients. Still, there are few reports of its use on the geriatric population (over 80 years of age) using a full-endoscopic foraminal decompression. Endoscopic Spine Surgery offers new treatment alternatives to even more complex pathologies, looking for the maximal reduction of injury to adjacent tissues and preserving the natural structure and function of the lumbar motion segment [9 - 12]. This chapter will cover the use of the minimally invasive Transforaminal Endoscopic Lumbar Foraminotomy for lumbar spinal stenosis in patients aged over 80 years.

RADICULOPATHY

One of the most common spine pain pathologies in geriatric patients is nerve root compression [6]. Many degenerated spine structures may lead to lumbar spinal stenosis (LSS) and the subsequent radiculopathy with radiating pain [1]. LSS is defined as the syndrome associated with narrowing the lumbar spinal canal and neural compression; it may have two origins: degenerative changes and developmental or congenital phenomena [13]. The degenerative type occurs mainly in older people starting around the fifth or sixth decade [1, 9, 12], and it is generally associated with arthritic changes in bony structures such as the intervertebral disc (loss of height), articular facets (hypertrophy), vertebral channel adjacent ligaments, or the presence of spondylolisthesis.

Previous to implementing any surgical alternative, all the medical options must have been tried, including weight loss. Once the surgical decision has been made to treat this pathology, it is advisable to start with procedures that preserve as much as possible the normal anatomy and function of adjacent tissues, *i.e.*, minimally invasive techniques including full endoscopic procedures [12, 14 - 16]. Although many conventional surgical alternatives have proven safe and effective [4, 17], open decompression implies disadvantages like severe damage in surrounding tissues, prolonged hospitalization, the need for general anesthesia, and slower recovery [9]. Nowadays, the less aggressive and safest option for foraminal stenosis treatment in geriatric patients is Transforaminal Endoscopic Lumbar Foraminotomy TELF, formerly called Endoscopic Lumbar Foraminoplasty (ELF) [18].

TRANSFORAMINAL ENDOSCOPIC LUMBAR FORAMINOTOMY

Transforaminal endoscopic lumbar foraminotomy (TELF) is defined as "the process of widening the foramen through endoscopic instruments" [18]. This full-endoscopic procedure allows to perform foraminal decompression with minimal invasion, nerve root mobilization and neurolysis, osteophyte ablation, disc collagen fiber tension, epidural scarring tissue liberation, and sequestered and extruded disc protrusion removal with a good exploration of the foramen, extraforaminal area, epidural and intradiscal space [19]. Because of its inherent benefits, TELF is an excellent alternative for the treatment of lumbar stenosis. Nevertheless, there are few reports of its use in the geriatric population. It is necessary to understand better the fundamental aspects of evolution, indications, advantages, surgical techniques, and, of course, to report the authors' results and compare them with other reports.

TELF EVOLUTION

Spinal endoscopic techniques underwent a remarkable development in the last 30 years, which has permitted to increase its range of indications. As far as its beginnings, we must highlight Kambin, who described the safe triangle in 1991 [20]. Later, in 1994, Knight in England [21], Siebert [22] and Hoogland [23] in Germany, and Yeung [24, 25] in the United States performed the first percutaneous endoscopic lumbar discectomies (PELD) with a transforaminal approach [26]. Martin Knight in 1994 [27] described the Endoscopic Laser

Foraminoplasty ELF: consisting in osseous and disc tissue decompression thereby improving intracanal visualization and access to the operating field. This method was accomplished by extending the foraminal window medially to the spinal channel. Knight's system used a holmium laser fiber with a lateral trigger under irrigation with saline solution.

In contrast, more recently, we use burring with high-speed instruments at the foraminal zone, which is not associated with exaggerated temperature increases [28]. Besides being a technique carried out in an awake patient under sedation and local anesthesia, these aspects diminish the possibility of an iatrogenic injury dramatically and ensure the integrity of the nerve root. Recently a panel of worldwide KOL's, including one researcher of our team authors, proposed an international consensus to unify the terms under a rationale and goal of every surgery. We define the endoscopic foraminal decompression as Transforaminal Endoscopic Lumbar Foraminotomy TELF [18].

TELF INDICATIONS

TELF in patients aged over 80 years is indicated in: lateral recess stenosis, epidural fibrosis, osteophytosis, spondylolytic spondylolisthesis, fixed listhesis, disc extrusion or sequestered disc fragment, and failed back surgery syndrome. Candidates are patients suffering from radiculopathy by compression and nerve root irritation with failure in the medical treatment of lumbar radiculopathy and claudication for a minimum of 12 weeks. In contrast, the use of TELF is not recommended and is not indicated in central extruded disc herniations, segmental instability, cauda equina syndrome, painless diabetic motor neuropathy, tumors, or any clinical findings that suggest a pathology different to a degenerative disc disease

ADVANTAGES AND DISADVANTAGES OF TELF

TELF in patients over 80 years aged offers a series of advantages that should be taken into account, such as less trauma to adjacent tissues, less blood loss, small incisions, decreased infection incidence, reduced postsurgical pain, a quick return to everyday life, and the surgery's outpatient nature and better cost-effectiveness. The surgical increase of the foraminal volume is the goal of the TELF procedure [21, 27]. From the technical point of view, it offers the surgeon direct and broader endoscopic visualization of the surgical zone and allows an adequate decompression. Among the disadvantages of the technique, we have the difficulty of repairing dural tears, a relatively long learning curve, the need for specialized tools and equipment, which creates the need for an initial infrastructure investment. Finally, it is necessary to have a surgical team highly trained in the procedure [28].

SURGICAL TECHNIQUE

The incision site in TELF for lateral recess stenosis is the same as that for the transforaminal approach. This approach's advantages include protection of posterior ligaments and bony structures, which produce a smaller incidence of postoperative instability, articular facet arthropathy, and narrowing of the disc space. The patient is positioned prone on a radiolucent table, and a biplanar fluoroscopic C-Arm is required [28, 29]. The hips should be placed in 60 to 90 degrees flexion. The surgeon is located on the affected level's symptomatic side with his assistant beside him.

A mark is made under fluoroscopic vision on the midline skin at the surgical intervention level or levels. The entry point is set between 8 and 12 centimeters from the midline, depending on the patient's physical complexion. We can achieve a more specific site measuring the most suitable angle to reach the foramen in an axial MRI view. A spinal needle is introduced at a 45 to 60 degrees angle concerning the horizontal plane and directed towards the disc's posterior third. The needle tip must be at the pedicular midline in the anteroposterior fluoroscopic view and at the lateral one's posterior vertebral line. This site corresponds to Kambin's safe triangle. Kambin, 1993 #71} In the case of L5-S1, if the iliac crest is too high, the needle entry site is medial to the iliac crest with the intervertebral disc with an angle of 10 to 30 degrees (Fig. **1**).

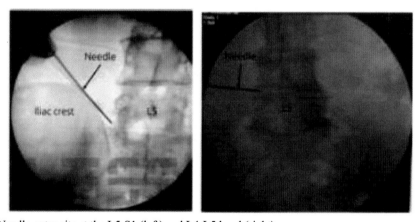

Fig. (1). Needle entry site at the L5-S1 (left) and L4-L5 level (right).

Once the needle is placed and its position has been checked, contrast media and methylene blue can be injected to obtain a discography. The purpose of doing this test during surgery is to evaluate the radiological pattern of the discal degeneration. On the other hand, methylene blue stain allows endoscopic differentiation between a healthy and a degenerated disc. A guide replaces the needle, and then a dilator with a 5.6 to 6.9 mm diameter is passed over it. The dilator makes it possible to gently dilate the muscular tissue from the skin to the annular disc and push away the exiting nerve root from the operating area (Fig. **2**).

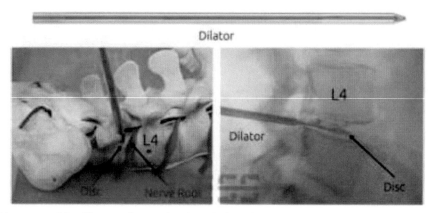

Fig. (2). Placement of the dilator on the annulus through the safe triangle.

A working cannula (sleeve) with a 7 to 8 mm diameter and a 145 to 185 mm length is passed over the dilator. The cutting instruments (trephine, burr, and rongeur) and the endoscope are passed through the sleeve's access channel (Fig. **3**).

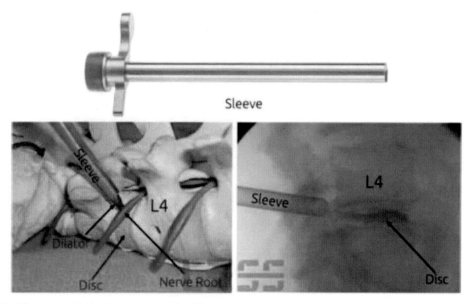

Fig. (3). Sleeves and their placement over the dilator.

After carefully removing the dilator, the endoscope is introduced through the sleeve. At this point, it is critical to have the assistance of the second surgeon, who must hold the sleeve firmly in order not to lose access or to damage adjacent structures ((Fig. **4**) - left). The commercially available endoscopic systems for spinal surgery are diverse. The authors use the Elliquence Transforaminal Spinal Endoscope TR100 (Elliquence LLC, NYC), with a lens of 30°, 181 mm in length, 7,0 mm in diameter, and with a 4,3 mm inner working channel ((Fig. **4**) - right).

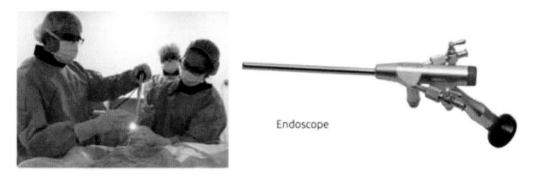

Fig. (4). a) Endoscope placement through the sleeve. **b)** Elliquence Transforaminal Spinal Endoscope TR100 with working channel (Elliquence LLC, NYC).

Once the endoscope is introduced, it is necessary to remember that the visual field is limited due to bleeding and an adipose layer covering the disc. This layer must be removed, and its vessels coagulated with the punch rongeur and radiofrequency probe. This maneuver makes it possible to remove the herniated disc, which is easily identified as previously stained with methylene blue. Once the field is clean without bleeding, and the endoscope is placed, the Kambin's safe triangle is identified (Fig. **4**). It corresponds to the working zone that permits a safe discectomy since, after being established, it allows permanent visualization of the dural sac, nerve root, annulus, and disc (Fig. **5**).

After identifying the safe triangle, the herniated disc is removed using a punch rongeur. This procedure is called mechanized discectomy and consists of removal of the extruded disc material – transforaminal and extraforaminal–. It is vital to remove the entire amount of the degenerated-herniated disc under endoscopic vision and radiologic assistance. Subsequently, it is necessary to decompress the nerve root, removing any perineural fibrosis thoroughly.

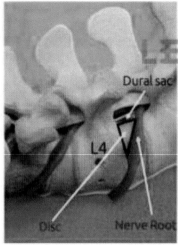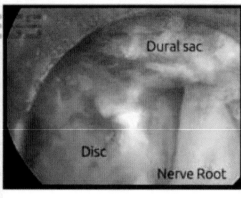

Fig. (5). Kambin's safe triangle anatomy: dural sac (zone 1), nerve root (zone 2) and annular disc (zone 3).

The initial cleaning of the extraforaminal zone is done with radiofrequency until reaching the foramen. We must ensure that all the elements causing nerve compression, traction, or irritation are removed under endoscopic vision. Nowadays, as a variant of the original Knight's technique using a laser [30], the authors prefer to do the foraminotomy through mechanical bone resection with a drill under endoscopic vision. This modification of the original technique is motivated by the high temperatures reached with the laser and the greater risk of injury they imply. The foraminal decompression is done using cutting burrs or with diamond tips, which are commercially available with or without hoods that protect neural structures. The burrs are connected to the shaver control, reaching 6,000 to 16,000 rpm (Fig. **6**).

To improve the surgery's safety, the procedure is done with saline solution irrigation, which besides diminishing temperature, provides a clear image of the foraminal structures. The superior and inferior facet joint surfaces are eggshelled out with burrs, trephine, and Kerrison forceps until the endoscope is allowed to enter the epidural space. The osteophytes present in the epidural space, in the facet joints, and the vertebral body must be removed. The nerves must be liberated from perineural and epidural fibrosis, and the yellow ligament and the superior foraminal ligaments must be removed to free the compressed structures. Some authors have described two types of foraminotomy [31]: the conventional and the extended endoscopic lumbar foraminotomy. The latter is used in herniated discs with severe caudal migration when the disc fragment is in close contact with the medial pedicle wall. It is necessary to remove a more comprehensive portion of the pedicle; it is recommended to use a trephine for this osteotomy.

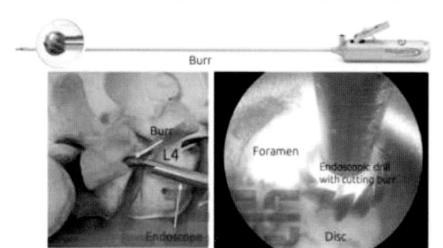

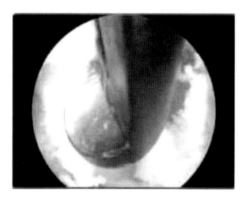

Fig. (6). Foraminal decompression by cutting burring and Kerrison.

Finally, it is recommended to examine the traversing and exiting nerve roots to ensure they are adequately decompressed medially and laterally along their course (Fig. **7**).

The instruments are withdrawn. The patient is asked to move the ankles to verify there is no neural injury. The epidural/foraminal area is infiltrated with a local anesthetic and a deposit corticosteroid. The skin incision is closed with a non-absorbable suture.

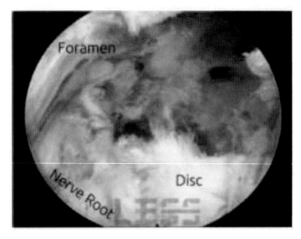

Fig. (7). Endoscopic view of the decompressed nerve root.

TELF POSTOPERATIVE CARE

After the procedure is accomplished, a neurological exam is done, especially evaluating sensitivity and mobility mainly of the extremity affected with radiated pain before surgery. The patient is discharged approximately 6 hours after surgery. The next day he/she is reexamined at an outpatient facility, and physical therapy protocol is established. Post-op pain is treated with common analgesics like acetaminophen and a non-steroidal anti-inflammatory drug.

CLINICAL SERIES

Lower extremity claudication associated with lumbar pain was the main indication for endoscopic surgery. Patients were examined to rule out vascular claudication. In neurogenic claudication, symptoms improve after changing position and rest, allowing the patient to continue walking. Vascular claudication requires that the patient lays down and raises the lower limbs to alleviate the pain. It is also associated with trophic skin and soft tissue changes. Radicular pain, paresthesias, and dysesthesias are other symptoms that should be explored thoroughly to identify and locate precisely the symptomatic area of neural compressions. In our center, we employ the following decision-making algorithm (Fig. **8**).

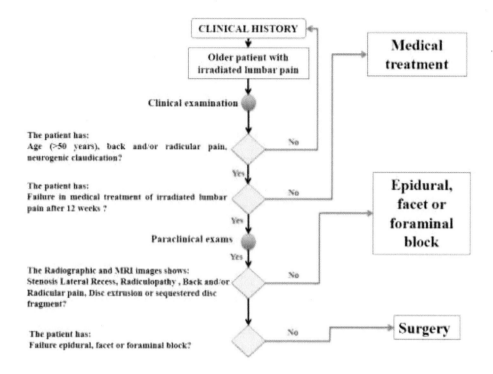

Fig. (8). Decision-making algorithm.

Between 1998 and 2018, 163 patients were selected for surgery employing our decision-making algorithm on whom we performed 301 TELF procedures. The mean age was 85.2 years ranging from 80 to 99 years. The diagnosis was determined by the correlation of clinical examination, plain film radiographs, and advanced imaging studies such as MRI. Moreover, the duration and onset of symptoms, comorbidities, prior treatments, and surgeries were recorded. The patients' functioning was graded with the visual analoge pain score (VAS) of leg pain and the Oswestry Disability Index (ODI).

The majority of patients had generalized multilevel degenerative spine disease. The most common surgical level was L4/5. The most common comorbidity was hypertension, which was recorded in 72% of patients. In our study, 92% of patients underwent treatment at more than one level on more than one occasion, emphasizing the staged management concept below. The principal diagnosis was foraminal stenosis in 124 patients (76%), followed by lateral recess stenosis (24%). All endoscopic surgeries in our geriatric patients were performed in our ambulatory surgery center. Typically, patients are recovered and observed for about 6 hours after the procedure. At the final two-year follow, clinical outcomes showed the VAS score to be reduced on average by five points, and the average ODI decreased by 35%. Ninety percent of patients were very satisfied with the treatment. We have twelve cases of readmission. Four were managed with medical therapy for dysesthesia, and eight cases had to undergo reoperation for failure to cure (5%). In one elderly patient, the surgery had to be terminated before its completion because he became hemodynamically unstable (2.5%).

DISCUSSION

Endoscopic lumbar surgery in the elderly is clearly of advantage in carefully selected patients. The incisions are smaller, and the surgery time is typically shorter and because not as much time is being spent on exposing the affected surgical levels or closing the wounds. Consequently, the anesthesia time is shorter, and patients can get through the surgery on a combination of local or epidural anesthesia and monitored anesthesia care (MAC) [32]. Hence, postanesthesia complications are also fewer, namely urinary retention, pulmonary atelectasis, nausea, and vomiting [33 - 37]. While this is all obvious to the unsuspecting reader, the hidden marvel in an endoscopic spinal surgery program is the patient selection and preoperative diagnostic protocol to decide which pathology to perform surgery on and, more importantly, which pathology to ignore [38]. Traditionally trained spine surgeons are accustomed to using image-based medical necessity criteria when establishing the indication for surgery [39]. The entire concept of minimally invasive endoscopic spinal surgery, however, revolves around simplifying and minimizing the extent of decompressive surgery to reduce the complications associated with traditional spine surgery while still delivering on significant clinical improvements to meet patients' expectations and gain their approval of the surgical outcome with high patient satisfaction scores [40]. So what to treat and what to ignore?

This question is by far from trivial and has been subject to clinical investigation. Validated preoperative diagnostic protocols by employing modern radiographic MRI [41 - 45] and CT [46] classifications systems focusing on stenosis in the lateral recess and the foraminal entry-, mid-and exit zone [39, 47, 48] and the adjunctive use of diagnostic spinal injections [49] have been published by Dowling *et al.* [38] They looked at which radiographic criteria to utilize when stratifying patients for which type of surgery. In short, the choice of surgical approach is based on analyzing the location of the compressive pathology: Transforaminal endoscopic approaches may be more suitable for neuroforaminal stenosis, and interlaminar decompression may be best suited for centrally located stenotic processes [38]. However, this stratification protocol leaves the endoscopic spine surgeon with the question of which level to select for endoscopic decompression when multiple levels are diseased. Again, this question seems trivial, but in fact, it is by far from it since L5 radiculopathy, for example, can arise from a traversing nerve root compression syndrome stemming from the L4/5 level or the exiting L5 nerve root from the L5/S1 level. As Lewandrowski *et al.* demonstrated, diagnostic injection protocols with just lidocaine may help improve the quality of the diagnostic information retrieved from the MRI review [49]. The MRI scan's positive predictive value to forecast a favorable outcome with transforaminal endoscopic decompression is, in reality, around 65 percent. Adding a diagnostic injection where the patient has a chance to verbalize to the surgeon from which level the radicular pain is emanating may be improved to 84% [50, 51]. Employing these protocols turns the patient-surgeon interaction into a shared decision-making scenario where both decide on the predominant pain generator and which other MRI findings to ignore. Defacto, applying these diagnostic protocols, uses the staged management style, which will result in high patient satisfaction in approximately 80% of the time [40]. Additional surgery may be required in the remaining 20% of patients, many of which are additional endoscopic decompressions on the opposite side of the same or at locations at an adjacent level [52, 53]. The need for future fusions within five years from the endoscopic index surgery with this approach is between 2.6 and 8.9% [52, 53]. Thus, it is extremely low compared to the numbers reported with traditional open spinal surgery [54, 55].

The majority of elderly patients are content with this clinical management style of their spinal stenosis related problems since it allows them to simplify their surgical treatment while delivering on meaningful functional improvements without the risk of exposure-related surgical sequelae and complications [54, 55], which in the elderly lead to higher readmission [56] - and higher utilization rates of medical services [57]. In short, two elements make a successful endoscopic spine surgery program work. First, clinical success hinges on simplifying the surgical treatment strategies to decrease the burden of perioperative risks and postoperative recovery on older patients who often suffer from multiple medical comorbidities, which would ordinarily render them, high-risk surgical candidates. Second, clinical success also hinges on the endoscopic spine surgeon's skill level and ability to deploy recent endoscopic equipment advancements effectively. These include endoscopic motorized shavers, drills, burs, and Kerrison rongeurs and graspers. The latter clearly emphasizes the need for surgeon training and to master the steep learning curve of the higher-end endoscopic spinal surgery decompression techniques [58 - 63]. For the readers of this chapter to be able to replicate the authors' clinical outcomes with these advanced endoscopic spinal surgery techniques in the elderly, this team of authors recommends increasing the complexity level of their application of endoscopic surgery in the elderly at a level that is commensurate with their equipment and skill level.

CONCLUSION

TELF is a safe and effective alternative for the treatment of lower back pain in older Individuals. The type of anesthesia and less tissue damage may be determinant factors for the safety of the technique. A successful TELF, like many other minimally invasive spine techniques, are positively related to good patient selection. It implies applying a strict pre-operative protocol based on clinical history, diagnostic images, and a psychological profile. Of course, implementing the proper training for this surgical procedure is another highly relevant factor for the technique's success. Finally, the authors have encountered very few complications in their patient series. Reported complications include inadequate compression of extruded disc material, nerve root lesions, wrong level surgery, hematomas, vascular damage, adjacent viscera injury, cerebrospinal fluid leakage, dural lesion, and excessive sedation [30].

CONSENT FOR PUBLICATION

Not applicable.

CONFLICT OF INTEREST

The authors declare no conflict of interest, financial or otherwise.

ACKNOWLEDGEMENTS

Declared none.

REFERENCES

[1]   Wong AY, Karppinen J, Samartzis D. Low back pain in older adults: risk factors, management options and future directions Scoliosis Spinal Disord 2017; 12: 14.
[http://dx.doi.org/10.1186/s13013-017-0121-3]

[2]   Ament JD, Thaci B, Yang Z, *et al.* Postoperative direct health care costs of lumbar discectomy are reduced with the use of a novel annular closure device in high-risk patients. Spine J 2019; 19(7): 1170-9.
[http://dx.doi.org/10.1016/j.spinee.2019.02.010] [PMID: 30776485]

[3]   Khanna K, Padegimas EM, Zmistowski B, Howley M, Verma K. Drivers of Medicare Reimbursement for Thoracolumbar Fusion: An Analysis of Data From The Centers For Medicare and Medicaid Services. Spine 2017; 42(21): 1648-56.
[http://dx.doi.org/10.1097/BRS.0000000000002171] [PMID: 28338572]

[4]   McGirt MJ, Parker SL, Hilibrand A, *et al.* Lumbar Surgery in the Elderly Provides Significant Health Benefit in the US Health Care System: Patient-Reported Outcomes in 4370 Patients From the N2QOD Registry. Neurosurgery 2015; 77(77) (Suppl. 4): S125-35.
[http://dx.doi.org/10.1227/NEU.0000000000000952] [PMID: 26378350]

[5]   Williamson E, Sanchez Santos MT, Morris A, *et al.* The Prevalence of Back and Leg Pain and the Cross-sectional Association With Adverse Health Outcomes in Community Dwelling Older Adults in England. Spine 2021; 46(1): 54-61.

[http://dx.doi.org/10.1097/BRS.0000000000003719] [PMID: 33315364]

[6]   Stewart Williams J, Ng N, Peltzer K, *et al.* Risk Factors and Disability Associated with Low Back Pain in Older Adults in Low- and Middle-Income Countries. Results from the WHO Study on Global AGEing and Adult Health (SAGE). PLoS One 2015; 10: e0127880.
[http://dx.doi.org/10.1371/journal.pone.0127880]

[7]   Vancampfort D, Stubbs B, Koyanagi A. Physical chronic conditions, multimorbidity and sedentary behavior amongst middle-aged and older adults in six low- and middle-income countries. Int J Behav Nutr Phys Act 2017; 14: 147.
[http://dx.doi.org/10.1186/s12966-017-0602-z]

[8]   Vancampfort D, Stubbs B, Veronese N, Mugisha J, Swinnen N, Koyanagi A. Correlates of physical activity among depressed older people in six low-income and middle-income countries: A community-based cross-sectional study. Int J Geriatr Psychiatry 2018; 33(2): e314-22.
[http://dx.doi.org/10.1002/gps.4796] [PMID: 28994143]

[9]   Lin YP, Wang SL, Hu WX, *et al.* Percutaneous Full-Endoscopic Lumbar Foraminoplasty and Decompression by Using a Visualization Reamer for Lumbar Lateral Recess and Foraminal Stenosis in Elderly Patients. World Neurosurg 2020; 136(136): e83-9.
[http://dx.doi.org/10.1016/j.wneu.2019.10.123] [PMID: 31866456]

[10]   Nellensteijn J, Ostelo R, Bartels R, Peul W, van Royen B, van Tulder M. Transforaminal endoscopic surgery for lumbar stenosis: a systematic review. Eur Spine J 2010; 19(6): 879-86.
[http://dx.doi.org/10.1007/s00586-009-1272-6] [PMID: 20087610]

[11]   Abbas J, Hamoud K, May H, *et al.* Degenerative lumbar spinal stenosis and lumbar spine configuration. Eur Spine J 2010; 19(11): 1865-73.
[http://dx.doi.org/10.1007/s00586-010-1516-5] [PMID: 20652366]

[12]   Abbas J, Hamoud K, Peled N, *et al.* Lumbar Schmorl's Nodes and Their Correlation with Spine Configuration and Degeneration Biomed Res Int 2018; 2018: 1574020.
[http://dx.doi.org/10.1155/2018/1574020]

[13]   Nellensteijn J, Ostelo R, Bartels R, Peul W, van Royen B, van Tulder M. Transforaminal endoscopic surgery for symptomatic lumbar disc herniations: a systematic review of the literature. Eur Spine J 2010; 19(2): 181-204.
[http://dx.doi.org/10.1007/s00586-009-1155-x] [PMID: 19756781]

[14]   Li H, Ou Y, Xie F, *et al.* Linical efficacy of percutaneous endoscopic lumbar discectomy for the treatment of lumbar spinal stenosis in elderly patients: a retrospective study. J Orthop Surg Res 2020; 15: 441.
[http://dx.doi.org/10.1186/s13018-020-01968-0]

[15]   Chen X, Qin R, Hao J, *et al.* Percutaneous endoscopic decompression *via* transforaminal approach for lumbar lateral recess stenosis in geriatric patients. Int Orthop 2019; 43(5): 1263-9.
[http://dx.doi.org/10.1007/s00264-018-4051-3] [PMID: 30027353]

[16]   Chung J, Kong C, Sun W, Kim D, Kim H, Jeong H. Percutaneous Endoscopic Lumbar Foraminoplasty for Lumbar Foraminal Stenosis of Elderly Patients with Unilateral Radiculopathy: Radiographic Changes in Magnetic Resonance Images. J Neurol Surg A Cent Eur Neurosurg 2019; 80(4): 302-11.
[http://dx.doi.org/10.1055/s-0038-1677052] [PMID: 30887488]

[17]   Ulrich NH, Kleinstück F, Woernle CM, *et al.* Clinical outcome in lumbar decompression surgery for spinal canal stenosis in the aged population: a prospective Swiss multicenter cohort study. Spine 2015; 40(6): 415-22.
[http://dx.doi.org/10.1097/BRS.0000000000000765] [PMID: 25774464]

[18]   Hofstetter CP, Ahn Y, Choi G, *et al.* AOSpine Consensus Paper on Nomenclature for Working-Channel Endoscopic Spinal Procedures. Global Spine J 2020; 10(2) (Suppl.): 111S-21S.
[http://dx.doi.org/10.1177/2192568219887364] [PMID: 32528794]

[19] Ramírez León JF. The motivators to endoscopic spine surgery implementation in Latin America. J Spine Surg 2020; 6(6) (Suppl. 1): S45-8.
[http://dx.doi.org/10.21037/jss.2019.09.12] [PMID: 32195414]

[20] Kambin P. Arthroscopic microdiscectomy of the lumbar spine. Clin Sports Med 1993; 12(1): 143-50.
[http://dx.doi.org/10.1016/S0278-5919(20)30463-4] [PMID: 8418975]

[21] Knight MT, Vajda A, Jakab GV, Awan S. Endoscopic laser foraminoplasty on the lumbar spine--early experience. Minim Invasive Neurosurg 1998; 41(1): 5-9.
[http://dx.doi.org/10.1055/s-2008-1052006] [PMID: 9565957]

[22] Siebert W. Percutaneous laser discectomy of cervical discs: preliminary clinical results. J Clin Laser Med Surg 1995; 13(3): 205-7.
[http://dx.doi.org/10.1089/clm.1995.13.205] [PMID: 10150647]

[23] Hoogland T. Percutaneous endoscopic discectomy. J Neurosurg 1993; 79(6): 967-8.
[PMID: 8246070]

[24] Yeung AT. Minimally Invasive Disc Surgery with the Yeung Endoscopic Spine System (YESS). Surg Technol Int 1999; 8(8): 267-77.
[PMID: 12451541]

[25] Yeung AT. The evolution of percutaneous spinal endoscopy and discectomy: state of the art. Mt Sinai J Med 2000; 67(4): 327-32.
[PMID: 11021785]

[26] Yeung AT. The Evolution and Advancement of Endoscopic Foraminal Surgery: One Surgeon's Experience Incorporating Adjunctive Techologies. SAS J 2007; 1(3): 108-17.
[http://dx.doi.org/10.1016/S1935-9810(07)70055-5] [PMID: 25802587]

[27] Knight MT, Goswami A, Patko JT, Buxton N. Endoscopic foraminoplasty: a prospective study on 250 consecutive patients with independent evaluation. J Clin Laser Med Surg 2001; 19(2): 73-81.
[http://dx.doi.org/10.1089/104454701750285395] [PMID: 11443793]

[28] Martínez CR, Lewandrowski KU, Rugeles Ortíz JG, Alonso Cuéllar GO, Ramírez León JF. Transforaminal Endoscopic Discectomy Combined With an Interspinous Process Distraction System for Spinal Stenosis. Int J Spine Surg 2020; 14(s3): S4-S12.
[http://dx.doi.org/10.14444/7121] [PMID: 33122183]

[29] Kim HS, Adsul N, Kapoor A, *et al.* A Mobile Outside-in Technique of Transforaminal Lumbar Endoscopy for Lumbar Disc Herniations. J Vis Exp 2018; 2018(138)
[http://dx.doi.org/10.3791/57999] [PMID: 30148483]

[30] Chiu JC, Negron F, Clifford T, Greenspan M, Princethal RA. Microdecompressive percutaneous endoscopy: spinal discectomy with new laser thermodiskoplasty for non-extruded herniated nucleosus pulposus. Surg Technol Int 1999; 8(8): 343-51.
[PMID: 12451548]

[31] Kambin P, Vaccaro A. Arthroscopic microdiscectomy. Spine J 2003; 3(3) (Suppl.): 60S-4S.
[http://dx.doi.org/10.1016/S1529-9430(02)00558-2] [PMID: 14589219]

[32] Abrão J. Anesthesia For Endoscopic Spine Surgery Of The Spine In An Ambulatory Surgery Center. Global Journal of Anesthesia & Pain Medicine 2020; 2020(3): 326-36. [GJAPM].
[http://dx.doi.org/10.32474/GJAPM.2020.03.000174]

[33] Vural C, Yorukoglu D. Comparison of patient satisfaction and cost in spinal and general anesthesia for lumbar disc surgery. Turk Neurosurg 2014; 24(3): 380-4.
[http://dx.doi.org/10.5137/1019-5149.JTN.8575-13.0] [PMID: 24848178]

[34] Ulutas M, Secer M, Taskapilioglu O, *et al.* General *versus* epidural anesthesia for lumbar microdiscectomy. J Clin Neurosci 2015; 22(8): 1309-13.
[http://dx.doi.org/10.1016/j.jocn.2015.02.018] [PMID: 26067543]

[35] McLain RF, Bell GR, Kalfas I, Tetzlaff JE, Yoon HJ. Complications associated with lumbar laminectomy: a comparison of spinal *versus* general anesthesia. Spine 2004; 29(22): 2542-7.
[http://dx.doi.org/10.1097/01.brs.0000144834.43115.38] [PMID: 15543071]

[36] Finsterwald M, Muster M, Farshad M, Saporito A, Brada M, Aguirre JA. Spinal *versus* general anesthesia for lumbar spine surgery in high risk patients: Perioperative hemodynamic stability, complications and costs. J Clin Anesth 2018; 46(46): 3-7.
[http://dx.doi.org/10.1016/j.jclinane.2018.01.004] [PMID: 29316474]

[37] De Rojas JO, Syre P, Welch WC. Regional anesthesia *versus* general anesthesia for surgery on the lumbar spine: a review of the modern literature. Clin Neurol Neurosurg 2014; 119(119): 39-43.
[http://dx.doi.org/10.1016/j.clineuro.2014.01.016] [PMID: 24635923]

[38] Dowling Á, Lewandrowski KU, da Silva FHP, Parra JAA, Portillo DM, Giménez YCP. Patient selection protocols for endoscopic transforaminal, interlaminar, and translaminar decompression of lumbar spinal stenosis. J Spine Surg 2020; 6(6) (Suppl. 1): S120-32.
[http://dx.doi.org/10.21037/jss.2019.11.07] [PMID: 32195421]

[39] Lewandrowski K-U. Pre-operative planning for endoscopic lumbar foraminal decompression–A prospective study. Eur Musculoskelet Rev 2008; 3: 46-51.

[40] Yeung A, Lewandrowski KU. Early and staged endoscopic management of common pain generators in the spine. J Spine Surg 2020; 6(6) (Suppl. 1): S1-5.
[http://dx.doi.org/10.21037/jss.2019.09.03] [PMID: 32195407]

[41] Lee GY, Lee JW, Choi HS, Oh KJ, Kang HS. A new grading system of lumbar central canal stenosis on MRI: an easy and reliable method. Skeletal Radiol 2011; 40(8): 1033-9.
[http://dx.doi.org/10.1007/s00256-011-1153-z] [PMID: 21286714]

[42] Lee S, Lee JW, Yeom JS, *et al.* A practical MRI grading system for lumbar foraminal stenosis. AJR Am J Roentgenol 2010; 194(4): 1095-8.
[http://dx.doi.org/10.2214/AJR.09.2772] [PMID: 20308517]

[43] Lønne G, Ødegård B, Johnsen LG, Solberg TK, Kvistad KA, Nygaard ØP. MRI evaluation of lumbar spinal stenosis: is a rapid visual assessment as good as area measurement? Eur Spine J 2014; 23(6): 1320-4.
[http://dx.doi.org/10.1007/s00586-014-3248-4] [PMID: 24573778]

[44] Sher I, Daly C, Oehme D, *et al.* Novel Application of the Pfirrmann Disc Degeneration Grading System to 9.4T MRI: Higher Reliability Compared to 3T MRI. Spine 2018; 2018(12/13)
[http://dx.doi.org/10.1097/BRS.0000000000002967] [PMID: 31205169]

[45] Yuan S, Zou Y, Li Y, Chen M, Yue Y. A clinically relevant MRI grading system for lumbar central canal stenosis. Clin Imaging 2016; 40(6): 1140-5.
[http://dx.doi.org/10.1016/j.clinimag.2016.07.005] [PMID: 27519125]

[46] Milette PC. Classification, diagnostic imaging, and imaging characterization of a lumbar herniated disk. Radiol Clin North Am 2000; 38(6): 1267-92.
[http://dx.doi.org/10.1016/S0033-8389(08)70006-X] [PMID: 11131632]

[47] Lee CK, Rauschning W, Glenn W. Lateral lumbar spinal canal stenosis: classification, pathologic anatomy and surgical decompression. Spine 1988; 13(3): 313-20.
[http://dx.doi.org/10.1097/00007632-198803000-00015] [PMID: 3388117]

[48] Lewandrowski KU. "Outside-in" technique, clinical results, and indications with transforaminal lumbar endoscopic surgery: a retrospective study on 220 patients on applied radiographic classification of foraminal spinal stenosis Int J Spine Surg 2014; 8
[http://dx.doi.org/10.14444/1026]

[49] Lewandrowski KU. Successful outcome after outpatient transforaminal decompression for lumbar foraminal and lateral recess stenosis: The positive predictive value of diagnostic epidural steroid injection. Clin Neurol Neurosurg 2018; 173(173): 38-45.

[http://dx.doi.org/10.1016/j.clineuro.2018.07.015] [PMID: 30075346]

[50]   Lewandrowski KU. Retrospective analysis of accuracy and positive predictive value of preoperative lumbar MRI grading after successful outcome following outpatient endoscopic decompression for lumbar foraminal and lateral recess stenosis. Clin Neurol Neurosurg 2019; 179(179): 74-80.
[http://dx.doi.org/10.1016/j.clineuro.2019.02.019] [PMID: 30870712]

[51]   Yeung AT, Lewandrowski KU. Retrospective analysis of accuracy and positive predictive value of preoperative lumbar MRI grading after successful outcome following outpatient endoscopic decompression for lumbar foraminal and lateral recess stenosis Clin Neurol Neurosurg 2019; 181: 52.
[http://dx.doi.org/10.1016/j.clineuro.2019.03.011]

[52]   Lewandrowski KU, Ransom NA. Five-year clinical outcomes with endoscopic transforaminal outside-in foraminoplasty techniques for symptomatic degenerative conditions of the lumbar spine. J Spine Surg 2020; 6(6) (Suppl. 1): S54-65.
[http://dx.doi.org/10.21037/jss.2019.07.03] [PMID: 32195416]

[53]   Yeung A, Lewandrowski KU. Five-year clinical outcomes with endoscopic transforaminal foraminoplasty for symptomatic degenerative conditions of the lumbar spine: a comparative study of *inside-out* versus *outside-in* techniques. J Spine Surg 2020; 6(6) (Suppl. 1): S66-83.
[http://dx.doi.org/10.21037/jss.2019.06.08] [PMID: 32195417]

[54]   Sebai MA, Kerezoudis P, Alvi MA, Yoon JW, Spinner RJ, Bydon M. Need for arthrodesis following facetectomy for spinal peripheral nerve sheath tumors: an institutional experience and review of the current literature. J Neurosurg Spine 2019; 31(1): 112-22.
[http://dx.doi.org/10.3171/2019.1.SPINE181057] [PMID: 30952137]

[55]   Yuan X, Wei C, Xu W, *et al.* Comparison of laminectomy and fusion vs laminoplasty in the treatment of multilevel cervical spondylotic myelopathy: A meta-analysis. Medicine (Baltimore) 2019; 98: e14971.
[http://dx.doi.org/10.1097/MD.0000000000014971]

[56]   Lewandrowski KU. Readmissions After Outpatient Transforaminal Decompression for Lumbar Foraminal and Lateral Recess Stenosis. Int J Spine Surg 2018; 12(3): 342-51.
[http://dx.doi.org/10.14444/5040] [PMID: 30276091]

[57]   Modhia U, Takemoto S, Braid-Forbes MJ, Weber M, Berven SH. Readmission rates after decompression surgery in patients with lumbar spinal stenosis among Medicare beneficiaries. Spine 2013; 38(7): 591-6.
[http://dx.doi.org/10.1097/BRS.0b013e31828628f5] [PMID: 23324923]

[58]   Morgenstern R, Morgenstern C, Yeung AT. The learning curve in foraminal endoscopic discectomy: experience needed to achieve a 90% success rate. SAS J 2007; 1(3): 100-7.
[http://dx.doi.org/10.1016/S1935-9810(07)70054-3] [PMID: 25802586]

[59]   Chaichankul C, Poopitaya S, Tassanawipas W. The effect of learning curve on the results of percutaneous transforaminal endoscopic lumbar discectomy. J Med Assoc Thai 2012; 95(95) (Suppl. 10): S206-12.
[PMID: 23451464]

[60]   Hsu HT, Chang SJ, Yang SS, Chai CL. Learning curve of full-endoscopic lumbar discectomy. Eur Spine J 2013; 22(4): 727-33.
[http://dx.doi.org/10.1007/s00586-012-2540-4] [PMID: 23076645]

[61]   Wang H, Huang B, Li C, *et al.* Learning curve for percutaneous endoscopic lumbar discectomy depending on the surgeon's training level of minimally invasive spine surgery. Clin Neurol Neurosurg 2013; 115(10): 1987-91.
[http://dx.doi.org/10.1016/j.clineuro.2013.06.008] [PMID: 23830496]

[62]   Xu H, Liu X, Liu G, Zhao J, Fu Q, Xu B. Learning curve of full-endoscopic technique through interlaminar approach for L5/S1 disk herniations. Cell Biochem Biophys 2014; 70(2): 1069-74.
[http://dx.doi.org/10.1007/s12013-014-0024-3] [PMID: 24839114]

[63]   Sharif S, Afsar A. Learning Curve and Minimally Invasive Spine Surgery. World Neurosurg 2018; 119(119): 472-8.
[http://dx.doi.org/10.1016/j.wneu.2018.06.094] [PMID: 29935319]

CHAPTER 12

Safety and Effectiveness of the Endoscopic Rhizotomy for the Treatment of Facet-Related Chronic Low Back Pain

Ralf Rothoerl[1,*], **Stefan Hellinger**[2], **Anthony Yeung**[3] and **Kai-Uwe Lewandrowski**[4,5,6]

[1] *Department of Neurosurgery, Isar Clinic, Munich, Germany*

[2] *Department of Orthopedic and Spine Surgery, Arabellaklinik, Munich, Germany*

[3] *Clinical Professor, University of New Mexico School of Medicine, Albuquerque, New Mexico Desert Institute for Spine Care, Phoenix, AZ, USA*

[4] *Center for Advanced Spine Care of Southern Arizona and Surgical Institute of Tucson, Tucson AZ, USA*

[5] *Associate Professor of Orthopaedic Surgery, Universidad Colsanitas, Bogota, Colombia, USA*

[6] *Visiting Professor, Department Orthopaedic Surgery, UNIRIO, Rio de Janeiro, Brazil*

Abstract: Lumbar spinal facet joints may be a significant source of chronic low back pain, with a reported prevalence of 7.7 to 75%. The clinical entity has been called facet joint syndrome. However, this syndrome and its therapies remain controversial as the clinical evidence for its treatment has been graded as weak. Intra- or periarticular injections have found acceptance as a diagnostic tool. Its etiology may be multifactorial, with degeneration of the joints' cartilage being the likely leading cause. This process incites an inflammatory response involving the synthesis of proinflammatory cytokines and metalloproteinases. Hence, local injections of glucocorticoids into the affected joint has become an accepted short-term treatment option but with weak long-term benefit. In this chapter, the authors review their clinical experience with the endoscopic rhizotomy when treating chronic low back pain due to facet syndrome. Its safety and effectiveness were evaluated in 84 patients, including 48 females and 36 males with a mean age of 65, ranging from 52 to 82. Patients were included in the study if they reported greater than 80% pain relief with lumbar medial branch blocks using ropivacaine on two separate occasions. Primary clinical outcome measures were the VAS BACK score and the Oswestry Disability Index (ODI). There were no adverse events and complications except one patient with a postoperative hematoma, which resolved with conservative care. At the final six months follow-up, the VAS scores were significantly lower (postop VAS 2.3; range 0 - 4) than before endoscopic rhizotomy (preop VAS mean 6.4; range 4-7; $p < 0.05$). The postoperative

---

* **Corresponding author Ralf Rothoerl:** Department of Neurosurgery, Isar Clinic, Munich, Germany; Tel: +49 89 1499036600; E-mail: ralf.rothoerl@isarklinikum.de

ODI of 24 (range 12 - 48) was significantly lower than its preoperative value 52 (range 42-67). The authors conclude that dorsal endoscopic rhizotomy is safe and effective for facet-related low back pain.

Keywords: Low back pain, Lumbar facet pain, Neurectomy, Rhizotomy.

INTRODUCION

The societal burden of chronic low-back pain (CLBP) is on the rise due to aging populations. The annualized prevalence is estimated to be between 3% to 10%. In the elderly, CLBP causes health care expenditures in other seemingly unrelated areas due to treatments of depression and poorly managed medical comorbidities due to immobilization [1]. The additional indirect cost of poorly managed CLBP due to lost wages is relevant to businesses and their employees. CLBP due to degenerative facet disease is often overlooked, notably when advanced imaging studies do not support standard treatments for compression of neural elements from a herniated disc or spinal stenosis in the central or lateral canal [2].

The etiology of CLBP from degeneration of the lumbar facet joints is believed to be related to the abundant innervation of the lumbar joint synovial membrane and joint capsule by nerve endings emanating from the medial branch of the dorsal ramus of the spinal nerve [3]. As the spinal nerve exits the lumbar neuroforamen, the posterior medial branch runs on the upper edge of the transverse process of the lower vertebral body and the lateral aspect of the superior articular process where it enters a fibro-osseous canal between the mammillary and the accessory processes. From there, it gives rise to fibers to facet joints, the muscles that attach to it [4]. It has been stipulated that facet degeneration produces increased stresses across the zygapophysial joint spaces. In turn, impingement of the synovial membrane folds reportedly stimulates the joint capsule's sensory receptors, causing inflammation [5] and pain *via* the medial branch [4]. The patient may complain of radiating pain not following a specific dermatome or localized mechanical low back pain [2].

The posterior branch of the spinal nerve exit from each lumbar neuroforamen also gives rise to the lateral branch, which may innervate the facet joint complex below, thus, creating abundant cross innervation [4, 6]. Therefore, ablation of the posterior medial branch as it runs on the upper edge of the lower vertebral body's transverse process and the lateral aspect of the superior articular process may result in incomplete pain relief [7]. Consequently, medial branch blocks have been employed to diagnostically determine whether the suspected facet joint complex is the pain generator relevant to the patient [8]. Unfortunately, these diagnostic blocks are not very accurate, with a false positive rate of 22% to 32% having been reported [9]. Therefore, many clinical investigators have proposed to perform at minimum two diagnostic injections with short- and long-acting local anesthetics to confirm the diagnosis and reduce the chance of a false positive response, which could prompt an unwarranted intervention. Some authors even go as far as only considering patients as true positive responders to diagnostic injections if their pain relief following the injections lasts as long as the expected half-life of a short- *Versus* long-acting local anesthetic [10]. If the response is consistent and the diagnosis is confirmed, additional treatments beyond the scope of non-steroidal anti-inflammatories, activity modifications, physical therapy, and other modalities can be considered. Repeated medial branch blocks may provide short-term pain without long-term benefit [11]. Typically, interventional pain management physicians perform needle-based percutaneous radiofrequency ablations with the reported longevity of the therapeutic benefit averaging three months because of the medial branch's regeneration and reinnervation of the painful facet joint complex [12]. In this chapter, the authors present their clinical experience with the endoscopically assisted rhizotomy, a surgically directly visualized facet joint denervation carried out with mechanical and radiofrequency ablation of the symptomatic facet joint.

ANATOMICAL BASIS FOR ANTERIOR & POSTERIOR COLUMN DENERVATION

Chronic low back pain related to anterior column degeneration is associated with Modic changes in the endplates and vertebral bodies [13]. Type I Modic changes appear more frequently associated with clinical symptoms [14 - 16] and have been successfully treated by denervation of the vertebral body's nerve supply. The innervation of the vertebral body was studied by Sherman *et al.* in 1963, who reported on a 'large solitary nerve trunk' tunneling into the posterior cortex that was communicating with the sinuvertebral nerve, which emanates from the ventral rami of the spinal nerves or nerves derived from the gray rami communicantes [17]. In 1997, Antonacci *et al.* corroborated this observation in a larger sample of the human vertebra by proving neurovascular bundles within the basivertebral foramen (BFV), and first using the term 'basivertebral nerves [18]. Later, they were associated with the vertebral osseous structures' microdamage, and their presence was confirmed with histopathological markers [19]. The innervation pathways linking endplate nociceptors to the basivertebral nerve trunk has been studied by Bailey *et al* [20]. They concluded that the vertebra courses' rich innervation along the intervertebral blood vessels toward the center of the vertebra from the branch out towards the endplates. These intimate structural interactions between the vertebral endplates and the intervertebral discs that axial back pain from multiple pain generators within the lumbar motion segment may be transmitted by the basivertebral nerve (BVN) [20 - 22]. The BVN accompanied by its vein and artery [16] enters the bone of the vertebral body *via* the midline of the posterior cortex *via* large, usually paired, neurovascular foramina that are located opposite from each other typically at the same distance from each endplate [23]. Sensitization of the BVN by neurotransmitters of the tachykinin family, such as substance P, have been associated with the transmission of pain signals [17, 24]. Transpedicular and extrapedicular approaches have been used to perform a radiofrequency ablation of this nerve [16, 21]. The laser has been employed *via* the transforaminal approach with epiduroscopy [23]. Knowingly or unknowingly, many surgeons may provide their patients with the benefit of posterior column denervation by the mere rhizotomy effect of their surgical exposure. Whenever the surgical exposure involves denuding the bone of any soft tissue attachments from the posterior elements, facet joints, transverse processes, an unintentional rhizotomy with mechanical tools or the monopolar electrocautery may be performed. Studies suggest that extensive monopolar electrocautery should be avoided to diminish injury to the radicular arteries [25] and to the spinal ganglia [26]. Therefore, bipolar continuous and more recently pulsed [27 - 31] radiofrequency ablation of the dorsal ramus tributaries has been the standard of care for decades. The medial branch emanates from the spinal nerve's dorsal ramus and runs posteriorly, medially, and caudally at the lateral aspect of the superior articular process of the lower vertebra adhering to the dorsal aspect of the root of the lower transverse process. The medial branch of the dorsal ramus enters a fibro-osseous canal formed by the mammilloaccessory ligament bridging the accessory with the mammillary process [32]. During medial branch ablation procedures, the lateral aspect of the superior articular process (SAP) and the root of the transverse process is targeted [33]. Anatomical studies show that the dorsal ramus gives to the medial, lateral branch, and the middle branch. The middle branch may share a common short trunk with the lateral branch [32 - 34]. However, the dorsal ramus of the L5 nerve root lacks the lateral branch [33, 34]. while others considered the middle branch as a subbranch of the lateral branch [35]. The skin, muscles, and ligaments attaching to the lateral aspect of the facet joints are innervated by the lateral ramus, which runs laterally, posteriorly, and caudally on the inferior aspect of the lower transverse process. The medial branch runs in the groove formed by the lower transverse process and the superior articular process. From there, it runs caudally and posteriorly to enter the fibro-osseous canal. At L5/S1, a groove is formed by the S1 SAP and the sacral ala in which the L5 dorsal ramus runs before giving rise to the lateral and the medial branches [35]. Typically, each lumbar facet joint is innervated by the medial branches from two adjacent spinal motion segments. It is sometimes from up to three motion segments providing the theoretical basis for performing a neurectomy at two to three levels simultaneously. The posterior column ablation *via* medial branch neurotomy is the subject of this chapter.

DIAGNOSTIC BLOCKS AS PROGNOSTICATOR OF OUTCOME

The strength of the clinical evidence in the prior literature supporting the use of therapeutic use intraarticular or periarticular facet joint injections with a steroid and a local anesthetic has been graded as weak [2, 8, 9, 11, 36 - 38]. However, such injections remain predominant clinical practice [1, 8, 39, 40]. Their diagnostic value though has been well recognized [41]. A patient's response of greater than 50% pain relief after facet joint injection or periarticular infiltration within three hours is commonly used as the diagnostic criterion to warrant thermal radiofrequency ablation at the same validated painful facet joint complex [42]. This recommendation has been further substantiated in a recent meta-analysis employed regression models to assess the correlation between response to diagnostic medial branch blocks and radiofrequency lesioning of the same joint while controlling for confounding variables [43]. Lee *et al.* included seven well-controlled clinical trials totaling 454 patients in their meta-analysis [43]. Radiofrequency denervation (231 patients) outcomes were compared to epidural steroid injections (223 patients), serving as control at one-year follow-up, demonstrating more significant improvements in back pain related outcome measures. A subgroup analysis of diagnostic injection responders consistently showed better back pain scores throughout the follow-up period than the control group. The authors' regression model demonstrated that the response to diagnostic medial branch blocks procedure was an excellent statistical prognosticator of the treatment effect.

RADIOFREQUENCY RHIZOTOMY

For lumbar facet joint rhizotomy, continuous radiofrequency (CRF) and pulsed radiofrequency (PRF) have been employed to sever the dorsal ramus's medial branch [44, 45]. Non-surgeons typically carry out this interventional procedure in an office- or ambulatory surgery center setting in an attempt to treat facet mediated axial back pain. This fluoroscopically guided radiofrequency lesioning may lack accuracy, and therefore pain relief may be short-lived [43]. Lim *et al.* demonstrated the benefit for pulsed radiofrequency ablation of the lumbar facet joint complex in twenty patients compared to 20 control patients treated with intraarticular steroid injections [31]. The authors explained that percutaneous pulsed radiofrequency ablation was as intraarticular steroid injections while avoiding steroids' harmful side effects. In 2020, consensus practice guidelines on lumbar facet joint pain interventions were formulated by a multispecialty, international working group following approval by the Board of Directors of the American Society of Regional Anesthesia and Pain Medicine [46]. A steering committee sent letters to 12 pain societies and the US Departments of Veterans Affairs and Defense. After internal committee discussions using a modified

Delphi method, 100% consensus was achieved on 17 questions approved by all but one society that dissented on the items questioning the number of blocks and the cut-off number considered a positive block before considering radiofrequency ablation. Nonetheless, the latter society also approved the entire final document, which detailed questions on the value of history and physical examination, imaging studies, conservative treatment, need for imaging to perform facet blocks, the diagnostic and prognostic value of medial branch blocks (MBB) and intra-articular (IA) injections, effects of sedation, and injectate volume on patient selection. Additional questions concerning the therapeutic value of facet blocks, the ideal cut-off value of a positive block with high predictive value, how many blocks are required before performing radiofrequency, electrodes' orientation, use of stimulation, and protocols to limit complications. Finally, participants were asked if clinical practice standards for repeat radiofrequency ablation should be changed. The consensus analysis revealed that lumbar medial branch radiofrequency ablation might provide benefit to well-selected individuals. Medial branch blocks were considered to have a high predictive value of favorable clinical outcome with the radiofrequency ablation than intraarticular injections. The consensus analysis stated that the use of stringent selection criteria could improve clinical outcomes and produce a higher percentage of false-negative patients escaping proper treatment [46].

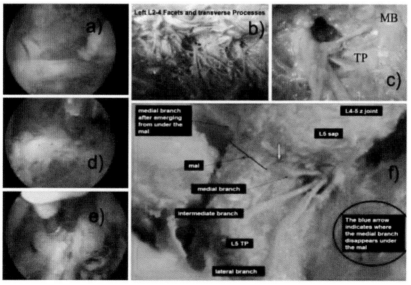

Fig. (1). Endoscopic visualizations **(a)** and cadaver dissections **(b, c and f)** of the dorsal ramus tributaries' relationship to the transverse processes and the superior articular process are shown. Endoscopic images of the medial branch during radiofrequency ablation of the medial branch **(d)** and mechanical transection of the lateral branch **(e)** are displayed.

ENDOSCOPIC FACET DEINNERVATION

The senior author has performed meticulous fresh cadaver dissection to determine the feasibility of the medial branch's direct endoscopic visualization, revealing that the dorsal ramus splits into the medial, intermediate, and lateral branches (Fig. **1**) [6]. Furthermore, his dissection findings were corroborated by others. Specifically, the dorsal ramus and its branches were shown to innervate the facet joints and the surrounding soft tissues and the paraspinal musculature, thereby contributing to non-discogenic axial back pain responsive to the medial branch blocks and rhizotomy [35].

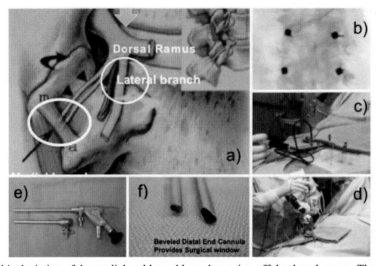

Fig. (2). Graphic depiction of the medial and lateral branch coming off the dorsal ramus. The medial branch runs posteriorly, medially, and caudally at the lateral aspect of the lower vertebra's superior articular process adhering to the dorsal aspect of the root of the lower transverse process. The medial branch of the dorsal ramus enters a fibro-osseous canal formed by the mammilloaccessory ligament bridging the accessory with the mammillary process **(a)**. Spinal needles are placed at the base of the transverse processes **(b, c)**, a lumbar rhizotomy endoscope **(e)** is placed after serial dilation of guidewires using a beveled working cannula **(f)** to aid in the visualization of the lateral aspect of the facet joint with the endoscope **(d)**.

The endoscopic rhizotomy may be performed with the patient in a prone position. A sterily draped fluoroscopy unit is brought into the field and used in the posterior-anterior (PA) and lateral (LAT) projection to identify and confirm the planes of the surgical level (Fig. **2**). A spinal needle is placed at the junction of the transverse process and the facet joint. A guidewire is introduced through the spinal needle after applying a 0.5 to 1 cc of 1% ropivacaine. A small 6 to 11 mm skin incision is then made around the guidewire. Serial dilators were then introduced and pushed onto the transverse process to directly place the endoscopic working cannula at the junction with the lumbar facet joint. The endoscope is then introduced for direct visualization of the facet joint capsule and the junction with the transverse process. Care is taken not to advance anteriorly and laterally. Slipping of the transverse process should be avoided in order to protect the nerve root at the neuroforamen or a penetrating injury to the retroperitoneal space. The next surgical step involves the removal of hypertrophic and inflamed tissue by opening of the joint capsule, irrigation as well as vaporization of the joint, and the RF ablation of pain-conducting nerves of the medial branch of dorsal ramus under direct endoscopic visualization. The same radiofrequency is also used for hemostasis. An endoscopic mechanical drill may be used in the abrasion of the medial branch in its fibro-osseous canal lateral to the SAP and formed by the mammillo-accessory ligament bridging the accessory with the mammillary process as it runs to the dorsal aspect of the root of the lower transverse process [32]. Both mechanical and radiofrequency ablation may be used in conjunction (Fig. **3**).

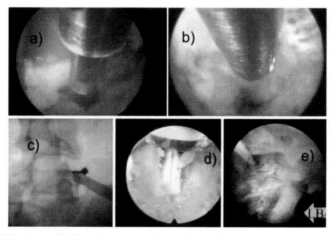

Fig. (3). Presented is the medial branch transsection with a radiofrequency probe **(a)** and ablation with a side-firing Holmium: YAG laser **(b)** during endoscopic visualizations **(c)**. The lateral branch's transsection can be done mechanically with rongeurs **(d)** or radiofrequency heat **(e)**.

At the completion of the procedure, the small skin incision is closed with a 3-0 absorbable monofilament suture after removing the endoscopic working cannula. If the diagnostic workup suggested multilevel involvement in the pain syndrome, adjacent levels were included in this denervation procedure to address any cross-innervation from adjacent cervical painful levels [47 - 53].

CLINICAL SERIES

From 2016 to 2018, we included 84 patients (48 females and 36 males, mean age 65 years range 52-82 years) diagnosed with lumbar facet-related chronic low back pain. Two diagnostic blocks confirmed the diagnosis (Table **1**).

Table 1. Demographics of patients treated with lumbar endoscopically assisted rhizotomy.

Age	-	Mean = 65 years	Range 52-82 years
Gender	Female	N= 48	57%
-	Male	N = 36	43%
Affected Level	L2/3	7.5%	-
-	L3/4	87%	-
-	L4/5	100%	-
-	L5/S1	100%	-
Grogan Classification	Grade 1	0%	-
-	Grade 2	12%	-
-	Grade 3	49%	-
-	Grade 4	39%	-

If the patients experienced pain relief of > 50% with two lumbar medial branch blocks using ropivacaine, they were recruited in the study. Patients' preoperative and postoperative VAS score, percentage of pain relief, and the Oswestry disability index were analyzed and compared. Possible complications were recorded. The inclusion criteria for endoscopic lumbar rhizotomy were:

1. Low back pain for more than three months,
2. failed six weeks of conservative treatment with physical therapy and non-steroidal anti-inflammatories (NSAIDs),
3. absence of overt neurological deficit,
4. advanced imaging studies demonstrating early-stage degenerative changes in the lumbar spine,
5. and more than 50% pain relief after diagnostic cervical medial branch block with 0.5 ml ropivacaine 5mg/ml.

Patients were excluded from the study if they had:

1. An infectious process,
2. fracture or any other traumatic injury,
3. a severe stenotic process in the spinal canal or foramen,
4. medical comorbidities including poorly controlled cardiopulmonary and hematological diseases, diabetes, and gastrointestinal ulcers,
5. age less than 18 years, and
6. women who were pregnant.

The authors established clinical protocol that essentially selected patients for the combination mechanical rhizotomy with opening and irrigation of the facet joint capsule followed by the pulsed radiofrequency ablation of at least one but more often two-level denervation procedure who were deemed not "bad enough" based on traditional image-based clinical treatment guidelines for a spinal fusion. These patients were typically at a loss with no definitive treatment being offered since they were deemed candidates for physical therapy, NSAIDs, and chronic pain management. The authors observed that many patients were frustrated with the lack of more definitive treatment. Therefore, patients were offered the denervation procedure described herein if they had a diagnostic medial branch block with at least 50% pain relief. The authors' patient selection was most likely suffering from hindsight [54, 55] and selection bias [56, 58]. They attempted to offer some treatment compassionately, particularly in those patients with significant disability, chronic pain, and unable to work and needed narcotics to control their pain. While patients were selected according to the inclusion/exclusion criteria, the authors did not attempt to distinguish between actual facet-related or discogenic axial low back pain with radiation into the gluteal region and possibly the leg *Versus* radicular pain from an inflamed or compromised lumbar nerve root whose extension was limited to the lower back without much radiation into the legs. In reality, it was impractical to make that distinction [59]. It was also irrelevant as a diagnostic injection with adequate pain relief was expected to be of high accuracy and positive predictive value, as observed and reported in other spine areas.

Grogan's criteria for facet arthropathy were used to grade as follows [60]: Grade 1, uniformly thick cartilage covering both articular surfaces completely; a uniform thin band of cortical bone. Grade 2, the cartilage covering the entire surface with eroded or irregular regions; a thin band of cortical bone extended into space from the articular surface. Grade 3, cartilage incompletely covering the articular surface, with the underlying bone exposed to the joint space; dense bone extended into the joint space but covering less than half the facet. Grade 4, complete absence of cartilage except for traces evident on the articular surface; the presence of osteophytes or dense cortical bone covered greater than half the facet joint. The Grogan grading is listed in Table **2**.

Table 2. Clinical outcome data of patients treated with lumbar endoscopically assisted rhizotomy.

-	Pre-operative	Follow-Up 1 year
VAS Back	7.2 range 5-10	2.3 range 0-5
ODI	52 range 42-67	24 range 12-48

There were no injuries to the lumbar nerve roots, wound complications, or excessive postoperative pain. One patient suffered from a conservatively treated hematoma. All patients were discharged from the hospital the next day. Analysis of the primary outcome measures that the VAS scores of pain postoperatively were significantly lower than that before endoscopic rhizotomy (VAS mean 6.4; range 4-7) before surgery and 2.3 (range 0-4 postoperatively; < 0.05). The ODI at six months follow-up was significantly lower than before surgery (mean 52 preoperatively range 42-67 *Versus* 24 postoperatively range 12-48). No complications were observed except for one conservatively treated hematoma (Fig. **4**).

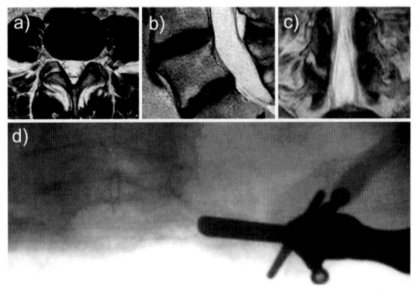

Fig. (4). Axial **(a)**, sagittal **(b)**, and coronal **(c)** T2-weighted MRI scans of an L4/5 painful right-sided facet joint complex is shown. This patient underwent endoscopically assisted rhizotomy after a diagnostic medial branch block employing a lumbar foraminoscope similar to the case shown at the L5/S1 level **(d)**.

DISCUSSION

Chronic lower back pain with or without radiation into the gluteal muscles or lower extremities can be disabling and incredibly frustrating to aging patients [61] who are told that there is no structural correlate on advanced imaging studies to explain their symptoms [62]. In those cases, the authors' endoscopic combination mechanical and radiofrequency denervation procedure is an attractive alternative to repetitive rounds of physical therapy, NSAIDs, and interventional and medical pain management. Real facet-related low back pain can be quite severe and may radiate into the gluteal muscles and the upper leg and muscular compartments and myofascial planes [62].

A significant proportion of the adult population has acute low-back pain at some stage of life. Although symptoms tend to resolve with either conservative treatment or without any treatment in most patients, there is a substantial group of patients who develop chronic pain [63]. In most cases, the cause of this chronic pain syndrome remains obscure, and there is no specific treatment available. In a large percentage of patients, a degenerated intervertebral disc seems to be the source of chronic low back pain. Studies on nerve blocks indicate that the prevalence of lumbar zygapophyseal joint pain among chronic low-back pain patients ranges from 15 to 40 percent [64]. Lumbar spinal facet joints were described in the medical literature as a source of low back pain in 1911 for the first time [65]. Since this first report, the so-called facet joint syndrome has become an accepted diagnosis, though still a controversial syndrome in the literature [1, 8, 66 - 71]. The Facet joint syndrome cannot be diagnosed clinically or radiologically, but it can be identified by using placebo-controlled local anesthesia to block the nerves supplying the painful joint.

The evidence comes from investigations reporting successful back pain relief following injections, either intraarticularly or periarticular [72]. The prevalence of lumbar pain due to painful facet joints, based on single diagnostic blocks, has a reported range from 7.7% to 75% in patients reporting back pain [73]. The facet joint syndrome is a degenerative process of the joint's cartilage. This process involves the immune system by initiating localized inflammatory responses. Such a reaction is followed by the synthesis of pro-inflammatory cytokines and metalloproteinases [74]. Because of the syndrome's inflammatory nature, local injections of glucocorticoids into the affected joint have become a standard treatment option. However, the results of various studies suggest that these injections have a limited value in the long-term treatment of patients suffering from chronic low back pain [75]. A controlled trial showed that corticosteroids' intraarticular injections did not significantly affect chronic pain in the cervical zygapophyseal joints [28]. Another treatment that has been advocated is percutaneous radiofrequency (RF) denervation. Since Shealy published his first article on radiofrequency denervation of the lumbar zygapophyseal joints in 1975 by Shealy 1975 [76], the technique has been modified and used with varying results [77 - 81]. Although the randomized controlled trials (RCTs) are published exclusively for lumbar and cervical pain, radiofrequency denervation is also used for example, in the management of sacroiliac joint pain [82, 83], thoracic zygapophyseal pain [84], trigeminal neuralgia [85 - 87], sympathetically maintained pain [88, 89], cervicogenic headaches [90], and intercostal neuralgia [91].

In a Cochrane review, several RCTs on chronic zygapophyseal joint pain were included [9, 92, 93]. The study population in van Kleef's study (n = 31) included patients with chronic low-back pain of more than 12 months duration and obtained at least 50 percent pain relief from a diagnostic dorsal ramus nerve block with a local anesthetic solution [92]. The inclusion criteria in Leclaire's study (n = 70) were patients with chronic low-back pain of longer than three months duration, who experienced significant pain relief for at least 24 hours during the week after intra-articular facet injection [93]. Van Kleef, and Leclaire, employed the modified Shealy technique [76], but they all induced a radiofrequency lesion at 80°C for 60 to 90 seconds. In the control group, electrodes were introduced in the radiofrequency lesion group, but no radiofrequency lesion was induced. Pain intensity was reported in all of the studies. Van Kleef and Leclaire assessed disorder-specific outcomes, whereas van Kleef also assessed generic functional status. Jacobson modified the classic radiofrequency technique by using parallel placement along either the posterior facet capsule or the facet joint's edges; the two electrodes create a bipolar lesion directed at the abnormal nerve endings in the facet joint capsule [94]. These additional lesions can be performed along with regular RFA of the recurrent branch or separately. This is a simple step with significant advantages, no added side effects, and, in preliminary cases, better initial and follow-up results.

In this chapter, the authors present their endoscopic version - a mechanical and modified radiofrequency technique validated by Jacobson [94], who reviewed the anatomy and innervation of the cervical facet joint and capsule in detail by showing that there is a more diffuse and extensive nerve supply extending into the capsule of the cervical facet joint than just those provided by the recurrent medial sensory branches that have been the focus of traditional radiofrequency lesioning. This chapter's authors stipulated that the spinal endoscope's direct visualization adds to the procedure's safety by allowing the surgeon to observe the ablation process on the video screen. Moreover, the additional use of endoscopic abrasion tools, including burrs or drills, may provide more durable pain relief due to the more thorough mechanical denervation effect.

Our endoscopic denervation protocol following a diagnostic injection with at least 50% reduction in the patient's symptoms was successfully employed in all of the 84 patients with a significant decrease in symptoms. The VAS scores of pain postoperatively were significantly lower than that before endoscopic rhizotomy (VAS mean 6.4 (range 4-7) prior surgery and 2.3 (range 0-4 postoperatively) P < 0.05). Patients suffered from minimal disability. Only one hematoma occurred and was treated conservatively. The authors combined endoscopic mechanical and pulsed radiofrequency ablation technique with the expectation that the therapeutic effect of endoscopic procedure is superior to percutaneous radiofrequency ablation. This has been recently demonstrated by Xue *et al.* These authors concluded that direct visualization of the medial branch during the endoscopic procedure provides a more targeted ablation with a lower risk of nerve root injury which could produce sensory loss in the corresponding dermatome [95]. This more aggressive long-segment denervation has been shown by Yeung *et al.* to be more durable with a lower nerve regeneration rate and better long-term efficacy [6]. While more effective than percutaneous facet rhizotomy, endoscopic mechanical and radiofrequency ablation of the facet joint complex may take longer than its percutaneous counterpart, be associated with a longer recovery due to the incision, and higher upfront cost. However, the latter will have to be formally investigated to see whether the long-term outcome analysis is associated with backend cost savings.

The most significant limitation of this case series study is that the authors had no way of determining whether their patients suffered from axial facet-related low back pain or suffered from radicular pain or both. The durability of the treatment benefit speaks for itself, with no additional denervation or decompression fusion procedures performed in any study patients. The most likely reason for more reliable pain relief with the endoscopic lumbar facet rhizotomy is the thorough disruption of the facet capsule's innervation. The dissection and irrigation of the facet capsule from medial to lateral and across adjacent levels are intended to ablate any cross-innervation. Besides durable and effective pain relief, the endoscopic combined mechanical and radiofrequency denervation procedure using the authors' direct posterior approach in their 2-year consecutive case series study was extremely safe with no injuries to the nerve roots or the paraspinal soft tissue. While the exact mechanisms of pain relief are not entirely known to the authors, it is conceivable that a combination of radicular and facet symptoms contributed to all patients' symptoms. The authors' theory is supportive of the additional pain relief they observed early on in the study with the addition of the laminotomy procedure. Therefore, the authors continued its use regardless of whether they did or did not fully understand how exactly that additional step in the denervation procedure provided additional benefit.

CONCLUSION

The surgical protocol the authors present in this book chapter is a time-proven in their hands. A formal clinical validation in more extensive clinical trials is indicated to mainstream the endoscopic combined mechanical and rhizotomy denervation of the lumbar facet joint complex.

CONSENT FOR PUBLICATION

Not applicable.

CONFLICT OF INTEREST

The authors declare no conflict of interest, financial or otherwise.

ACKNOWLEDGEMENT

Declared none.

REFERENCES

[1] Manchikanti L, Boswell MV, Singh V, *et al.* Prevalence of facet joint pain in chronic spinal pain of cervical, thoracic, and lumbar regions. BMC Musculoskelet Disord 2004; 5: 15.
[http://dx.doi.org/10.1186/1471-2474-5-15]

[2] Cohen SP, Huang JH, Brummett C. Facet joint pain--advances in patient selection and treatment. Nat Rev Rheumatol 2013; 9(2): 101-16.
[http://dx.doi.org/10.1038/nrrheum.2012.198] [PMID: 23165358]

[3] Li ZZ, Hou SX, Shang WL, Song KR, Wu WW. Evaluation of endoscopic dorsal ramus rhizotomy in managing facetogenic chronic low back pain. Clin Neurol Neurosurg 2014; 126(126): 11-7.
[http://dx.doi.org/10.1016/j.clineuro.2014.08.014] [PMID: 25194305]

[4] Saito T, Steinke H, Hammer N, *et al.* Third primary branch of the posterior ramus of the spinal nerve at the thoracolumbar region: a cadaveric study. Surg Radiol Anat 2019; 41(8): 951-61.
[http://dx.doi.org/10.1007/s00276-019-02258-z] [PMID: 31119410]

[5] Mattei TA, Goulart CR, McCall TD. Pathophysiology of regression of synovial cysts of the lumbar spine: the 'anti-inflammatory hypothesis'. Med Hypotheses 2012; 79(6): 813-8.
[http://dx.doi.org/10.1016/j.mehy.2012.08.034] [PMID: 23021571]

[6] Yeung A, Gore S. Endoscopically guided foraminal and dorsal rhizotomy for chronic axial back pain based on cadaver and endoscopically visualized anatomic study. Int J Spine Surg 2014; 8
[http://dx.doi.org/10.14444/1023]

[7] Cohen I, Rittenberg JD. Factors Associated with Successful Outcomes with Lumbar Medial Branch Radiofrequency Neurotomy. Curr Phys Med Rehabil Rep 2015; 3(2): 173-80.
[http://dx.doi.org/10.1007/s40141-015-0088-z]

[8] Manchikanti L, Kaye AD, Boswell MV, *et al.* A Systematic Review and Best Evidence Synthesis of the Effectiveness of Therapeutic Facet Joint Interventions in Managing Chronic Spinal Pain. Pain Physician 2015; 18(4): E535-82.
[http://dx.doi.org/10.36076/ppj.2015/18/E535] [PMID: 26218948]

[9] Lakemeier S, Lind M, Schultz W, *et al.* A comparison of intraarticular lumbar facet joint steroid injections and lumbar facet joint radiofrequency denervation in the treatment of low back pain: a randomized, controlled, double-blind trial. Anesth Analg 2013; 117(1): 228-35.
[http://dx.doi.org/10.1213/ANE.0b013e3182910c4d] [PMID: 23632051]

[10] Hafezi-Nejad N, Guermazi A, Roemer FW, Eng J, Zikria B, Demehri S. Long term use of analgesics and risk of osteoarthritis progressions and knee replacement: propensity score matched cohort analysis of data from the Osteoarthritis Initiative. Osteoarthritis Cartilage 2016; 24(4): 597-604.
[http://dx.doi.org/10.1016/j.joca.2015.11.003] [PMID: 26564576]

[11] Sae-Jung S, Jirarattanaphochai K. Outcomes of lumbar facet syndrome treated with oral diclofenac or methylprednisolone facet injection: a randomized trial. Int Orthop 2016; 40(6): 1091-8.
[http://dx.doi.org/10.1007/s00264-016-3154-y] [PMID: 26987980]

[12] Kim MH, Kim SW, Ju CI, Chae KH, Kim DM. Effectiveness of Repeated Radiofrequency Neurotomy for Facet joint Syndrome after Microscopic Discectomy. Korean J Spine 2014; 11(4): 232-4.
[http://dx.doi.org/10.14245/kjs.2014.11.4.232] [PMID: 25620983]

[13] Kääpä E, Luoma K, Pitkäniemi J, Kerttula L, Grönblad M. Correlation of size and type of modic types 1 and 2 lesions with clinical symptoms: a descriptive study in a subgroup of patients with chronic low back pain on the basis of a university hospital patient sample. Spine 2012; 37(2): 134-9.
[http://dx.doi.org/10.1097/BRS.0b013e3182188a90] [PMID: 21415809]

[14] Rahme R, Moussa R. The modic vertebral endplate and marrow changes: pathologic significance and relation to low back pain and segmental instability of the lumbar spine. AJNR Am J Neuroradiol 2008; 29(5): 838-42.
[http://dx.doi.org/10.3174/ajnr.A0925] [PMID: 18272564]

[15] Albert HB, Sorensen JS, Christensen BS, Manniche C. Antibiotic treatment in patients with chronic low back pain and vertebral bone edema (Modic type 1 changes): a double-blind randomized clinical controlled trial of efficacy. Eur Spine J 2013; 22(4): 697-707.
[http://dx.doi.org/10.1007/s00586-013-2675-y] [PMID: 23404353]

[16] Becker S, Hadjipavlou A, Heggeness MH. Ablation of the basivertebral nerve for treatment of back pain: a clinical study. Spine J 2017; 17(2): 218-23.
[http://dx.doi.org/10.1016/j.spinee.2016.08.032] [PMID: 27592808]

[17] Antonacci MD, Mody DR, Heggeness MH. Innervation of the human vertebral body: a histologic study. J Spinal Disord 1998; 11(6): 526-31.
[http://dx.doi.org/10.1097/00002517-199812000-00013] [PMID: 9884299]

[18] Antonacci MD, Hanson DS, Leblanc A, Heggeness MH. Regional variation in vertebral bone density and trabecular architecture are influenced by osteoarthritic change and osteoporosis. Spine 1997; 22(20): 2393-401.
[http://dx.doi.org/10.1097/00007632-199710150-00014] [PMID: 9355221]

[19] Antonacci MD, Mody DR, Rutz K, Weilbaecher D, Heggeness MH. A histologic study of fractured human vertebral bodies. J Spinal Disord Tech 2002; 15(2): 118-26.
[http://dx.doi.org/10.1097/00024720-200204000-00005] [PMID: 11927820]

[20] Bailey JF, Liebenberg E, Degmetich S, Lotz JC. Innervation patterns of PGP 9.5-positive nerve fibers within the human lumbar vertebra. J Anat 2011; 218(3): 263-70.
[http://dx.doi.org/10.1111/j.1469-7580.2010.01332.x] [PMID: 21223256]

[21] Khalil JG, Smuck M, Koreckij T, et al. A prospective, randomized, multicenter study of intraosseous basivertebral nerve ablation for the treatment of chronic low back pain. Spine J 2019; 19(10): 1620-32.
[http://dx.doi.org/10.1016/j.spinee.2019.05.598] [PMID: 31229663]

[22] Truumees E, Macadaeg K, Pena E, et al. A prospective, open-label, single-arm, multi-center study of intraosseous basivertebral nerve ablation for the treatment of chronic low back pain. Eur Spine J 2019; 28(7): 1594-602.
[http://dx.doi.org/10.1007/s00586-019-05995-2] [PMID: 31115683]

[23] Kim HS, Adsul N, Yudoyono F, et al. Transforaminal Epiduroscopic Basivertebral Nerve Laser Ablation for Chronic Low Back Pain Associated with Modic Changes: A Preliminary Open-Label Study. Pain Res Manag 2018.
[http://dx.doi.org/10.1155/2018/6857983]

[24] Hirsch C, Ingelmark BE, Miller M. The anatomical basis for low back pain. Studies on the presence of sensory nerve endings in ligamentous, capsular and intervertebral disc structures in the human lumbar spine. Acta Orthop Scand 1963; 33(33): 1-17.
[http://dx.doi.org/10.3109/17453676308999829] [PMID: 13961170]

[25] Aydin MD, Yildirim OS, Gundogdu C, Onder A, Okur A. Thrombogenetic effect of facet denervation using in disc surgery on spinal radicular arteries: an experimental study. Minim Invasive Neurosurg 2006; 49(6): 328-30.
[http://dx.doi.org/10.1055/s-2006-954825] [PMID: 17323257]

[26] Aydin MD, Dane S, Gundogdu C, Gursan N. Neurodegenerative effects of monopolar

electrocauterization on spinal ganglia in lumbar disc surgery. Acta Neurochir (Wien) 2004; 146(10): 1125-9.
[http://dx.doi.org/10.1007/s00701-004-0300-x] [PMID: 15744848]

[27] Chang MC. Effect of bipolar pulsed radiofrequency on refractory chronic cervical radicular pain: A report of two cases. Medicine (Baltimore) 2017; 96: e6604.
[http://dx.doi.org/10.1097/MD.0000000000006604]

[28] Choi GS, Ahn SH, Cho YW, Lee DG. Long-term effect of pulsed radiofrequency on chronic cervical radicular pain refractory to repeated transforaminal epidural steroid injections. Pain Med 2012; 13(3): 368-75.
[http://dx.doi.org/10.1111/j.1526-4637.2011.01313.x] [PMID: 22296730]

[29] Choi GS, Ahn SH, Cho YW, Lee DK. Short-term effects of pulsed radiofrequency on chronic refractory cervical radicular pain. Ann Rehabil Med 2011; 35(6): 826-32.
[http://dx.doi.org/10.5535/arm.2011.35.6.826] [PMID: 22506211]

[30] Ding Y, Li H, Hong T, *et al.* Efficacy of Pulsed Radiofrequency to Cervical Nerve Root for Postherpetic Neuralgia in Upper Extremity. Front Neurosci 2020; 14: 377.
[http://dx.doi.org/10.3389/fnins.2020.00377]

[31] Lim JW, Cho YW, Lee DG, Chang MC. Comparison of Intraarticular Pulsed Radiofrequency and Intraarticular Corticosteroid Injection for Management of Cervical Facet Joint Pain. Pain Physician 2017; 20(6): E961-7.
[PMID: 28934800]

[32] Bogduk N, Long DM. The anatomy of the so-called "articular nerves" and their relationship to facet denervation in the treatment of low-back pain. J Neurosurg 1979; 51(2): 172-7.
[http://dx.doi.org/10.3171/jns.1979.51.2.0172] [PMID: 156249]

[33] Bogduk N, Wilson AS, Tynan W. The human lumbar dorsal rami. J Anat 1982; 134(Pt 2): 383-97.
[PMID: 7076562]

[34] Bogduk N. The innervation of the lumbar spine. Spine 1983; 8(3): 286-93.
[http://dx.doi.org/10.1097/00007632-198304000-00009] [PMID: 6226119]

[35] Shuang F, Hou S-X, Zhu J-L, *et al.* Clinical Anatomy and Measurement of the Medial Branch of the Spinal Dorsal Ramus. Medicine (Baltimore) 2015; 94(52): e2367-7.
[http://dx.doi.org/10.1097/MD.0000000000002367] [PMID: 26717379]

[36] Boswell MV, Shah RV, Everett CR, *et al.* Interventional techniques in the management of chronic spinal pain: evidence-based practice guidelines. Pain Physician 2005; 8(1): 1-47.
[http://dx.doi.org/10.36076/ppj.2006/9/1] [PMID: 16850041]

[37] Lee DW, Huston C. Fluoroscopically-Guided Cervical Zygapophyseal Therapeutic Joint Injections May Reduce the Need for Radiofrequency. Pain Physician 2018; 21(6): E661-5.
[PMID: 30508997]

[38] Mazmudar A, Nayak R, Patel AA. Therapeutic Facet Joint Interventions in the Lumbar Spine: An Economic Value Perspective. Clin Spine Surg 2020; 33(10): 411-7.
[http://dx.doi.org/10.1097/BSD.0000000000001046] [PMID: 32657844]

[39] Snidvongs S, Taylor RS, Ahmad A, *et al.* Facet-joint injections for non-specific low back pain: a feasibility RCT. Health Technol Assess 2017; 21(74): 1-130.
[http://dx.doi.org/10.3310/hta21740] [PMID: 29231159]

[40] Wu T, Zhao WH, Dong Y, Song HX, Li JH. Effectiveness of Ultrasound-Guided *Versus* Fluoroscopy or Computed Tomography Scanning Guidance in Lumbar Facet Joint Injections in Adults With Facet Joint Syndrome: A Meta-Analysis of Controlled Trials. Arch Phys Med Rehabil 2016; 97(9): 1558-63.
[http://dx.doi.org/10.1016/j.apmr.2015.11.013] [PMID: 26705882]

[41] Boswell MV, Colson JD, Sehgal N, Dunbar EE, Epter R. A systematic review of therapeutic facet joint interventions in chronic spinal pain. Pain Physician 2007; 10(1): 229-53.

[http://dx.doi.org/10.36076/ppj.2007/10/229] [PMID: 17256032]

[42]   Walter SG, Schildberg FA, Rommelspacher Y. Endoscopic Sacrolumbar Facet Joint Denervation in Osteoarthritic and Degenerated Zygapophyseal Joints. Arthrosc Tech 2018; 7(12): e1275-9.
[http://dx.doi.org/10.1016/j.eats.2018.08.014] [PMID: 30591874]

[43]   Lee CH, Chung CK, Kim CH. The efficacy of conventional radiofrequency denervation in patients with chronic low back pain originating from the facet joints: a meta-analysis of randomized controlled trials. Spine J 2017; 17(11): 1770-80.
[http://dx.doi.org/10.1016/j.spinee.2017.05.006] [PMID: 28576500]

[44]   Rimmalapudi VK, Kumar S. Lumbar Radiofrequency Rhizotomy in Patients with Chronic Low Back Pain Increases the Diagnosis of Sacroiliac Joint Dysfunction in Subsequent Follow-Up Visits. Pain Res Manag > 2017.
[http://dx.doi.org/10.1155/2017/4830142]

[45]   Leon JF, Ortiz JG, Fonseca EO, Martinez CR, Cuellar GO. Radiofrequency Neurolysis for Lumbar Pain Using a Variation of the Original Technique. Pain Physician 2016; 19(3): 155-61.
[http://dx.doi.org/10.36076/ppj/2019.19.155] [PMID: 27008289]

[46]   Cohen SP, Bhaskar A, Bhatia A, *et al.* Consensus practice guidelines on interventions for lumbar facet joint pain from a multispecialty, international working group. Reg Anesth Pain Med 2020; 45(6): 424-67.
[http://dx.doi.org/10.1136/rapm-2019-101243] [PMID: 32245841]

[47]   Kallakuri S, Li Y, Chen C, Cavanaugh JM. Innervation of cervical ventral facet joint capsule: Histological evidence. World J Orthop 2012; 3(2): 10-4.
[http://dx.doi.org/10.5312/wjo.v3.i2.10] [PMID: 22470845]

[48]   Yin W, Willard F, Dixon T, Bogduk N. Ventral innervation of the lateral C1-C2 joint: an anatomical study. Pain Med 2008; 9(8): 1022-9.
[http://dx.doi.org/10.1111/j.1526-4637.2008.00493.x] [PMID: 18721172]

[49]   Zhou HY, Chen AM, Guo FJ, Liao GJ, Xiao WD. Sensory and sympathetic innervation of cervical facet joint in rats. Chin J Traumatol 2006; 9(6): 377-80.
[PMID: 17096935]

[50]   Casatti CA, Frigo L, Bauer JA. Origin of sensory and autonomic innervation of the rat temporomandibular joint: a retrograde axonal tracing study with the fluorescent dye fast blue. J Dent Res 1999; 78(3): 776-83.
[http://dx.doi.org/10.1177/00220345990780031001] [PMID: 10096453]

[51]   Yoshida N, Nishiyama K, Tonosaki Y, Kikuchi S, Sugiura Y. Sympathetic and sensory innervation of the rat shoulder joint: a WGA-HRP tracing and CGRP immunohistochemical study. Anat Embryol (Berl) 1995; 191(5): 465-9.
[http://dx.doi.org/10.1007/BF00304431] [PMID: 7625615]

[52]   Wiberg M, Widenfalk B. An anatomical study of the origin of sympathetic and sensory innervation of the elbow and knee joint in the monkey. Neurosci Lett 1991; 127(2): 185-8.
[http://dx.doi.org/10.1016/0304-3940(91)90790-Z] [PMID: 1881630]

[53]   Widenfalk B, Wiberg M. Origin of sympathetic and sensory innervation of the temporo-mandibular joint. A retrograde axonal tracing study in the rat. Neurosci Lett 1990; 109(1-2): 30-5.
[http://dx.doi.org/10.1016/0304-3940(90)90533-F] [PMID: 1690367]

[54]   Zwaan L, Monteiro S, Sherbino J, Ilgen J, Howey B, Norman G. Is bias in the eye of the beholder? A vignette study to assess recognition of cognitive biases in clinical case workups. BMJ Qual Saf 2017; 26(2): 104-10.
[http://dx.doi.org/10.1136/bmjqs-2015-005014] [PMID: 26825476]

[55]   Henriksen K, Kaplan H. Hindsight bias, outcome knowledge and adaptive learning. Qual Saf Health Care 2003; 12(12) (Suppl. 2): ii46-50.

[http://dx.doi.org/10.1136/qhc.12.suppl_2.ii46] [PMID: 14645895]

[56]   Noseworthy PA, Attia ZI, Brewer LC, *et al.* Assessing and Mitigating Bias in Medical Artificial Intelligence: The Effects of Race and Ethnicity on a Deep Learning Model for ECG Analysis. Circ Arrhythm Electrophysiol 2020; 13: e007988.
        [http://dx.doi.org/10.1161/CIRCEP.119.007988]

[57]   Sibbald M, Sherbino J, Ilgen JS, *et al.* Correction to: Debiasing *versus* knowledge retrieval checklists to reduce diagnostic error in ECG interpretation. Adv Health Sci Educ Theory Pract 2019; 24(3): 441-2.
        [http://dx.doi.org/10.1007/s10459-019-09884-7] [PMID: 30915640]

[58]   Sibbald M, Cavalcanti RB. The biasing effect of clinical history on physical examination diagnostic accuracy. Med Educ 2011; 45(8): 827-34.
        [http://dx.doi.org/10.1111/j.1365-2923.2011.03997.x] [PMID: 21752079]

[59]   Ahn Y, Lee SH. Outcome predictors of percutaneous endoscopic lumbar discectomy and thermal annuloplasty for discogenic low back pain. Acta Neurochir (Wien) 2010; 152(10): 1695-702.
        [http://dx.doi.org/10.1007/s00701-010-0726-2] [PMID: 20607314]

[60]   Grogan J, Nowicki BH, Schmidt TA, Haughton VM. Lumbar facet joint tropism does not accelerate degeneration of the facet joints. AJNR Am J Neuroradiol 1997; 18(7): 1325-9.
        [PMID: 9282864]

[61]   Mehling WE, Gopisetty V, Bartmess E, *et al.* The prognosis of acute low back pain in primary care in the United States: a 2-year prospective cohort study. Spine 2012; 37(8): 678-84.
        [http://dx.doi.org/10.1097/BRS.0b013e318230ab20] [PMID: 22504516]

[62]   Schwarzer AC, Aprill CN, Derby R, Fortin J, Kine G, Bogduk N. The prevalence and clinical features of internal disc disruption in patients with chronic low back pain. Spine 1995; 20(17): 1878-83.
        [http://dx.doi.org/10.1097/00007632-199509000-00007] [PMID: 8560335]

[63]   Croft PR, Macfarlane GJ, Papageorgiou AC, Thomas E, Silman AJ. Outcome of low back pain in general practice: a prospective study. BMJ 1998; 316(7141): 1356-9.
        [http://dx.doi.org/10.1136/bmj.316.7141.1356] [PMID: 9563990]

[64]   Schwarzer AC, Aprill CN, Derby R, Fortin J, Kine G, Bogduk N. The false-positive rate of uncontrolled diagnostic blocks of the lumbar zygapophysial joints. Pain 1994; 58(2): 195-200.
        [http://dx.doi.org/10.1016/0304-3959(94)90199-6] [PMID: 7816487]

[65]   Goldthwait JE. The lumbosacral articulation. An explanation of many cases of lumbago, sciatica, and paraplegia. Boston Med Surg J 1911; 164(11): 365-72.
        [http://dx.doi.org/10.1056/NEJM191103161641101]

[66]   Badgley CE. The articular facets in relation to low-back pain and sciatic radiation. 1941; 23: 481-96.

[67]   Carrera GF, Haughton VM, Syvertsen A, Williams AL. Computed tomography of the lumbar facet joints. Radiology 1980; 134(1): 145-8.
        [http://dx.doi.org/10.1148/radiology.134.1.7350594] [PMID: 7350594]

[68]   Helbig T, Lee CK. The lumbar facet syndrome. Spine 1988; 13(1): 61-4.
        [http://dx.doi.org/10.1097/00007632-198801000-00015] [PMID: 3381141]

[69]   Manchikanti L, Helm Ii S, Singh V, Hirsch JA. Accountable interventional pain management: a collaboration among practitioners, patients, payers, and government. Pain Physician 2013; 16(6): E635-70.
        [http://dx.doi.org/10.36076/ppj.2013/16/E635] [PMID: 24284849]

[70]   Nachemson AL. Newest knowledge of low back pain. A critical look. Clin Orthop Relat Res 1992; 279: 8-20.
        [http://dx.doi.org/10.1097/00003086-199206000-00003] [PMID: 1534725]

[71]   Raskin SP. Degenerative changes of the lumbar spine: assessment by computed tomography.

Orthopedics 1981; 4(2): 186-95.
[http://dx.doi.org/10.3928/0147-7447-19810201-13] [PMID: 24822600]

[72]   Lewinnek GE, Warfield CA. Facet joint degeneration as a cause of low back pain. Clin Orthop Relat Res 1986; 213(&NA;): 216-22.
[http://dx.doi.org/10.1097/00003086-198612000-00031] [PMID: 2946505]

[73]   Dreyer SJ, Dreyfuss PH. Low back pain and the zygapophysial (facet) joints. Arch Phys Med Rehabil 1996; 77(3): 290-300.
[http://dx.doi.org/10.1016/S0003-9993(96)90115-X] [PMID: 8600875]

[74]   Igarashi A, Kikuchi S, Konno S, Olmarker K. Inflammatory cytokines released from the facet joint tissue in degenerative lumbar spinal disorders. Spine 2004; 29(19): 2091-5.
[http://dx.doi.org/10.1097/01.brs.0000141265.55411.30] [PMID: 15454697]

[75]   Carette S, Marcoux S, Truchon R, *et al.* A controlled trial of corticosteroid injections into facet joints for chronic low back pain. N Engl J Med 1991; 325(14): 1002-7.
[http://dx.doi.org/10.1056/NEJM199110033251405] [PMID: 1832209]

[76]   Shealy CN. Percutaneous radiofrequency denervation of spinal facets. Treatment for chronic back pain and sciatica. J Neurosurg 1975; 43(4): 448-51.
[http://dx.doi.org/10.3171/jns.1975.43.4.0448] [PMID: 125787]

[77]   Andersen KH, Mosdal C, Vaernet K. Percutaneous radiofrequency facet denervation in low-back and extremity pain. Acta Neurochir (Wien) 1987; 87(1-2): 48-51.
[http://dx.doi.org/10.1007/BF02076015] [PMID: 2960131]

[78]   Cho J, Park YG, Chung SS. Percutaneous radiofrequency lumbar facet rhizotomy in mechanical low back pain syndrome. Stereotact Funct Neurosurg 1997; 68(1-4 Pt 1): 212-7.
[http://dx.doi.org/10.1159/000099926] [PMID: 9711719]

[79]   Dreyfuss P, Halbrook B, Pauza K, Joshi A, McLarty J, Bogduk N. Efficacy and validity of radiofrequency neurotomy for chronic lumbar zygapophysial joint pain. Spine 2000; 25(10): 1270-7.
[http://dx.doi.org/10.1097/00007632-200005150-00012] [PMID: 10806505]

[80]   Göçer AI, Cetinalp E, Tuna M, Ildan F, Bağdatoğlu H, Haciyakupoğlu S. Percutaneous radiofrequency rhizotomy of lumbar spinal facets: the results of 46 cases. Neurosurg Rev 1997; 20(2): 114-6.
[http://dx.doi.org/10.1007/BF01138194] [PMID: 9226670]

[81]   Mehta M, Sluijter ME. The treatment of chronic back pain. A preliminary survey of the effect of radiofrequency denervation of the posterior vertebral joints. Anaesthesia 1979; 34(8): 768-75.
[http://dx.doi.org/10.1111/j.1365-2044.1979.tb06410.x] [PMID: 160757]

[82]   Ferrante FM, King LF, Roche EA, *et al.* Radiofrequency sacroiliac joint denervation for sacroiliac syndrome. Reg Anesth Pain Med 2001; 26(2): 137-42.
[http://dx.doi.org/10.1053/rapm.2001.21739] [PMID: 11251137]

[83]   Vallejo R, Benyamin RM, Kramer J, Stanton G, Joseph NJ. Pulsed radiofrequency denervation for the treatment of sacroiliac joint syndrome. Pain Med 2006; 7(5): 429-34.
[http://dx.doi.org/10.1111/j.1526-4637.2006.00143.x] [PMID: 17014602]

[84]   Stolker RJ, Vervest AC, Groen GJ. Percutaneous facet denervation in chronic thoracic spinal pain. Acta Neurochir (Wien) 1993; 122(1-2): 82-90.
[http://dx.doi.org/10.1007/BF01446991] [PMID: 8333313]

[85]   Kanpolat Y, Berk C, Savas A, Bekar A. Percutaneous controlled radiofrequency rhizotomy in the management of patients with trigeminal neuralgia due to multiple sclerosis. Acta Neurochir (Wien) 2000; 142(6): 685-9.
[http://dx.doi.org/10.1007/s007010070113] [PMID: 10949444]

[86]   Mathews ES, Scrivani SJ. Percutaneous stereotactic radiofrequency thermal rhizotomy for the treatment of trigeminal neuralgia. Mt Sinai J Med 2000; 67(4): 288-99.
[PMID: 11021779]

[87]   Kanpolat Y, Savas A, Bekar A, Berk C. Percutaneous controlled radiofrequency trigeminal rhizotomy for the treatment of idiopathic trigeminal neuralgia: 25-year experience with 1,600 patients. Neurosurgery 2001; 48(3): 524-32.
        [http://dx.doi.org/10.1097/00006123-200103000-00013] [PMID: 11270542]

[88]   Rocco AG. Radiofrequency lumbar sympatholysis. The evolution of a technique for managing sympathetically maintained pain. Reg Anesth 1995; 20(1): 3-12.
        [PMID: 7727325]

[89]   Manchikanti L. The role of radiofrequency in the management of complex regional pain syndrome. Curr Rev Pain 2000; 4(6): 437-44.
        [http://dx.doi.org/10.1007/s11916-000-0067-6] [PMID: 11060589]

[90]   Sjaastad O, Stolt-Nielsen A, Blume H, Zwart JA, Fredriksen TA. Cervicogenic headache. Long-term results of radiofrequency treatment of the planum nuchale. Funct Neurol 1995; 10(6): 265-71.
        [PMID: 8837990]

[91]   Stolker RJ, Vervest AC, Groen GJ. The treatment of chronic thoracic segmental pain by radiofrequency percutaneous partial rhizotomy. J Neurosurg 1994; 80(6): 986-92.
        [http://dx.doi.org/10.3171/jns.1994.80.6.0986] [PMID: 8189279]

[92]   van Kleef M, Barendse GA, Kessels A, Voets HM, Weber WE, de Lange S. Randomized trial of radiofrequency lumbar facet denervation for chronic low back pain. Spine 1999; 24(18): 1937-42.
        [http://dx.doi.org/10.1097/00007632-199909150-00013] [PMID: 10515020]

[93]   Leclaire R, Fortin L, Lambert R, Bergeron YM, Rossignol M. Radiofrequency facet joint denervation in the treatment of low back pain: a placebo-controlled clinical trial to assess efficacy. Spine 2001; 26(13): 1411-6.
        [http://dx.doi.org/10.1097/00007632-200107010-00003] [PMID: 11458140]

[94]   Jacobson RE, Palea O, Granville M. Bipolar Radiofrequency Facet Ablation of the Lumbar Facet Capsule: An Adjunct to Conventional Radiofrequency Ablation for Pain Management. Cureus 2017; 9: e1635.
        [http://dx.doi.org/10.7759/cureus.1635]

[95]   Xue Y, Ding T, Wang D, *et al.* Endoscopic rhizotomy for chronic lumbar zygapophysial joint pain J Orthop Surg Res 2020; 15: 4.
        [http://dx.doi.org/10.1186/s13018-019-1533-y]

CHAPTER 13

Visualized Endoscopic Radiofrequency Ablation of Sinuvertebral Nerve and Basivertebral Nerve for Chronic Discogenic Back Pain

Pang Hung Wu[1,2], **Hyeun Sung Kim**[1,*] and **Il-Tae Jang**[1]

[1] *Department of Neurosurgery, Nanoori Hospital, Gangnam, Seoul, South Korea*

[2] *National University Health System, Jurong Health Campus, Orthopaedic Surgery, Singapore*

Abstract: Chronic discogenic back pain is a leading cause of disability in man. Degenerative disc disease and its associated pathological neurotization of the sinuvertebral and basivertebral nerve are some of the mechanisms that lead to lower back pain. The use of radiofrequency ablation to denervate pathological sensitized sinuvertebral and basivertebral nerve has been described to decrease pain in patients with degenerative disc disease. Radiofrequency energy system can be introduced into the region of sinuvertebral and basivertebral nerve *via* inside out and outside in technique through fluoroscopic and/or endoscopic guidance. This chapter discusses the methods of outside-in-endoscopic guided radiofrequency ablation of sinuvertebral and basivertebral nerves.

Keywords: Basivertebral nerve, Chronic discogenic back pain, Degenerative disc disease, Neurotization, Radiofrequency energy system, Sinuvertebral nerve.

INTRODUCTION

Lower back pain affects 70-85% of people during their lifetime, and recurred back pain episodes are as high as 85% [1]. Multiple factors can contribute to lower back pain, including degenerative disc disease, facet arthritis, lumbar prolapsed intervertebral disc, lumbar spondylolysis, and spondylolisthesis. Most of the time, more than one concurrent factor may lead to lower back pain. Management of degenerative disc disease ranges from conservative management, restorative therapy, reconstructive therapy, and surgery [2]. A normal intervertebral disc is avascular, aneural, and mechanically stable.

---

* **Corresponding author Hyeun-Sung Kim:** Department of Neurosurgery, Nanoori Hospital, Gangnam, Seoul, South Korea; Tel: +82-10-2440-2631; E-mail: neurospinekim@gmail.com

Disruption of the intervertebral disc's mechanical and anatomical structure leads to an inflammatory response with the generation with its secreted cytokines and vascular factors, which leads to neurotization of the diseased disc [3]. This pathological neurotization leads to the sensitization of native sinuvertebral and basivertebral nerves around the disc. These nerves send pain signals to the central nervous system. They are leading to hyperalgesia and allodynia of normal and increased load to the affected disc [4]. Radiofrequency ablation of these pathological nerves can provide sustained relief for patients who suffer from lower back pain [5].

RATIONALE

Pathoanatomical and Pathophysiological Considerations of Degenerated Lumbar Intervertebral Disc Structural Degeneration

Necrosis of chondrocyte-like cells in the nucleus is a natural process with an accelerating rate (with age 2% at birth to 50% in adulthood). This degeneration and necrosis accelerate during pathological processes such as prolapsed intervertebral disc (PID). Structural changes in the spinal column include syndesmophyte formation, osteophyte at the facet joint, decreased disc height, and stiffening of the intervertebral disc (IVD) [5]. Degenerative disc disease results from complex multifactorial etiology interplay of structural changes, genetics, trauma, environmental factors, and aging.

Triggers for accelerated degeneration: In the literature, several trigger events are attributed to DDD progression. They are: 1) alteration of coronal and sagittal parameters, 2) ligamentous laxity and muscle imbalance, 3) excessive mechanical load or repetitive and chronic exposure to high mechanical load, 4) predisposing genetics vulnerability, 5) smoking, obesity, and diabetes mellitus 6) Nutritional deficiency [5].

Inflammatory Cascade, Neuronal Sensitization and Pathologic Neuronization of the Disc

Inflammatory response plays a crucial role in the induction of hyperalgesia of the disc. Animals experiments showed that exposure of the ruptured nucleus could lead to increase inflammation around the ruptured area [4]. We found significant neovascularization and adhesive tissue around the region of disc degeneration, sinuvertebral, and basivertebral nerve region.

Anatomy of Sinuvertebral Nerve and Basiverebral Nerve (BVN)

Dr. Hubert von Luschka described the sinuvertebral nerve (SVN) in 1850 as a sympathetic nerve derived from the spinal nerve. There are extensive intersegmental anastomoses with extension to posterior annulus fibrosus. The sinuvertebral nerve is derived by combining the somatic root from the ventral ramus and autonomic root by grey ramus. It supplies both proprioceptive and pain fibers to join at grey ramus communicans. After joining grey ramus communicans, it has a recurrent course to the spinal canal through intervertebral foramen along the upper portion of the pedicle cephalad to the corresponding disc. It gives rise to an ascending branch, which goes intraosseous to provide an increase to Basivertebral Nerve. Basivertebral nerve (BVN) is a nerve in pairs as branches from SVN, which provides nociceptive transmission for endplates, which enters the vertebral body from the central vascular foramen around the endplates. It arises from the ascending branch of sinuvertebral nerves, which goes intraosseous and give rise to Basivertebral Nerves near the upper medial pedicle [5, 6]. Sinuvertebral nerve also gives out a descending branch that supplies adjacent to the posterior longitudinal ligament and disc. This is the region which we target for sinuvertebral nerve radiofrequency ablation (Fig. **1**) [7].

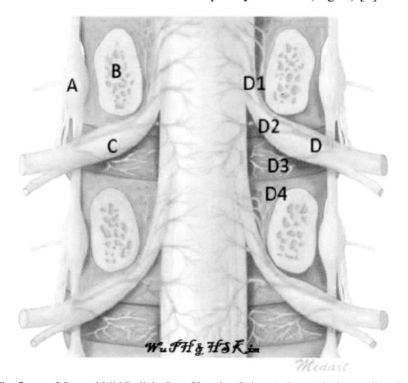

Fig. (1). The figure of Coronal Mid Pedicle Cut of Lumbar Spine. A: Sympathetic ganglion, B: Pedicle, C: Dorsal Root Ganglion, D: Sinuvertebral Nerve giving rise to branches D1: Ascending branch, which goes intraosseous and gives rise to Basivertebral Nerve near the pedicle D4, D2: Descending Branch supplying adjacent to Posterior longitudinal ligament and disc, D3: Direct branches to intervertebral disc.

Current Radiofrequency Ablation Approaches For Denervation

There are two common paths for radiofrequency ablation (RFA) for pathologically sensitized sinuvertebral and basivertebral nerve. The intradiscal method and extra-discal approach. The intradiscal approach utilizes a fluoroscopic transforaminal approach with herniotomy and a small amount of disc removal (manual discectomy) to create a path of access for the radiofrequency probe. The radiofrequency ablation was performed with the probe at specific spots guided by fluoroscopy (nucleus ablation and annulus modulation) [8]. Extra discal approach is popularized by Kim and Wu *et al.* with endoscopic guided targeted access to an area of peridiscal region of sinuvertebral and basivertebral nerves. The location of sinuvertebral and basivertebral nerves have typical features of neovascularization and adhesion of various grades. Upon early contact with radiofrequency ablation, the patient will have twitching of the buttock and possibly the leg (Kim's Twitch). Upon completion of radiofrequency ablation, the leg's twitching would not recur even if the radiofrequency ablation is applied on the same spot. Details of the technique would be discussed in the next segments [5]. There are two parts to this procedure. First, we provide space and access to the spinal canal, providing appropriate exposure to the region of SVN and BVN. The second is for thermal shrinkage of disc bulge/protrusion.

Diagnostic Procedure For Candidates Suitable For Radiofrequency Ablation Of Pathological Nerves

Lower back pain tends to have multifactorial causes. Careful and meticulous patient selection is paramount to the success of this procedure. Patient with discogenic back pain typically presents with mechanical lower back pain, which radiates to the affected buttock and sometimes even the affected dermatome. There is no sign of numbness of weakness suggestive of nerve compression. MRI performed showed degenerative disc disease with or without annular tear with high signal intensity zone (HIZ) signal changes without significant neural compression. A provocative discogram is performed to confirm discogenic back pain is the primary source of pain. For our chapter, we exclude cases of patients who have a concurrent herniated disc and spinal stenosis.

Anesthesia and Positioning

Our patients underwent general anesthesia, and a single dose of intravenous antibiotics was given. The patient's face was placed in a commercial anesthesia pillow foam supporting bony prominence with space created for eyes, nose, and mouth. The patient positioned prone on the Wilson frame on top of the radiolucent operating table with thorax and abdomen free of external pressure.

The patient's arms were tucked longitudinally and padded next to the patient. The hips and knees were flexed slightly with padding.

SURGICAL STEPS

Transforaminal Approach

The surgeon stands on the same side of the painful back and leg. The skin is marked to the lumbar spine's corresponding degenerated disc level defined under the fluoroscopic guidance of anteroposterior (AP) and lateral view. We use manual palpation and fluoroscopic guidance to mark the skin start point for the approach. The skin incision chosen should aim for the most distal and dorsal end of Kambin's triangle on the target intervertebral disc in a slight 5- 10° cephalad caudal direction 25-35° to horizontal in the axial plane with 12-14 cm from the midline of the lumbar spinous process (Fig. **2**). The projected trajectory shown in fluoroscopy should land on the HIZ seen on MRI. Local anesthesia under monitored sedation is given in the standard fashion. We may use indigo carmine if there is planned discectomy, but if the primary intention is only for RFA, then indigo carmine is optional. We performed a mobile outside-in technique [9]. Skin incision made with serial dilation is done and docked with the open beveled working cannula. We use an endoscope with a 30° viewing angle, 7.3 mm outer diameter, and 4.7 mm working channel, 251 mm length transforaminal endoscope. The procedure was performed under continuous irrigation with normal saline at hydraulic pressures not exceeding 25 mm Hg. We try to minimize the endoscopically guided foraminoplasty as far as possible unless there is concomitant foraminal or lateral recess stenosis. After docking on the most distal and dorsal point of Kambin's triangle, a small amount of discectomy is done under endoscopic visualization with fluoroscopic guidance to provide space for access to the region of SVN and BVN. SVN exposure is required to create space 3-5mm caudal to the center of the distal aspect of annulus.

To provide RFA to SVN, we need to remove the degenerated disc dorsal portion annulus in the HIZ region [10]. Posterior longitudinal ligament should be preserved while doing the annuolotomy. SVN region is commonly just caudal to the center of the annulus. SVN is identified, and RFA is applied. After completion of SVN RFA. We proceed to the BVN region, the location at the upper medial part of the pedicle. We usually need some dorsal portion of annulotomy to gain access to the upper medial aspect of the pedicle. Both SVN and BVN region typically shows neovascularization and adhesive inflammatory granulation tissues. On the initial application of RFA, Kim's twitch is observed; upon completion of RFA to SVN, Kim's twitch subsides.

The patient is no longer twitching in the lower extremity in response to the RFA [5]. No drain is required for this procedure, and the patient can mobilize within the same day.

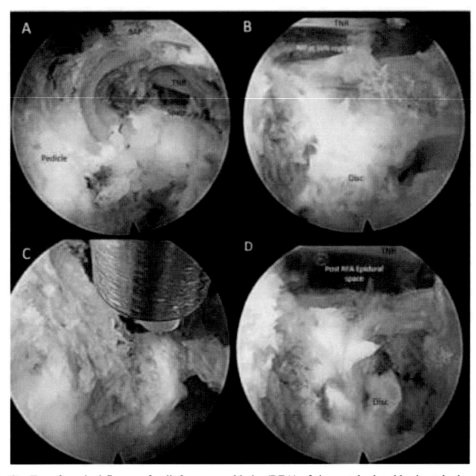

Fig. (2). Transforaminal figures of radiofrequency ablation(RFA) of sinuvertebral and basivertebral nerves. Fig. (**2A**): After the mobile outside-in technique, drilling the base of superior articular process (SAP) and pedicle, traversing nerve root(TNR), and epidural space is exposed and disc space-separated posterior longitudinal ligament. Fig. (**2B**): Granulation tissue medial to the upper portion of the pedicle with neovascularization (NV) marked the basivertebral nerve site. Fig. (**2C**): RFA is applied to the upper medial part of the pedicle at the basivertebral Nerve region. Fig. (**2D**): Post RFA application, the granulation tissue is ablated with free nerve root pulsation under endoscopic fluid hydrostatic pressure.

Interlaminar Approach

The procedure is done under regional or general anesthesia. The endoscope is docked on the intervertebral disc line's junction and medial to the facet joint on the superficial flavum under fluoroscopic guidance. Serial dilation is done and anchored with an open beveled working cannula. An endoscope with a 30°

viewing angle, 7.3 mm outer diameter and 4.7 mm working channel, 251 mm length is inserted. A shorter length endoscope with a small diameter can be used as well. To minimize ligament disruption, the ligamentum flavum splitting technique using a blunt probe and working cannula to hold the split ligamentum flavum apart is used to perform the procedure (Fig. **3**). We gain access to the region of SVN and BVN by retracting the neural elements out of harm's way with the help of a working cannula. We advance and rotate the working cannula counterclockwise on the left and clockwise on the right when we attempt to retract the traversing and exiting nerve root. We can gently medialize the working cannula once we retract the nerve out of harm's way to expose the SVN in the region of caudal to the disc. After SVN RFA completion, we can move the working cannula to the region of BVN in the upper and medial portion of the pedicle to complete BVN RFA. Similar findings of neovascularization and adhesion, as well as Kim's twitch, is seen in this technique for affirmation of the locations of SVN and BVN. Unlike the transforaminal approach, we do not need to do annulotomy in this approach.

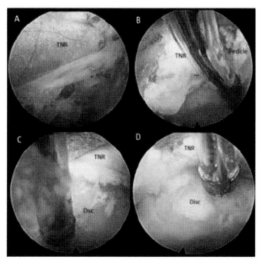

Fig. (3). Interlaminar approach to radiofrequency ablation. Fig. (**3A**): Epidural fat in the lateral recess adjacent to the traversing nerve root (TNR). Fig. (**3B**): Working cannula retraction of traversing nerve root to expose the pedicle's upper medial part for basivertebral nerve RFA. Fig. (**3C**): Retract the traversing nerve root medially to expose the disc for thermal shrinkage of bulging dis. Fig. (**3D**): RFA applied to the area of sinuvertebral nerve just caudal to the disc space.

Thermal Shrinkage Of Bulging Degenerative Disc.

Upon completion of SVN and BVN radiofrequency ablation, thermal energy is applied to degenerated disc annulus to shrink the bulging degenerative disc.

Skin Closure And Postoperative Rehabilitation Protocol

No drain is required. Skin is closed in layers with tissue glue to the skin. The patient can be prescribed with a brace for comfort and soft tissue recovery. They mobilized on the same day and can be discharged from the hospital.

Key Feature Of Radiofrequency Ablation Technique

There are three critical differences in endoscopic RFA of SVN and BVN compared to percutaneous RFA described ubiquitously in literature.

1. Transforaminal or interlaminar approach through the epidural space in peridiscal region dorsal and caudal to the posterior annulus in epidural space for SVN and adjacent to pedicle BVN as compared to intradiscal for percutaneous RFA.
2. Direct visualization of granulation tissue, neovascularization, and adhesive tissue in the region of SVN and BVN.
3. Clinical response of Kim's twitch upon RFA application to SVN and BVN, which disappears when SVN and BVN had been ablated.

POTENTIAL RISKS

The procedure's potential risks include wrong-level surgery, excessive discal resection leading to instability for transforaminal approach, exiting nerve root injury (dysesthesia, motor, and sensory deficit) in the transforaminal approach, dura tear and direct nerve root injury in both approaches, recurrence of SVN and BVN pain, and the progression of degeneration.

CLINICAL SERIES

In Nanoori Hospital Gangnam, Seoul, the Republic of Korea, 36 levels of Endoscopic RFA of SVN and BVN were performed in 30 patients from 1st June 2016 to 1st June 2018. Out of which 11 patients underwent one level(L4/5), 15 patients underwent one level L5/S1, and four patients underwent multi-level RFA., 6 cases were done with the transforaminal approach. Additional cases were performed with the interlaminar method. Overall preoperative, 1week, six months, and final follow up. All except 2 had the clinical sign of Kim's twitch. The 2 cases without Kim's twitch had less improvement in VAS and ODI scores. VAS score and ODI for preoperative, one week, six months, and final follow-up in the first patient was VAS(6,4,4,4), ODI (64,42,38,38), respectively. The second patient was VAS (8,4,3,4) and ODI (80,36,32,38), respectively, with a fair MacNab score for both cases. There was a statistically significant improvement in VAS score with mean and range of preoperative, one week, six months, and at final follow up of 7.37 (6–8), 2.96 (2–4), 1.97 (1–4), and 1.67 (1–4), respectively. Using a paired T-test, the VAS score mean differences between 1 week, six months, and at final follow-up with preoperative were 4.4 ± 1.0, 5.5 ± 1.2, and 5.7 ± 1.3, respectively ($p < 0.0001$). There was a statistically significant improvement in ODI score with mean and range of preoperative, one week, six months and at final follow up are 73.83 (62–86), 28.07 (20–42), 23.47 (18–38), and 21.13 (2–38) The mean improvement of ODI at 1week, six months and final follow up compared with preoperative values are 45.8 ± 8.7, 50.4 ± 8.2 and 52.7 ± 10.3, $p < 0.0001$. MacNab's criteria showed excellent outcomes in 17 cases, good outcomes in 11 patients, and fair outcomes in another two.

DISCUSSION

Chronic lower back pain is one of the significant causes of disability around the world [11]. Pain generators in lower back pain can be from facet arthropathy, degenerative disc disease, and related discogenic and Modic changes related back problems, spinal stenosis, and spinal instability [2]. Patient selection is key to a successful procedure outcome. Patients with yellow flags such as workmen compensation, psychiatric history, financial gain from disability, and patients with physical findings that displayed positive Waddell signs are best to be excluded for endoscopic RFA. Patients who have mechanical discogenic back pain would benefit from a preoperative diagnostic discogram. Those who had failed conservative treatment with positive discogram and well counseled for risk and benefits of endoscopic RFA SVN and BVN are candidates for this procedure [2].

Percutaneous RFA to HIZ zone and the adjacent region has good clinical efficacy [8]. However, the needle trajectory is key to the procedure, and being fluoroscopic guided, there is an element of uncertainty whether the RFA is applied to the correct target. Hence, the surgeon/pain specialist who performs the procedure tends to RFA a broader region than the target zone's expected area to achieve an effective RFA. Endoscopic RFA had been applied to the sacroiliac joint with good clinical efficacy. The sacroiliac joint being more superficial and external to epidural space, is a favorable region for endoscopic RFA [12].

Endoscopic RFA, introduced in this chapter, provided an option to improve the visualization and efficacy in achieving the target region of SVN and BVN. Proposing an RFA procedure without the need for decompression, we advise minimizing bony and soft tissue trauma by minimizing foraminoplasty in the transforaminal approach and using the ligamentum splitting technique in the interlaminar approach. Minimal removal of bone and soft tissue helps in the preservation of bony structures and preventing epidural scarring. With the clear visualization of neural structures, the RFA can be applied safely and effectively to the specific region with neural structures protected out of harm's way by the open beveled working cannula. RFA can be applied directly at projected SVN and BVN regions with Kim's twitch's clinical response. These procedural steps ensure consistency and reproducibility.

This procedure's main limitation is the lack of long-term data and the scarcity of literature on this technique and its results. Despite our success from long-term effects with a mean follow-up of 14.9 (6-31) months, from our RFA experience in the sacroiliac joint and medial branch, there is a possible recurrence of pain after successful RFA in the initial few months to years [13]. More studies and scientific understanding of SVN and BVN pathophysiology, neurotization, and pathoanatomy is required. The science behind pathological nerve regeneration after RFA needs to be better understood to give a better insight into the treatment of this group of pathologies.

TECHNICAL PEARLS

In the authors' opinion, there are the following surgical pearls of the procedures:

1. Preoperative evaluation should aim to localize the area of pain to be discogenic or Modic changes related pain secondary to degenerative disc disease. MRI findings of degenerative disc disease with Modic changes and high-intensity zone (HIZ). Patients with positive discograms are good candidates for Endoscopic RFA.
2. Concurrent spinal conditions such as spinal stenosis and disc herniation takes precedence over RFA of SVN and BVN. They can be treated in the same setting as endoscopic decompression and discectomy
3. Spinal instability is a relative contraindication to RFA SVN and BVN. These patients would benefit from fusion.
4. Endoscopic drilling and foraminoplasty should be limited to avoid spinal instability in endoscopic RFA. Mobile outside in or direct inside out technique is the preferred method of transforaminal approach.
5. Sinuvertebral nerves branches to the disc where RFA is applied are located in the region caudal to the distal dorsal part of the annulus in the paracentral region
6. Basivertebral nerve branches arise from the ascending branch of the sinuvertebral nerve near the upper medial pedicle.
7. Open beveled working cannula is used to retract and protect neural elements out of harms' way
8. Area of granulation and neovascularization is observed in the region of pathological neurotization of SVN and BVN, RFA is applied directly at these regions

9. Kim's twitch corresponds favorably at the correct area of RFA application.

CONCLUSION

Endoscopic RFA is a minimally invasive precise, and safe treatment strategy for discogenic back pain secondary to sinuvertebral and basivertebral nerves pathological sensitization.

CONSENT FOR PUBLICATION

Not applicable.

CONFLICT OF INTEREST

The authors declare no conflict of interest, financial or otherwise.

ACKNOWLEDGEMENT

Declared none.

REFERENCES

[1] Fritzell P, Hägg O, Jonsson D, Nordwall A. Cost-effectiveness of lumbar fusion and nonsurgical treatment for chronic low back pain in the Swedish Lumbar Spine Study: a multicenter, randomized, controlled trial from the Swedish Lumbar Spine Study Group. Spine 2004; 29(4): 421-34.
[http://dx.doi.org/10.1097/01.BRS.0000102681.61791.12] [PMID: 15094539]

[2] Wu PH, Kim HS, Jang I-T. Intervertebral Disc Diseases PART 2: A Review of the Current Diagnostic and Treatment Strategies for Intervertebral Disc Disease. Int J Mol Sci 2020; 21(6): 2135.
[http://dx.doi.org/10.3390/ijms21062135] [PMID: 32244936]

[3] Simon J, McAuliffe M, Shamim F, Vuong N, Tahaei A. Discogenic low back pain. Phys Med Rehabil Clin N Am 2014; 25(2): 305-17.
[http://dx.doi.org/10.1016/j.pmr.2014.01.006] [PMID: 24787335]

[4] Risbud MV, Shapiro IM. Role of cytokines in intervertebral disc degeneration: pain and disc content. Nat Rev Rheumatol 2014; 10(1): 44-56.
[http://dx.doi.org/10.1038/nrrheum.2013.160] [PMID: 24166242]

[5] Kim HS, Wu PH, Jang I-T. Lumbar Degenerative Disease Part 1: Anatomy and Pathophysiology of Intervertebral Discogenic Pain and Radiofrequency Ablation of Basivertebral and Sinuvertebral Nerve Treatment for Chronic Discogenic Back Pain: A Prospective Case Series and Review of Literature. Int J Mol Sci 2020; 21(4): 1483.
[http://dx.doi.org/10.3390/ijms21041483] [PMID: 32098249]

[6] Fischgrund JS, Rhyne A, Franke J, *et al.* Intraosseous Basivertebral Nerve Ablation for the Treatment of Chronic Low Back Pain: 2-Year Results From a Prospective Randomized Double-Blind Sham-Controlled Multicenter Study. Int J Spine Surg 2019; 13(2): 110-9.
[http://dx.doi.org/10.14444/6015] [PMID: 31131209]

[7] Cavanaugh JM, Ozaktay AC, Yamashita T, Avramov A, Getchell TV, King AI. Mechanisms of low back pain: a neurophysiologic and neuroanatomic study. Clin Orthop Relat Res 1997; 335: 166-80.
[http://dx.doi.org/10.1097/00003086-199702000-00016] [PMID: 9020216]

[8] Kumar N, Kumar A, Siddharth MS, *et al.* Annulo-nucleoplasty using Disc-FX in the management of

lumbar disc pathology: early results. International journal of spine surgery 2014.
[http://dx.doi.org/10.14444/1018]

[9]   Kim HS, Adsul N, Kapoor A, *et al.* A Mobile Outside-in Technique of Transforaminal Lumbar Endoscopy for Lumbar Disc Herniations. J Vis Exp 2018; (138):
[http://dx.doi.org/10.3791/57999] [PMID: 30148483]

[10]   Kim HS, Kashlan ON, Singh R, *et al.* Percutaneous Transforaminal Endoscopic Radiofrequency Ablation of the Sinuvertebral Nerve in an Olympian with a Left L5 Pedicle/Pars Interarticularis Fracture-Associated Left L5-S1 Disk Desiccation. World Neurosurg X 2019; 3: 100032.
[http://dx.doi.org/10.1016/j.wnsx.2019.100032] [PMID: 31225524]

[11]   Vos T, Flaxman ADP, Naghavi M, *et al.* Years lived with disability (YLDs) for 1160 sequelae of 289 diseases and injuries 1990-2010: a systematic analysis for the Global Burden of Disease Study 2010. Lancet 2012; 380(9859): 2163-96.
[http://dx.doi.org/10.1016/S0140-6736(12)61729-2] [PMID: 23245607]

[12]   Ibrahim R, Telfeian AE, Gohlke K, Decker O. Endoscopic Radiofrequency Treatment of the Sacroiliac Joint Complex for Low Back Pain: A Prospective Study with a 2-Year Follow-Up. Pain Physician 2019; 22(2): E111-8.
[PMID: 30921988]

[13]   Choi EJ, Choi YM, Jang EJ, *et al.* Neural Ablation and Regeneration in Pain Practice. Korean J Pain 2016; 29: 3-11.
[http://dx.doi.org/10.3344/kjp.2016.29.1.3]

CHAPTER 14

Endoscopic Resection of Schwannoma in the Psoas Major Muscle

Yan Yuqu[1], **Bu Rongqiang**[1], **Zhang Xifeng**[1,*] and **An Sixing**[1]

[1] *Department of Orthopedics, First Medical Center, PLA General Hospital, Beijing, 100853, China*

Abstract: Surgical treatment of benign tumors of the spine when required is still aggressive compared to the lack of malignancy of the underlying disease process. While such lesions rarely cause systemic problems, grow slowly, and rarely degenerate into the malignant lesions or metastasize, their open surgical treatment rivals that done for malignant lesions causing tremendous exposure-related collateral damage from tissue dissections, blood loss, and scarring of the surgical corridor. Endoscopic spinal surgery techniques offer an attractive alternative to gain access and visualize areas deep to the spine that ordinarily would require complicated anterior, posterior, or even combined approaches to decompress and stabilize iatrogenic instability. In this chapter, the authors present an exemplary case of applying endoscopy to treating benign nerve sheath tumors of the lumbar spine – a schwannoma.

Keywords: Benign tumor, Endoscopic decompression, Lumbar nerve compression.

INTRODUCTION

Degenerative conditions of the spine are the most common reason patients seek spine surgeons' attention to alleviate pain and improve function. At the heart of every spinal surgery is neural element decompression and, in some cases, stabilization of the spine when dictated by the underlying disease or when the decompression induces instability [1]. It is only understandable that endoscopic spine surgery is venturing out of the degenerative arena [2 - 13] into other spine surgery areas where infections and tumors may be the underlying cause of pain and disability. In this chapter, the authors present such an example where a tumorous paraspinal lesion was treated with full endoscopic techniques.

---

[*] **Corresponding author Zhang Xifeng:** Department of Orthopedics, First Medical Center, PLA General Hospital, Beijing, 100853, China; Tel: +86 (10) 8821 9862; E-mail: xifengzhang301@163.com

Kai-Uwe Lewandrowski, Jorge Felipe Ramírez León, Anthony Yeung, Hyeun-Sung Kim, Xifeng Zhang, Gun Choi, Stefan Hellinger and Álvaro Dowling (Eds.)

EXEMPLARY CASE

The patient is a 76-year-old female with a chief complaint of pain and numbness radiating into the left lower extremity for three years, which was recently aggravated for the last three months before presenting to our hospital. Most recently, the patient's complaint included pain and numbness in the buttock, now radiating to the left heel. She had tried several traditional Chinese Medicine modalities, including acupuncture, massage, and physiotherapy, none of which were effective. At its worst, the patient had symptoms at rest, which were slightly relieved by standing up and ambulation. The physical examination did not reveal any apparent abnormalities. There were negative upper motor neuron signs. The lumbar MRI scan produced at admission to our hospital did not show any obvious abnormalities within the spinal canal or the foramina. However, there were circular patterns with a mixed-signal in the left psoas major muscle at the L3-4 level, which seemed to be emanating from the left spinal canal (Figs. **1** and **2**). Because of failed non-operative care and the worrisome lesion in the left psoas major muscle, the indication for an excisional biopsy was determined. To minimize the collateral damage to reaching the psoas muscle, an endoscopic approach under local anesthesia under videoendoscopic and fluoroscopic control was planned.

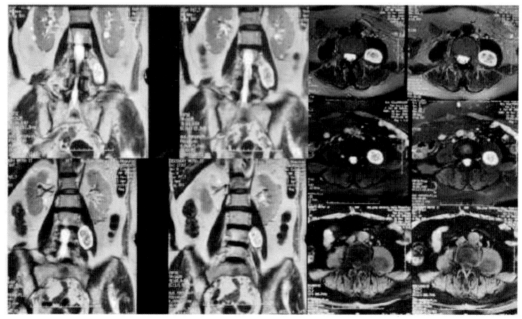

Fig. (1). Coronal and axial T1- and T2-weighted MRI scans of the patient diagnosed with a Schwannoma in the left psoas major likely emanating from the L3/4 level.

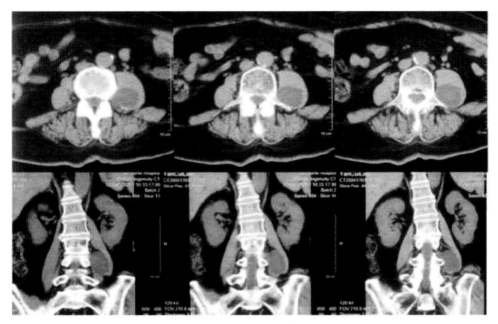

Fig. (2). CT examination of lumbar spine shows a space occupying lesion in the psoas major muscle on the left side at the lumbar 3-4 level.

SURGICAL PROCEDURE

The patient was placed on a Wilson frame in the prone position and prepped and draped in standard surgical fashion. The L4 vertebral body was marked employing intraoperative fluoroscopy. The lesion was approached approximately 5 – 6 cm from the midline on the left side The needle entry point was infiltrated with local anesthesia using 20 ml of 2% lidocaine mixed with 40 ml 0.9% sodium chloride. Under fluoroscopic confirmation, a spinal needle was vertically inserted about 6 cms to the left of the L4 transverse process. A guidewire was inserted through the spinal needle, which was then removed. After serial dilation, the working cannula was placed onto the L4 transverse process. The endoscope was inserted to directly visualize the space-occupying lesion within the left psoas major muscle.

After initial exploration and dissection, a 2.5 x 3 cm mass could clearly be demarcated from the surrounding area. A soft and light yellow mass was seen. The surrounding muscle tissue was dissected of the mass using a disposable radiofrequency probe under direct endoscopic visualization. Pituitary rongeurs were also used during the dissection. After excisional biopsy of the lesion was completed, the wound was thoroughly irrigated and the endoscopic instruments were withdrawn after wich the wound was closed with a single stitch. Some representative intraoperative images are shown in Figs. (**3 - 5**).

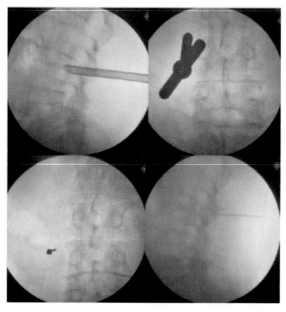

Fig. (3). Intraoperative fluoroscopy images illustrated the targeting and working cannula placement to access a space occupying lesion in the psoas major muscle on the left side at the lumbar 3-4 level.

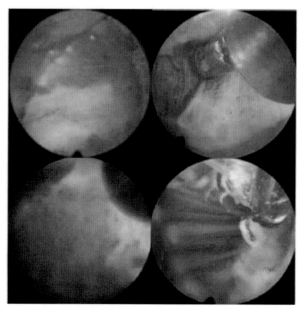

Fig. (4). Intraoperative endoscopic images of the space occupying lesion in the psoas major muscle on the left side at the lumbar 3-4 level. The mass was yellow in color and easily dissected of the surrounding muscle tissue with a radiofrequency probe.

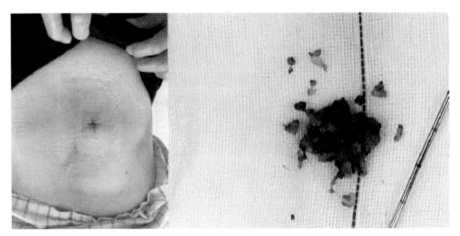

Fig. (5). The paraspinal incision to access the lesion in the psoas major muscle on the left side at the lumbar 3-4 level and the removed tissue obtained during the excisional biopsy which eventually was diagnosed as a Schwannoma.

The histopathological diagnosis of the mass of left psoas major muscle was neurogenic tumor, considered as schwannoma, with a total size of 1.8 x 1.5 x 0.5 cm. Immunohistochemical staining revealed: CD34 (-), CD117 (-), S0X-10 (+),S-100 (+), Bcl-2(+),CD99 (+), CD68 (+) Desmin (-), SMA (-), Ki-67 (+ <5%).

There were no postoperative complications are additional treatments required and the patients symptoms were relieved after the surgery. The immediate postoperative MRI scan showed postsurgical edema in the area previously occupied by the tumor (Fig. **6**), which had reduced substantially 3 months after surgery (Fig. **7**).

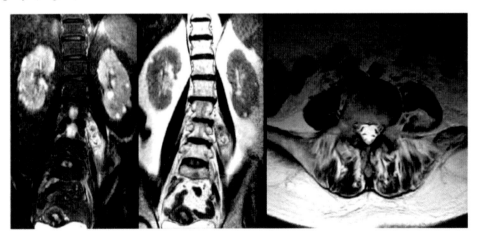

Fig. (6). The immediate postoperative sagittal (left) and axial (right) MRI scan show a high signal in the area occupied previously by the lesion in the psoas major muscle on the left side at the lumbar 3-4 level.

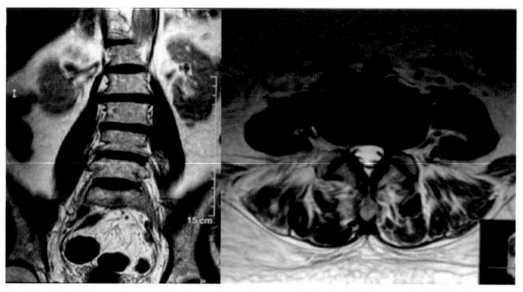

Fig. (7). The MRI scan three months after endoscopic removal of the left-sided paraspinal L3/4 schwannoma shows marked reduction of the high-signal area in the left sided psoas major muscle both on the coronoal (left) and axial (right) scan.

DISCUSSION

The space-occupying lesion in the left psoas major muscle later identified as a Schwannoma caused pain and neurological symptoms [14, 15]. In the past, the patient presented in our case presentation would have likely have had open surgery as no other means of accessing the tumor were available [16]. As demonstrated by our tumor case, spinal endoscopy was used for an excisional biopsy done for appropriate staging and histopathological diagnosis. It also turned out to be the definitive treatment as the lesion turned out to be a benign nerve sheath tumor – a schwannoma. This case highlights the versatility and utility of the endoscopic spinal surgery techniques in as much as their application is not limited to degenerative conditions of the spine. Tumorous and infectious lesions may also be accessed and at least biopsied to determine further treatment [14, 17 - 19]. Endoscopic culture and lavage would have also been a possible outcome of our case since spinal infection with a paraspinal phlegmon also had to be considered in the differential diagnosis. In case of infection, endoscopic lavage and placement of a pigtail drainage catheter would have certainly been possible. The authors have performed it for tuberculosis of the spine as previously reported by others [20 - 22].

The technical caveats of this case are worth discussing. Under local anesthesia, a portion of the transverse process bone was removed to access the tumor below.

Ideally, the schwannoma is dissected cleanly of the involved nerve root, which in our case likely was the exiting L3 nerve root. Symptoms immediately improved postoperatively. Our patient was somewhat unusual since schwannomas are more common in the head and neck area. Schwannomas are benign nerve sheath tumors and do not spread. However, they can become quite sizable and, as in our case, compress neural elements and other spinal structures due to their sheer size. Malignant degeneration into neurofibrosarcomas is very uncommon [15]. The treatment is surgical removal to achieve symptom relief as in our patient. Care must be taken not to take down the involved nerve root [16] – something that is easier said than done and speaks for the surgeon authors' technical skill level – involved in the treatment of this patient with the endoscopic surgical techniques. Thankfully, the postoperative pathology results were reported as schwannoma, a benign tumor from the nerve sheath [23], which meant that the excisional biopsy was also the definitive care for this patient. Tumor staging must be followed, and contamination of the surrounding areas with tumor cells must be avoided not to propagate the spread of tumor cells. If the postoperative pathological results had shown a malignant tumor, further detailed staging workup with thoracic, abdominal, and pelvis CT scan would have been needed to establish an accurate diagnosis and staging required for definitive surgical and adjuvant therapies as dictated by the histopathology.

CONCLUSION

Endoscopic spinal surgery techniques may not only be applied to the treatment of degenerative conditions of the spine. As shown by our case example, the endoscope may also be useful in diagnosing and treating tumorous lesions emanating from the spine and its structures. Our case of treating a benign nerve sheath tumor – a schwannoma – with endoscopic surgical technique speaks to the authors' skill level. It exemplifies their quest to apply this skill set beyond the current assortment of accepted clinical indications.

CONSENT FOR PUBLICATION

Not applicable.

CONFLICT OF INTEREST

The authors declare no conflict of interest, financial or otherwise.

ACKNOWLEDGEMENTS

Declared none.

REFERENCES

[1]   Sebai MA, Kerezoudis P, Alvi MA, Yoon JW, Spinner RJ, Bydon M. Need for arthrodesis following facetectomy for spinal peripheral nerve sheath tumors: an institutional experience and review of the current literature. J Neurosurg Spine 2019; 31(1): 112-22.
[http://dx.doi.org/10.3171/2019.1.SPINE181057] [PMID: 30952137]

[2]   Yoshimoto M, Miyakawa T, Takebayashi T, *et al.* Microendoscopy-assisted muscle-preserving interlaminar decompression for lumbar spinal stenosis: clinical results of consecutive 105 cases with more than 3-year follow-up. Spine 2014; 39(5): E318-25.
[http://dx.doi.org/10.1097/BRS.0000000000000160] [PMID: 24365896]

[3]   Yang Y, Liu B, Rong LM, *et al.* Microendoscopy-assisted minimally invasive transforaminal lumbar interbody fusion for lumbar degenerative disease: short-term and medium-term outcomes. Int J Clin Exp Med 2015; 8(11): 21319-26.
[PMID: 26885072]

[4]   Ishimoto Y, Yamada H, Curtis E, *et al.* Spinal Endoscopy for Delayed-Onset Lumbar Radiculopathy Resulting from Foraminal Stenosis after Osteoporotic Vertebral Fracture: A Case Report of a New Surgical Strategy. Case Rep Orthop 2018; 2018: 1593021.
[http://dx.doi.org/10.1155/2018/1593021]

[5]   Kim HS, Adsul N, Kapoor A, *et al.* A Mobile Outside-in Technique of Transforaminal Lumbar Endoscopy for Lumbar Disc Herniations. J Vis Exp 2018; 2018(138)
[http://dx.doi.org/10.3791/57999] [PMID: 30148483]

[6]   Kim JE, Choi DJ. Unilateral biportal endoscopic decompression by 30° endoscopy in lumbar spinal stenosis: Technical note and preliminary report. J Orthop 2018; 15(2): 366-71.
[http://dx.doi.org/10.1016/j.jor.2018.01.039] [PMID: 29881155]

[7]   Gao K, Yang H, Yang LQ, Hu MQ. [Application of intervertebral foramen endoscopy BEIS technique in the lumbar spine surgery failure syndrome over 60 years old]. Zhongguo Gu Shang 2019; 32(7): 647-52. [Application of intervertebral foramen endoscopy BEIS technique in the lumbar spine surgery failure syndrome over 60 years old].
[http://dx.doi.org/10.3969/j.issn.1003-0034.2019.07.012] [PMID: 31382724]

[8]   Heo DH, Lee DC, Park CK. Comparative analysis of three types of minimally invasive decompressive surgery for lumbar central stenosis: biportal endoscopy, uniportal endoscopy, and microsurgery. Neurosurg Focus 2019; 46: E9.
[http://dx.doi.org/10.3171/2019.2.FOCUS197]

[9]   Komatsu J, Iwabuchi M, Endo T, *et al.* Clinical outcomes of lumbar diseases specific test in patients who undergo endoscopy-assisted tubular surgery with lumbar herniated nucleus pulposus: an analysis using the Japanese Orthopaedic Association Back Pain Evaluation Questionnaire (JOABPEQ). Eur J Orthop Surg Traumatol 2019; 2019.
[http://dx.doi.org/10.1007/s00590-019-02574-5] [PMID: 31595359]

[10]   Lewandrowski K-U. The strategies behind "inside-out" and "outside-in" endoscopy of the lumbar spine: treating the pain generator. J Spine Surg 2020; 6(S1) (Suppl. 1): S35-9.
[http://dx.doi.org/10.21037/jss.2019.06.06] [PMID: 32195412]

[11]   Xin Z, Huang P, Zheng G, *et al.* Using a percutaneous spinal endoscopy unilateral posterior interlaminar approach to perform bilateral decompression for patients with lumbar lateral recess stenosis. Asian J Surg 2019; 2019
[http://dx.doi.org/10.1016/j.asjsur.2019.08.010] [PMID: 31594687]

[12]   Lewandrowski KU. The strategies behind "inside-out" and "outside-in" endoscopy of the lumbar spine: treating the pain generator. J Spine Surg 2020; 6(6) (Suppl. 1): S35-9.
[http://dx.doi.org/10.21037/jss.2019.06.06] [PMID: 32195412]

[13]   Lewandrowski KU, Dowling A, Calderaro AL, *et al.* Dysethesia due to irritation of the dorsal root ganglion following lumbar transforaminal endoscopy: Analysis of frequency and contributing factors.

Clin Neurol Neurosurg 2020; 197: 106073.
[http://dx.doi.org/10.1016/j.clineuro.2020.106073]

[14] Suratwala SJ, Kondra K, Cronin M, Leone V. Malignant peripheral nerve sheath tumor of the sciatic nerve presenting with leg pain in the setting of lumbar scoliosis and spinal stenosis. Spine Deform 2020; 8(2): 333-8.
[http://dx.doi.org/10.1007/s43390-019-00013-3] [PMID: 31925758]

[15] Lee MT, Panbehchi S, Sinha P, Rao J, Chiverton N, Ivanov M. Giant spinal nerve sheath tumours - Surgical challenges: case series and literature review. Br J Neurosurg 2019; 33(5): 541-9.
[http://dx.doi.org/10.1080/02688697.2019.1567678] [PMID: 30836023]

[16] Safaee MM, Lyon R, Barbaro NM, *et al.* Neurological outcomes and surgical complications in 221 spinal nerve sheath tumors. J Neurosurg Spine 2017; 26(1): 103-11.
[http://dx.doi.org/10.3171/2016.5.SPINE15974] [PMID: 27472744]

[17] Zou F, Guan Y, Jiang J, *et al.* Factors Affecting Postoperative Neurological Deficits After Nerve Root Resection for the Treatment of Spinal Intradural Schwannomas. Spine 2016; 41(5): 384-9.
[http://dx.doi.org/10.1097/BRS.0000000000001248] [PMID: 26919412]

[18] Miura T, Nakamura K, Tanaka H, Kawaguchi H, Takeshita K, Kurokawa T. Resection of cervical spinal neurinoma including affected nerve root: recovery of neurological deficit in 15 cases. Acta Orthop Scand 1998; 69(3): 280-2.
[http://dx.doi.org/10.3109/17453679809000930] [PMID: 9703403]

[19] Schultheiss R, Gullotta G. Resection of relevant nerve roots in surgery of spinal neurinomas without persisting neurological deficit. Acta Neurochir (Wien) 1993; 122(1-2): 91-6.
[http://dx.doi.org/10.1007/BF01446992] [PMID: 8333314]

[20] Macke JJ, Engel AJ, Sawin PD, *et al.* Tuberculosis of the cervical spine. Orthopedics 2015; 38: 280: 332-285.
[http://dx.doi.org/10.3928/01477447-20150504-01]

[21] Ben Hamida MK, Benmohamed O, Bekkay MA, *et al.* Tuberculosis of the cervical spine. Tunis Med 2019; 97(3): 512-5.
[PMID: 31729729]

[22] Yuan B, Zhao Y, Zhou S, *et al.* Treatment for tuberculosis of the subaxial cervical spine: a systematic review. Arch Orthop Trauma Surg 2020; 2020
[http://dx.doi.org/10.1007/s00402-020-03572-7] [PMID: 32776174]

[23] Sharma GK, Eschbacher JM, Uschold TD, Theodore N. Neuroblastoma-like schwannoma of lumbar spinal nerve root. J Neurosurg Spine 2010; 13(1): 82-6.
[http://dx.doi.org/10.3171/2010.3.SPINE09251] [PMID: 20594022]

CHAPTER 15

Endoscopic Uninstrumented Transforaminal Lumbar Interbody Fusion with Allograft for Surgical Management of Endstage Degenerative Vacuum Disc Disease

Álvaro Dowling[1,2,*], **James Gerald Hernández Bárcenas**[3] and **Kai-Uwe Lewandrowski**[4,5,6]

[1] *Endoscopic Spine Clinic, Santiago, Chile*

[2] *Department of Orthopaedic Surgery, USP, Ribeirão Preto, Brazil*

[3] *Orthopedic Surgeon/Spine Surgeon. Regional Hospital of High Specialty of Bajío, León, Guanajuato, México Endoscopic Spine Clinic, Santiago, Chile*

[4] *Center for Advanced Spine Care of Southern Arizona and Surgical Institute of Tucson, Tucson AZ, USA*

[5] *Associate Professor of Orthopaedic Surgery, Universidad Colsanitas, Bogota, Colombia, USA*

[6] *Visiting Professor, Department Orthpoaedic Surgery, UNIRIO, Rio de Janeiro, Brazil*

Abstract: Not every patient with painful end-stage degenerative disc disease is a candidate for instrumented fusion surgery or wants it regardless of whether it is carried out through open, mini-open, or minimally invasive incisions. The authors were intrigued by their anecdotal observation that elderly patients with painful vacuum discs serendipitously found during endoscopic decompression went on to successful fusion and enjoyed substantial long-term pain relief. Therefore, we investigated the feasibility of a transforaminal endoscopic decompression and un-instrumented lumbar interbody fusion procedures with cancellous bone allograft. A total of 29 patients had their vacuum discs directly visualized with a modified hybrid transforaminal technique employing procedural components of both the outside-in and the inside-out technique. Intraoperative endoscopic visualization of a painful, hollow collapsed, rigid intervertebral disc space allowed grafting it with cancellous allograft chips. In addition to the two-year radiographic assessment of fusion, patients were evaluated with VAS, ODI, and modified MacNab criteria. At the final follow-up, mean VAS and ODI scores reduced from 7.34 ± 1.63 and 50.03 ± 10.64 preoperatively to 1.62 ± 1.741 and 6.69 ± 4.294 postoperatively ($p < 0.0001$). According to Macnab criteria, excellent and good clinical outcomes were obtained in 34.5% and 62.1% of patients, respectively. Only one patient had minimal improvement from "Poor" preoperatively to "Fair" postoperatively. Computed tomography assessment of interbody fusion at the last

*** Corresponding author Álvaro Dowling:** Endoscopic Spine Clinic, Santiago, Chile and Department of Orthopaedic Surgery, USP, Ribeirão Preto, Brazil; Tel: +569 659 47260; E-mail: adowling@dws.cl

follow-up showed successful fusion in 91.4% of patients. Based on these study observations, the authors concluded that an un-instrumented interbody fusion by packing a hollow interspace with cancellous bone allograft chips could be an adjunct to endoscopic foraminal lateral recess decompression select patients with validated painful, collapsed, and rigid motion segments.

Keywords: Allograft, Endoscopic lumbar decompression, Interbody fusion.

INTRODUCTION

A vacuum phenomenon is often seen on plain radiographs in patients with painful end-stage lumbar degenerative disc disease [1 - 20]. Recently, this radiographic finding has been correlated with directly visualized pathology often seen during routine lumbar endoscopy [10]. Patients often complain of a combination of mechanical back pain and neurogenic claudication [11, 13, 17, 18]. Naturally, this condition usually occurs in the elderly, often lacking general health status. Medical comorbidities often prohibit extensive spinal decompression and reconstructive fusion procedures. However, longer life expectancies and cumulative disability from spinal stenosis bring these types of patients routinely back into the office for evaluation and re-evaluation in search of less aggressive yet effective ways to treat their spinal stenosis-related walking endurance problems with less burdensome treatment [21 - 24]. While these visits can be frustrating for both the surgeon and the patient as seemingly nothing is getting done, the debate about what to do with these geriatric patients in their 80ies and 90ies remains [25].

In the elderly, the lumbar spine is often vertically collapsed, deformed, and may show radiographic signs of instability [11, 26 - 28]. Mechanical back pain is often combined with claudication symptoms making it increasingly difficult to get around. Many of these patients become increasingly dependent on assistive devices and, in the worst cases, on others' help. In many patients, painful collapsed lumbar motion segments may be associated with or vertical and anterolateral instability. Facet joints disease may also be involved [26]. This process can lead to the motion segment's complete structural failure and the loss of its biological function. Pfirrmann *et al.* published on the MRI appearance of advanced disc degeneration [27]. The vacuum phenomenon is often seen on plain radiographs, or CT scan images represent progressive intervertebral disc degeneration [14, 28]. This vacuum sign suggests complete disintegration of the nucleus pulposus tissue. Its underlying cause is unknown [18]. Patients' symptoms are often attributable to this type of severe disc degeneration because of associated stenosis in the central and lateral spinal canal, instability, and deformity [12]. Ongoing vertical collapse with spontaneous fusion may stabilize the spine but could also add to mechanical axial low back pain [29 - 33].

In the elderly, instrumented fusion surgeries are often not wanted by patients or prevented by the complexity of their poorly managed medical comorbidities. While the stenosis-related symptoms can easily be addressed with the various endoscopic decompression techniques, the empty vacuum disc is often left untreated. Hence, patients may continue to suffer from back pain since pain generators residing inside the intervertebral disc space remain untreated. This shortcoming of the endoscopic foraminal or lateral recess decompression provided the rationale for the authors' feasibility investigation of achieving more sustainable and reliable relief of low back pain by performing a concomitant interbody fusion with allograft bone chips. The authors expected that the addition of this simplified interbody fusion procedure by decorticating the endplates under direct endoscopic visualization and placing bone graft into the hollow vacuum disc interspace would provide patients with more reliable and longer-lasting pain relief.

The "insight-out" transforaminal endoscopic decompression technique is one of the initial techniques developed by many of the earlier key opinion leader spine surgeons – two of them are co-editor of this Bentham text on spinal endoscopy. While many surgeons have advocated other endoscopic techniques, the time-proven "insight-out" technique has afforded the authors of this chapter the ability to visualize the interior of an empty intervertebral disc space that they often encountered serendipitously during routine transforaminal endoscopic surgery. The video-endoscopic examination of an end-stage degenerative vacuum disc and direct visualization of pain generators within it has provided the conceptual basis for the authors' study on the clinical benefit of placing bone graft inside such a painful vacuum disc that can be easily validated with diagnostic provocative- and analgesia injections [34 - 38] either preoperatively or intraoperatively in the sedated yet awake patient [39 - 45]. The placement of bone graft into a vacuum disc space does not add much complexity to the endoscopic decompression surgery. In this chapter, the authors report clinical outcomes with the percutaneous transforaminal endoscopic decompression with the report on the feasibility of an un-instrumented interbody fusion with impaction of bone allograft into the lumbar interspace through the endoscopic working cannula as an alternative to more complex spinal procedures for those patients who are either unsuitable for or unwilling to undergo these more burdensome surgeries.

POSITION, ANESTHESIA & ACCESS PLANING

As with routine lumbar endoscopy, the patients are placed in a prone position on a lordotic frame under local anesthesia and sedation in all patients. The access trajectories for the transforaminal approach are also described in great detail in the peer-reviewed literature and several chapters of this Bentham book series on spinal endoscopy [39 - 45]. For those surgeons who do not routinely perform the "insight-out technique, originally popularized by Yeung [46 - 48], the key steps of the un-instrumented interbody fusion procedure is the use a foraminoplasty in patients with or without lateral stenosis to facilitate the placement of the endoscopic working cannula inside the hollow vacuum disc space.

PEARLS OF THE SURGICAL TECHNIQUE

Patients routinely consented to the endoscopic interbody fusion during their preoperative visits should the participating surgeon authors find a hollow vacuum disc during the endoscopic decompression operation. The authors advocate the transforaminal approach and employ the "inside out" technique or a combination of these two whenever required. A recent publication has summarized the surgical steps of this hybridized endoscopic technique that the authors specifically developed for patients with painful vacuum discs [10, 11, 49]. Without repeating common knowledge of the transforaminal endoscopic technique, a few details of the surgical procedural steps seem worth mentioning in this chapter. The authors employed the "outside-in-in" technique [50, 51]. After completing the transforaminal decompression, which routinely involved a foraminoplasty, the authors carefully inspected the intervertebral disc's posterior annulus to look for annular tears or delamination from the endplate or any delamination or any delamination other unstable disc fragments. After an initial discectomy, as dictated by the direct visualization of the herniated disc impinging the symptomatic neural elements, the authors always explored the interior of the surgical disc space, mainly if a vacuum disc is found intraoperatively. The purpose of this routine intradiscal exploration is to remove any devitalized tissue delaminated from the endplates and inspection the posterior annulus. This portion of the annulus is in direct contact with the dural sac and entrapped disc herniations, or painful, inflamed annular tears within it may be painful.

The foraminoplasty is needed to create a large enough surgical corridor to the disc space to accommodate the working cannula. A bone graft may require subtotal or total resection of the superior and inferior articular processes. The authors prefer power drills, Kerrisons, and chisels to accomplish this bony resection, which can be quite extensive in patients with hypertrophic facet joints. Another consideration of a generous foraminoplasty under continuous endoscopic visualization is a lower dysesthesia rate as the exiting and traversing nerve roots may not be as aggressively compressed or manipulated [52 - 54]. Once the working cannula has been safely placed into the disc space, this surgical compartment between two adjacent vertebral bodies of the disease motion segment can be inspected and further prepared for the fusion. The spinal endoscope and its working cannula may be moved around in the disc space and aimed at any intradiscal painful pathology identified during this portion of the surgery. The authors recommend copiously irrigating the disc space before placing approximately 15 to 30 cc of the allograft chips. Initially, a bone graft should be placed on the far-side opposite of the annulotomy. The graft should be impacted with a mallet through a funnel system to avoid graft dislodgement or resorption. The bone allograft may also be enriched with bone marrow concentrate and activated platelet-derived growth factor (PRP). The suggested enrichment procedure involves the aspiration of approximately 30 ccs of autologous bone marrow from the iliac crest, which typically contains an average of ~200,000/μL cells known to release platelet-derived growth factor (PRP), transforming growth factor-β, vascular endothelial growth factor, and others (Fig. 1) [55, 56].

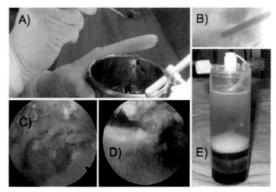

Fig. (1). The bone graft was placed through the endoscopic working cannula and compacted into the intervertebral disc space **(A)**, starting anteriorly **(B)**. After completing the grafting procedure, the traversing nerve root **(C)** should be inspected videoendoscopically to ensure no bone graft is compromising the root. Following the endplate preparation **(D)**, 15 to 30 cc cancellous allograft chips were enriched with bone marrow concentrate and activated platelet-derived growth factor (PRP) with a commercially available system **(E)**.

CLINICAL SERIES

The authors' feasibility study included 29 patients 16 of whom were male and another 13 were female. All patients indicated sciatica or claudication due to MRI-supported herniated disc or degenerative disc disease-induced spinal stenosis associated with severe low back pain. Additional inclusion criteria were dysesthesias, decreased motor function and failed non-operative treatment, including physical therapy and transforaminal. Patients were excluded from entering the study if there was higher than grade 1 spondylolisthesis with overt instability on extension/flexion views or severe central spinal stenosis as defined by a cross-sectional area of less than 100 mm2 on axial advanced imaging [57, 58]. Patients with a history of trauma, recent infection, or evidence of metastatic disease were also not treated with the authors' un-instrumented interbody fusion protocol. A history of previous spine surgery was not necessarily a contraindication to the authors. Many of these patients needed surgery for recurrent stenosis either at the index level or another adjacent level.

Every study patient had a unilateral single-level operation. As expected, the L4/5 level (13/29) and the L5/S1 level (13/29) were the most frequently operated levels. The indication for surgery was lumbar disc herniation (23/29) in most patients, three of which had surgery for a recurrent disc herniation. The remaining patients with vacuum disc underwent surgery for mechanical low back pain. Surveillance radiographs to monitor the fusion were taken periodically throughout the postoperative follow-up. All study patients had radiographs taken at their two-year follow-up appointment. Clinical outcomes were measured with the visual analog score (VAS) for leg pain [59], which improved from 7.34 ± 1.63 preoperatively to 1.62 ± 1.741 postoperatively ($p < 0.01$). Functional improvements were measured with the Oswestry Disability Index (ODI) [60], which improved from 50.03 ± 10.64 preoperatively to 6.69 ± 4.294 postoperatively ($p < 0.01$). Macnab outcome analysis [61] showed that 69% of patients ranked themselves as "Fair" and 31% as "Poor" preoperatively. The scoreboard flipped postoperatively to 34.5% of patients reporting "Excellent," and 62.1% of them reporting "Good" clinical outcomes (Table **1**).

Table 1. Pre- and postoperative outcome measures.

Paired Samples Test	Paired Differences					t	df	Sig. (2-tailed)
-	Mean	Std. Deviation	Std. Error Mean	95% Confidence Interval of the Difference		t	df	Sig. (2-tailed)
	-	-	-	Lower	Upper	-	-	-
VAS Preop – VAS Postop	5.724	2.520	.468	4.766	6.683	12.233	28	.000
ODI Preop – ODI Postop	43.345	9.689	1.799	39.659	47.030	24.091	28	.000
Paired Samples Statistics	-	-	-	-	**Macnab**	-	-	-
	Mean	N	Std Dev	Std Error	Preop	Fair	20	69.0%
VAS Preop	7.34	29	1.632	.303	-	Poor	9	31.0%
VAS Postop	1.62	29	1.741	.323	Postop	Excellent	10	34.5%
	-	-	-	-	-	Good	18	62.1%
ODI Preop	50.03	29	10.635	1.975	-	Fair	1	3.4%
ODI Postop	6.69	29	4.294	.797	-	-	29	-

FUSION ASSESSMENT

The assessment of the success of the endoscopic un-instrumented interbody spinal fusion is essential in the merit-based evaluation of this simplified fusion procedure intended for a highly selected group of patients. For this purpose, the authors used any routine postoperative radiographic study available butt ideally dynamic motion radiographs and computerized tomography scans. The Brantigan, Steffee, Fraser – BSF – classification was employed to assess the bone graft-host interface [62 - 64]. Moreover, this classification takes the presence of new bone formation, resorption, and bone remodeling into account. Briefly, a BSF-1 grade was assigned if postoperative radiographic studies showed loss of disc space height, anterolateral slippage, bone graft resorption, or lucency around the periphery of the graft suggested pseudoarthrosis. A BSF-2 was assigned to any postoperative radiographic study showing solid bone growing into the spacer from each vertebral endplate with some central lucency. Bridging bone bridges occupying at least half of the fusion area was graded as a BSF-3 grade. Most patients' fusion (23/29) was deemed successful as they were assigned a BSF-3 grade. The remaining six patients were given a BSF-2 grade and reported Excellent or Good Macnab outcomes. There were no pseudoarthrosis patients (BSF 1 grade). There was only one 41-year-old patient whose clinical outcome was rated as "Fair" because of extrusion of part of the bone graft leading to recurrent S1 radiculopathy. These symptoms were ultimately resolved with supportive care and interventional care measures, including several transforaminal epidural steroid injections. This patient's final postoperative CT scan was graded as a BSF-3 (Fig. **2**).

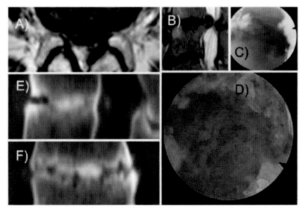

Fig. (2). Axial **(a)** and sagittal **(b)** T2-weighted preoperative lumbar MRI images at the L4/5 level. The endplate decortication was visualized endoscopically **(C)**. Growth factor enriched bone graft was impacted into the interspace **(D)**. Successful BSF-3 graded fusion was demonstrated on sagittal **(E)**, coronal **(F)** CT images 12 months after surgery.

DISCUSSION

The authors were able to demonstrated the feasibility of a simplified endoscopic fusion patients with end-stage degenerative vacuum disc disease. In a select group of patients suffering from disabling mechanical low back pain and claudication symptoms the addition of the endoscopic interspace grafting following a transforaminal decompression does not expand the scope beyond what would be considered appropriate for an outpatient surgery center setting. Generally, the authors observed favorable clinical outcomes with impaction of cancellous bone allograft chips into the hollow lumbar intervertebral disc space. All but 1 of the 29 patients and excellent and good Macnab outcomes. This simplified fusion when applied in select patients with rigid collapsed degenerative lumbar motion segments without a cage may be considered an alternative to more complex spinal surgeries. This may be of particular relevance to the elderly where multiple medical comorbidities are common [65].

Clinical outcomes with the intervertebral disc augmentation with cancellous bone allograft were favorable. Although many postoperative images showed incomplete interbody fusion, patients did well and reported a substantial reduction in pain scores while enjoying a short convalescence period without serious complications. This team of authors stipulated that the procedure may be a valuable adjunct to the endoscopic decompression procedure. The method appears attractive because of its simplicity and the use of biological grafting material. In highly selected, our endoscopic fusion procedure without any other supplemental implant is a benign procedure. The procedure can be done in an outpatient ASC setting without adding too much human and capital infrastructure. The authors intend to perform a future formal cost-benefit analysis to highlight better the indications and benefits of this type of endoscopic fusion procedure.

CONCLUSION

Endoscopic transforaminal decompression and interbody fusion with cancellous bone allograft chips is an attractive alternative to open lumbar surgery, which works well in select elderly patients with single-level end-stage vacuum disc. This combined procedure addresses herniated disc- and claudication symptoms and disabling mechanical low back pain due to severe advanced lumbar disc degeneration. The authors' clinical results show the feasibility of achieving an excellent safety profile and favorable clinical outcomes with this simplified fusion procedure. Its merits should be further investigated.

CONSENT FOR PUBLICATION

Not applicable.

CONFLICT OF INTEREST

The authors declare no conflict of interest, financial or otherwise.

ACKNOWLEDGEMENTS

Declared none.

REFERENCES

[1]   An KC, Kong GM, Park DH, Baik JM, Youn JH, Lee WS. Response to: Comparison of Posterior Lumbar Interbody Fusion and Posterolateral Lumbar Fusion in Monosegmental Vacuum Phenomenon within an Intervertebral Disc. Asian Spine J 2016; 10(5): 984.
[http://dx.doi.org/10.4184/asj.2016.10.5.984] [PMID: 27790332]

[2]   An KC, Kong GM, Park DH, Baik JM, Youn JH, Lee WS. Comparison of Posterior Lumbar Interbody Fusion and Posterolateral Lumbar Fusion in Monosegmental Vacuum Phenomenon within an Intervertebral Disc. Asian Spine J 2016; 10(1): 93-8.
[http://dx.doi.org/10.4184/asj.2016.10.1.93] [PMID: 26949464]

[3]   Anda S, Dale LG, Vassal J. Intradural disc herniation with vacuum phenomenon: CT diagnosis. Neuroradiology 1987; 29(4): 407.
[http://dx.doi.org/10.1007/BF00348927] [PMID: 3627428]

[4]   Anda S, Støvring J, Rø M. CT of extraforaminal disc herniation with associated vacuum phenomenon. Neuroradiology 1988; 30(1): 76-7.
[http://dx.doi.org/10.1007/BF00341949] [PMID: 3357572]

[5]   Chevrot A, Pillon B, Revel M, Moutounet J, Pallardy G. [The radiological phenomenon of lumbar vacuum-disc (author's transl)]. J Radiol Electrol Med Nucl 1978; 59(4): 267-70. [The radiological phenomenon of lumbar vacuum-disc (author's transl)].
[PMID: 660575]

[6]   Dowling Á, Bárcenas JGH, Lewandrowski KU. Transforaminal endoscopic decompression and uninstrumented allograft lumbar interbody fusion: A feasibility study in patients with end-stage vacuum degenerative disc disease. Clin Neurol Neurosurg 2020; 196106002
[http://dx.doi.org/10.1016/j.clineuro.2020.106002] [PMID: 32562950]

[7]   Ford LT, Gilula LA, Murphy WA, Gado M. Analysis of gas in vacuum lumbar disc. AJR Am J Roentgenol 1977; 128(6): 1056-7.
[http://dx.doi.org/10.2214/ajr.128.6.1056] [PMID: 414544]

[8]   Latif AB. [Vacuum phenomenon in the intervertebral disc]. Magy Traumatol Orthop Helyreallito Seb 1991; 34(4): 297-300. [Vacuum phenomenon in the intervertebral disc].
[PMID: 1685543]

[9]   Lee CH, Cho JH, Hyun SJ, Yoon SH, Kim KJ, Kim HJ. Symptomatic gas-containing herniated disc with the vacuum phenomenon: mechanism and treatment. Case report. Neurol Med Chir (Tokyo) 2012; 52(2): 106-8.
[http://dx.doi.org/10.2176/nmc.52.106] [PMID: 22362295]

[10]   Lewandrowski KU, León JFR, Yeung A. Use of "Inside-Out" Technique for Direct Visualization of a Vacuum Vertically Unstable Intervertebral Disc During Routine Lumbar Endoscopic Transforaminal Decompression-A Correlative Study of Clinical Outcomes and the Prognostic Value of Lumbar

Radiographs. Int J Spine Surg 2019; 13(5): 399-414.
[http://dx.doi.org/10.14444/6055] [PMID: 31741829]

[11]   Lewandrowski KU, Zhang X, Ramírez León JF, de Carvalho PST, Hellinger S, Yeung A. Lumbar vacuum disc, vertical instability, standalone endoscopic interbody fusion, and other treatments: an opinion based survey among minimally invasive spinal surgeons. J Spine Surg 2020; 6(S1) (Suppl. 1): S165-78.
[http://dx.doi.org/10.21037/jss.2019.11.02] [PMID: 32195425]

[12]   Liao JC, Lu ML, Niu CC, Chen WJ, Chen LH. Surgical outcomes of degenerative lumbar spondylolisthesis with anterior vacuum disc: can the intervertebral cage overcome intradiscal vacuum phenomenon and enhance posterolateral fusion? J Orthop Sci 2014; 19(6): 851-9.
[http://dx.doi.org/10.1007/s00776-014-0618-z] [PMID: 25104604]

[13]   Lin TY, Liao JC, Tsai TT, *et al.* The effects of anterior vacuum disc on surgical outcomes of degenerative *versus* spondylolytic spondylolisthesis: at a minimum two-year follow-up. BMC Musculoskelet Disord 2014; 15(1): 329.
[http://dx.doi.org/10.1186/1471-2474-15-329] [PMID: 25277044]

[14]   Murata K, Akeda K, Takegami N, Cheng K, Masuda K, Sudo A. Morphology of intervertebral disc ruptures evaluated by vacuum phenomenon using multi-detector computed tomography: association with lumbar disc degeneration and canal stenosis. BMC Musculoskelet Disord 2018; 19(1): 164.
[http://dx.doi.org/10.1186/s12891-018-2086-7] [PMID: 29793459]

[15]   Murata Y, Kanaya K, Wada H, *et al.* L5 Radiculopathy due to Foraminal Stenosis Accompanied With Vacuum Phenomena of the L5/S Disc on Radiography Images in Extension Position. Spine 2015; 40(23): 1831-5.
[http://dx.doi.org/10.1097/BRS.0000000000001067] [PMID: 26208231]

[16]   Pak KI, Hoffman DC, Herzog RJ, Lutz GE. Percutaneous intradiscal aspiration of a lumbar vacuum disc herniation: a case report. HSS J 2011; 7(1): 89-93.
[http://dx.doi.org/10.1007/s11420-010-9168-x] [PMID: 22294964]

[17]   Raines JR. Intervertebral disc fissures (vacuum intervertebral disc). Am J Roentgenol Radium Ther Nucl Med 1953; 70(6): 964-6.
[PMID: 13104729]

[18]   Schweitzer ME, el-Noueam KI. Vacuum disc: frequency of high signal intensity on T2-weighted MR images. Skeletal Radiol 1998; 27(2): 83-6.
[http://dx.doi.org/10.1007/s002560050342] [PMID: 9526773]

[19]   Soffler C, Karpenstein H, Kramer M. Tierarztl Prax Ausg K Klientiere Heimtiere 2014; 42(2): 88-93. [The intervertebral vacuum phenomenon as a computed-tomographic finding in the dog and its significance as an indicator for surgical treatment of vertebral disc herniations].
[http://dx.doi.org/10.1055/s-0038-1623746]

[20]   Viswanathan VK, Subramanian S. Letter: Comparison of Posterior Lumbar Interbody Fusion and Posterolateral Lumbar Fusion in Monosegmental Vacuum Phenomenon within an Intervertebral Disc. Asian Spine J 2016; 10(5): 982-3.
[http://dx.doi.org/10.4184/asj.2016.10.5.982] [PMID: 27790331]

[21]   Benoist M, Parent H, Nizard M, Lassale B, Deburge A. Lumbar discal herniation in the elderly: long-term results of chymopapain chemonucleolysis. Eur Spine J 1993; 2(3): 149-52.
[http://dx.doi.org/10.1007/BF00301413] [PMID: 20058468]

[22]   Chung J, Kong C, Sun W, Kim D, Kim H, Jeong H. Percutaneous Endoscopic Lumbar Foraminoplasty for Lumbar Foraminal Stenosis of Elderly Patients with Unilateral Radiculopathy: Radiographic Changes in Magnetic Resonance Images. J Neurol Surg A Cent Eur Neurosurg 2019; 80(4): 302-11.
[http://dx.doi.org/10.1055/s-0038-1677052] [PMID: 30887488]

[23]   Imajo Y, Taguchi T, Neo M, *et al.* Complications of spinal surgery for elderly patients with lumbar spinal stenosis in a super-aging country: An analysis of 8033 patients. J Orthop Sci 2017; 22(1): 10-5.

[http://dx.doi.org/10.1016/j.jos.2016.08.014] [PMID: 27646205]

[24]   Rosen DS, O'Toole JE, Eichholz KM, *et al.* Minimally invasive lumbar spinal decompression in the elderly: outcomes of 50 patients aged 75 years and older. Neurosurgery 2007; 60(3): 503-9.
[http://dx.doi.org/10.1227/01.NEU.0000255332.87909.58] [PMID: 17327795]

[25]   Jasper GP, Francisco GM, Telfeian AE. A retrospective evaluation of the clinical success of transforaminal endoscopic discectomy with foraminotomy in geriatric patients. Pain Physician 2013; 16(3): 225-9.
[PMID: 23703409]

[26]   Luk KD, Chow DH, Holmes A. Vertical instability in spondylolisthesis: a traction radiographic assessment technique and the principle of management. Spine 2003; 28(8): 819-27.
[http://dx.doi.org/10.1097/01.BRS.0000058941.55208.14] [PMID: 12698127]

[27]   Pfirrmann CW, Metzdorf A, Zanetti M, Hodler J, Boos N. Magnetic resonance classification of lumbar intervertebral disc degeneration. Spine 2001; 26(17): 1873-8.
[http://dx.doi.org/10.1097/00007632-200109010-00011] [PMID: 11568697]

[28]   Lee JH, Han IH, Kim DH, *et al.* Spine Computed Tomography to Magnetic Resonance Image Synthesis Using Generative Adversarial Networks : A Preliminary Study. J Korean Neurosurg Soc 2020; 63(3): 386-96.
[http://dx.doi.org/10.3340/jkns.2019.0084] [PMID: 31931556]

[29]   Adogwa O, Parker SL, Bydon A, Cheng J, McGirt MJ. Comparative effectiveness of minimally invasive *versus* open transforaminal lumbar interbody fusion: 2-year assessment of narcotic use, return to work, disability, and quality of life. J Spinal Disord Tech 2011; 24(8): 479-84.
[http://dx.doi.org/10.1097/BSD.0b013e3182055cac] [PMID: 21336176]

[30]   Crawford CH III, Smail J, Carreon LY, Glassman SD. Health-related quality of life after posterolateral lumbar arthrodesis in patients seventy-five years of age and older. Spine 2011; 36(13): 1065-8.
[http://dx.doi.org/10.1097/BRS.0b013e3181e8afa0] [PMID: 21217437]

[31]   Hsu KY, Zucherman JF, Hartjen CA, *et al.* Quality of life of lumbar stenosis-treated patients in whom the X STOP interspinous device was implanted. J Neurosurg Spine 2006; 5(6): 500-7.
[http://dx.doi.org/10.3171/spi.2006.5.6.500] [PMID: 17176013]

[32]   Nunley PD, Patel VV, Orndorff DG, Lavelle WF, Block JE, Geisler FH. Interspinous Process Decompression Improves Quality of Life in Patients with Lumbar Spinal Stenosis. Minim Invasive Surg 2018; 20181035954
[http://dx.doi.org/10.1155/2018/1035954] [PMID: 30057811]

[33]   Sobottke R, Röllinghoff M, Siewe J, *et al.* Clinical outcomes and quality of life 1 year after open microsurgical decompression or implantation of an interspinous stand-alone spacer. Minim Invasive Neurosurg 2010; 53(4): 179-83.
[http://dx.doi.org/10.1055/s-0030-1263108] [PMID: 21132610]

[34]   el-Khoury GY, Renfrew DL. Percutaneous procedures for the diagnosis and treatment of lower back pain: diskography, facet-joint injection, and epidural injection. AJR Am J Roentgenol 1991; 157(4): 685-91.
[http://dx.doi.org/10.2214/ajr.157.4.1832511] [PMID: 1832511]

[35]   Geurts JW, Kallewaard JW, Richardson J, Groen GJ. Targeted methylprednisolone acetate/hyaluronidase/clonidine injection after diagnostic epiduroscopy for chronic sciatica: a prospective, 1-year follow-up study. Reg Anesth Pain Med 2002; 27(4): 343-52.
[PMID: 12132057]

[36]   Lewandrowski KU. Successful outcome after outpatient transforaminal decompression for lumbar foraminal and lateral recess stenosis: The positive predictive value of diagnostic epidural steroid injection. Clin Neurol Neurosurg 2018; 173: 38-45.
[http://dx.doi.org/10.1016/j.clineuro.2018.07.015] [PMID: 30075346]

[37] MacVicar J, King W, Landers MH, Bogduk N. The effectiveness of lumbar transforaminal injection of steroids: a comprehensive review with systematic analysis of the published data. Pain Med 2013; 14(1): 14-28.
[http://dx.doi.org/10.1111/j.1526-4637.2012.01508.x] [PMID: 23110347]

[38] Valat JP. Epidural corticosteroid injections for sciatica: placebo effect, injection effect or anti-inflammatory effect? Nat Clin Pract Rheumatol 2006; 2(10): 518-9.
[http://dx.doi.org/10.1038/ncprheum0286] [PMID: 17016473]

[39] Gold MI, Watkins WD, Sung YF, *et al.* Remifentanil *versus* remifentanil/midazolam for ambulatory surgery during monitored anesthesia care. Anesthesiology 1997; 87(1): 51-7.
[http://dx.doi.org/10.1097/00000542-199707000-00007] [PMID: 9232133]

[40] Hertzog JH, Campbell JK, Dalton HJ, Hauser GJ. Propofol anesthesia for invasive procedures in ambulatory and hospitalized children: experience in the pediatric intensive care unit. Pediatrics 1999; 103(3)E30
[http://dx.doi.org/10.1542/peds.103.3.e30] [PMID: 10049986]

[41] Hua W, Zhang Y, Wu X, *et al.* Full-Endoscopic Visualized Foraminoplasty and Discectomy Under General Anesthesia in the Treatment of L4-L5 and L5-S1 Disc Herniation. Spine 2019; 44(16): E984-91.
[http://dx.doi.org/10.1097/BRS.0000000000003014] [PMID: 31374002]

[42] Li Z, Long H, Huang F, Zhang Y, Xu J, Wang X. Impact of Epidural *Versus* General Anesthesia on Major Lumbar Surgery in Elderly Patients. Clin Spine Surg 2019; 32(1): E7-E12.
[http://dx.doi.org/10.1097/BSD.0000000000000708] [PMID: 30222620]

[43] O'Shea JP, Sarwat MA, Sutcliffe CJ. Asleep-Awake-Asleep general anesthesia for open cervical rhizotomy: case report and description of the technique. J Neurosurg Anesthesiol 2000; 12(4): 356-8.
[http://dx.doi.org/10.1097/00008506-200010000-00008] [PMID: 11147384]

[44] Singhal NR, Jones J, Semenova J, *et al.* Multimodal anesthesia with the addition of methadone is superior to epidural analgesia: A retrospective comparison of intraoperative anesthetic techniques and pain management for 124 pediatric patients undergoing the Nuss procedure. J Pediatr Surg 2016; 51(4): 612-6.
[http://dx.doi.org/10.1016/j.jpedsurg.2015.10.084] [PMID: 26700690]

[45] Taylor E, Ghouri AF, White PF. Midazolam in combination with propofol for sedation during local anesthesia. J Clin Anesth 1992; 4(3): 213-6.
[http://dx.doi.org/10.1016/0952-8180(92)90068-C] [PMID: 1610577]

[46] Yeung AT. Minimally Invasive Disc Surgery with the Yeung Endoscopic Spine System (YESS). Surg Technol Int 1999; 8: 267-77.
[PMID: 12451541]

[47] Yeung AT. The evolution of percutaneous spinal endoscopy and discectomy: state of the art. Mt Sinai J Med 2000; 67(4): 327-32.
[PMID: 11021785]

[48] Tsou PM, Yeung AT. Transforaminal endoscopic decompression for radiculopathy secondary to intracanal noncontained lumbar disc herniations: outcome and technique. Spine J 2002; 2(1): 41-8.
[http://dx.doi.org/10.1016/S1529-9430(01)00153-X] [PMID: 14588287]

[49] Lewandrowski KU, Yeung A. Lumbar Endoscopic Bony and Soft Tissue Decompression With the Hybridized Inside-Out Approach: A Review And Technical Note. Neurospine 2020; 17 (Suppl. 1): S34-43.
[http://dx.doi.org/10.14245/ns.2040160.080] [PMID: 32746516]

[50] Lewandrowski KU. "Outside-in" technique, clinical results, and indications with transforaminal lumbar endoscopic surgery: a retrospective study on 220 patients on applied radiographic classification of foraminal spinal stenosis. Int J Spine Surg 2014; 8: 8.

[http://dx.doi.org/10.14444/1026] [PMID: 25694915]

[51]   Lewandrowski KU. The strategies behind "inside-out" and "outside-in" endoscopy of the lumbar spine: treating the pain generator. J Spine Surg 2020; 6(S1) (Suppl. 1): S35-9.
[http://dx.doi.org/10.21037/jss.2019.06.06] [PMID: 32195412]

[52]   Lewandrowski KU, Ransom NA. Five-year clinical outcomes with endoscopic transforaminal outside-in foraminoplasty techniques for symptomatic degenerative conditions of the lumbar spine. J Spine Surg 2020; 6(S1) (Suppl. 1): S54-65.
[http://dx.doi.org/10.21037/jss.2019.07.03] [PMID: 32195416]

[53]   Lin YP, Wang SL, Hu WX, *et al.* Percutaneous Full-Endoscopic Lumbar Foraminoplasty and Decompression by Using a Visualization Reamer for Lumbar Lateral Recess and Foraminal Stenosis in Elderly Patients. World Neurosurg 2020; 136: e83-9.
[http://dx.doi.org/10.1016/j.wneu.2019.10.123] [PMID: 31866456]

[54]   Yeung A, Lewandrowski KU. Five-year clinical outcomes with endoscopic transforaminal foraminoplasty for symptomatic degenerative conditions of the lumbar spine: a comparative study of *inside-out* versus *outside-in* techniques. J Spine Surg 2020; 6(S1) (Suppl. 1): S66-83.
[http://dx.doi.org/10.21037/jss.2019.06.08] [PMID: 32195417]

[55]   Vavken J, Vavken P, Mameghani A, Camathias C, Schaeren S. Platelet concentrates in spine fusion: meta-analysis of union rates and complications in controlled trials. Eur Spine J 2016; 25(5): 1474-83.
[http://dx.doi.org/10.1007/s00586-015-4193-6] [PMID: 26298478]

[56]   Feiz-Erfan I, Harrigan M, Sonntag VK, Harrington TR. Effect of autologous platelet gel on early and late graft fusion in anterior cervical spine surgery. J Neurosurg Spine 2007; 7(5): 496-502.
[http://dx.doi.org/10.3171/SPI-07/11/496] [PMID: 17977190]

[57]   Sengupta DK, Herkowitz HN. Lumbar spinal stenosis. Treatment strategies and indications for surgery. Orthop Clin North Am 2003; 34(2): 281-95.
[http://dx.doi.org/10.1016/S0030-5898(02)00069-X] [PMID: 12914268]

[58]   Yuan S, Zou Y, Li Y, Chen M, Yue Y. A clinically relevant MRI grading system for lumbar central canal stenosis. Clin Imaging 2016; 40(6): 1140-5.
[http://dx.doi.org/10.1016/j.clinimag.2016.07.005] [PMID: 27519125]

[59]   Reed CC, Wolf WA, Cotton CC, Dellon ES. A visual analogue scale and a Likert scale are simple and responsive tools for assessing dysphagia in eosinophilic oesophagitis. Aliment Pharmacol Ther 2017; 45(11): 1443-8.
[http://dx.doi.org/10.1111/apt.14061] [PMID: 28370355]

[60]   Fairbank JC, Pynsent PB. The Oswestry Disability Index. Spine 2000; 25(22): 2940-52.
[http://dx.doi.org/10.1097/00007632-200011150-00017] [PMID: 11074683]

[61]   Macnab I. The surgery of lumbar disc degeneration. Surg Annu 1976; 8: 447-80.
[PMID: 936011]

[62]   Brantigan JW, Steffee AD. A carbon fiber implant to aid interbody lumbar fusion. Two-year clinical results in the first 26 patients. Spine 1993; 18(14) (Suppl.): 2106-7.
[http://dx.doi.org/10.1097/00007632-199310001-00030] [PMID: 8272967]

[63]   Brantigan JW, Steffee AD, Geiger JM. A carbon fiber implant to aid interbody lumbar fusion. Mechanical testing. Spine 1991; 16(6) (Suppl.): S277-82.
[http://dx.doi.org/10.1097/00007632-199106001-00020] [PMID: 1862425]

[64]   Brantigan JW, Steffee AD, Lewis ML, Quinn LM, Persenaire JM. Lumbar interbody fusion using the Brantigan I/F cage for posterior lumbar interbody fusion and the variable pedicle screw placement system: two-year results from a Food and Drug Administration investigational device exemption clinical trial. Spine 2000; 25(11): 1437-46.
[http://dx.doi.org/10.1097/00007632-200006010-00017] [PMID: 10828927]

[65]   Stopa BM, Robertson FC, Karhade AV, *et al.* Predicting nonroutine discharge after elective spine surgery: external validation of machine learning algorithms. J Neurosurg Spine 2019; 31(5): 1-6.
[http://dx.doi.org/10.3171/2019.5.SPINE1987] [PMID: 31349223]

CHAPTER 16

Full Endoscopic Endplate Decortication and Vertebral Mobilization Technique of Transforaminal Lumbar Interbody Fusion for Degenerative Spondylolisthesis

Ji-Yeon Kim[1], Hyeun Sung Kim[1,*] and Jang Il-Tae[1]

[1] Department of Neurosurgery, Nanoori Hospital, Gangnam, Seoul, South Korea

Abstract: There are two kinds of endoscopic lumbar interbody fusion. One approach is a transforaminal approach using uniportal endoscopic surgery [6-8], and the other is a posterolateral approach like MIS TLIF using uniportal or biportal endoscopic surgery. The transkambin approach is similar to transforaminal uniportal endoscopic lumbar discectomy through the Kambin triangle through which also the endplate preparation and cage insertion are done. The posterolateral endoscopic TLIF techniques are similar to MIS TLIF using a tubular retractor system and mainly used by the surgeons who practice biportal endoscopic surgery. Because of the paucity of literature describing the uniportal endoscopic posterolateral approach for transforaminal interbody fusion (Endo-TLIF), we describe in this chapter the technique of full endoscopic endplate denudation and adhesion releasing technique of endoscopic transforaminal lumbar interbody fusion for degenerative spondylolisthesis and degenerative scoliosis.

Keywords: Endoscopic, Endplate Preparation, Fusion, Transforaminal Interbody Fusion.

INTRODUCTION

The aging population has increased the incidence of symptomatic degenerative spinal diseases such as degenerative spinal stenosis, spondylolisthesis, and degenerative disc disease [1]. Minimal invasive (MIS) spine surgery has the advantages of early recovery and normal structure preservations. The technical advancements in endoscopic spine surgery have led to more minimally invasive options for lumbar spine surgery [2]. Endoscopic lumbar interbody fusion has been attempted [3 - 5]. There are two kinds of endoscopic lumbar interbody fusion. According to the approaching route or corridors, one approach is a

* **Corresponding author Hyeun Sung Kim:** Department of Neurosurgery, Nanoori Hospital, Gangnam, South Korea; E-mail: neurospinekim@gmail.com

Kai-Uwe Lewandrowski, Jorge Felipe Ramírez León, Anthony Yeung, Hyeun-Sung Kim, Xifeng Zhang, Gun Choi, Stefan Hellinger and Álvaro Dowling (Eds.)

transforaminal approach using uniportal endoscopic surgery [6 - 8], and the other is a posterolateral approach like MIS TLIF using uniportal or biportal endoscopic surgery [3, 9, 10] (Figs. **1A** and **1B**). The transkambin approach is similar to transforaminal uniportal endoscopic lumbar discectomy through the Kambin triangle. Endplate preparation and cage insertion were performed *via* Kambin's triangle [6]. The posterolateral endoscopic TLIF techniques are similar to MIS TLIF using a tubular retractor system and mainly used by the surgeons who practice biportal endoscopic surgery. A paucity of literature describes the uniportal endoscopic posterolateral approach for transforaminal interbody fusion (Endo-TLIF). Kim and Wu *et al.* reported the clinical and computer tomographic study with technical note using the uniportal full endoscopic posterolateral transforaminal lumbar interbody fusion with endoscopic disc drilling preparation technique for symptomatic foraminal stenosis [3]. As the methods of the Endo-TLIF have developed, surgical indications have extended to most lumbar degenerative conditions, including spondylolisthesis and scoliosis.

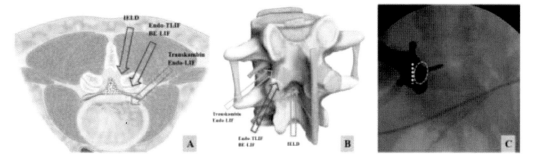

Fig. (1). Three routes of Endoscopy were illustrated on the axial plane **(A)** and the 3D vertebral model **(B)**. IELD is an interlaminar endoscopic lumbar discectomy, Endo-TLIF is uniportal full endoscopic posterolateral transforaminal lumbar interbody fusion, BE-LIF is biportal endoscopic lumbar interbody fusion, Transkambin EndoLIF is uniporal transforaminal transkambin approach endoscopic lumbar interbody fusion. Docking position of left L5-S1 Endo-TLIF **(C).** The incision (dotted white line) was made over the left L5 pedicle (dotted green circle), and the working cannula was docked on the pars interarticularlis of right L5-S1.

In this chapter, we elaborate on the technique of full endoscopic endplate denudation and adhesion releasing technique of endoscopic transforaminal lumbar interbody fusion for degenerative spondylolisthesis and degenerative scoliosis, which decreases the endplate injury during endplate preparation by denudation technique and increase the mobility of the index segment for deformity correction by releasing the adhesions in the intravertebral disc space.

RATIONALE

Anatomical Considerations During Endo-TLIF Surgery

Uniportal transforaminal endoscopic fusion surgery is performed within a small safe corridor of Kambin's triangle [11]. It has to use a narrow-width cage to fit through the narrow safety corridor not to injure the exiting nerve root. In the uniportal full endoscopic posterolateral route transforaminal interbody fusion, the complete resection of the ipsilateral facet joint created enough space for the sizable interbody cage used in microscopic tubular transforaminal lumbar interbody fusion [1] (Figs. **1A** and **1B**).

Direct Bilateral and Contralateral Decompression of Central Spinal Canal and Nerve Roots with Endo-TLIF

Endo-TLIF has the advantages of both MIS fusion and endoscopic surgery. This technique is based on conventional MIS TLIF procedures [12] so that Endo-TLIF can perform direct decompression of neural structure [1 - 3]. Unilateral laminotomy for bilateral decompression is one of the advantages of the uniportal full endoscopic approach [13]. The contralateral nerve root could be fully decompressed through the inside-out and outside-in techniques [4, 5, 14]. The outside-in technique is defined as bony de¬compression of cephalad lamina, caudal lamina, inferior articu¬lar process, and superior articular process ("outside") to the ex¬tent that is sufficient for complete release of ligamentum flavum before removal of ligamentum en-bloc with a blunt instrument in the last part of the procedure to expose the spinal canal ("in"). This technique is commonly known as over the top decompression technique. [1, 4.15] The inside-out technique, on the other hand, involved bony decompression of the lamina, inferior articular process, and superior articular process with the early splitting of ligamentum flavum to get into the spinal canal ("inside") before releasing ligamentum flavum from within the spinal canal with concurrent bony decompression ("out") [5, 6]. Also, indirect decompression of the contralateral foramen can be achieved by reducing spondylolisthesis and restoration of the collapsed disc space by inserting a large-sized cage [7]. In the case that indirect decompression is insufficient, contralateral direct foraminotomy could be done by Endo-TLIF [16].

Concepts of Full Endoscopic Adhesion Releasing Technique with Endoscopic Drill

In a severe collapsed disc space, large syndesmophytes or a calcified disc may obstruct the disc space's entry due to extreme disc adhesion in the annulus portion of the intravertebral disc space. In these cases, it is difficult to open up the annulus by Endo-TLIF procedures because of the limited endoscopic surgical instruments compared to microscopic MIS TLIF or biportal endoscopic TLIF. The radiofrequency ablator, forceps, plasma coagulators, blunt probe, and drill are usually used in combination to open the annulus. The 3.5~4.5 mm endoscopic diamond burr could be used to resect the syndesmophytes in cases of severe disc adhesion (Fig. **4C**). Segmental mobility of the index level would be increased by the disc adhesion releasing technique with an endoscopic drill. Such increased segmental mobility allows more significant restoration of disc height even in severe collapsed intervertebral disc space.

Concepts of Full Endoscopic Endplate Denudation Technique

After annulus opening, endplate preparation for interbody fusion under endoscopic vision is performed using a mixture of the endoscopic drill, forceps, a blunt bent probe, and plasma coagulator. The optimal fusion bed preparation would be done by denuding the endplate cartilage with punctate bleeding of subchondral bone but not breaching the cortex of the endplate to prevent endplate injury (Fig. **4D**). As the distal tip of the endoscope advance to the intervertebral disc space, we can denudate the disc and cartilage from the posterior annulus to the anterior annulus just short of the anterior longitudinal ligament under direct magnified endoscopic visualization [1, 3] (Fig. **4E**). Also, the curette is not used in the process of endplate preparation to prevent endplate violations. To avoid subsidence, the well-prepared endplate is critical to withstand the high pressure between the inserted large interbody cage and an endplate. Kim and Wu *et al.* reported the Endo-TLIF case series with 12 months mean follow-up period [3.16]. No subsidence occurred compared to the 6% rate of subsidence resulting from transforaminal interbody fusion [8].

Concepts of Large-sized Interbody Cage Insertion Using the Harrison Cage Glider

There are advantages of the use of the larger interbody cage during Endo-TLIF. 1) the proper Cobb angle correction by insertion of the large cage in the lateral wedging site (Figs. **5A - H**). 2) The versatility in using various commercially available transforaminal lumbar interbody fusion cages available compared with the limited kinds of cages used in the transforaminal endoscopic approach *via* Kambin's triangle. 3) more bone graft materials could be packed in the disc space and the cage to enhance interbody fusion [1, 7]. It is technically difficult to safely insert the large interbody cage by the endoscopic procedures, so it is necessary for several components during the large cage insertion [1, 3, 7]. 1) the complete resection of the ipsilateral facet joint created enough space for a sizeable interbody cage used in microscopic tubular transforaminal lumbar interbody fusion (Fig. **3**). 2) the Harrison cage glider protects the exiting and traversing roots while gently retracting the neural structures to provide enough space for the cage. (Figs. **2C - G**) 3) Increased segmental mobility by disc adhesion releasing technique allows larger sized interbody cage insertion even in severe collapsed intervertebral disc space. The Harrison cage glider is a specially designed instrument by Harrison (Hyeun-Sung) Kim [1]. The tailored tip could be positioned in the dorsal one-third of the intervertebral space and bilaterally divided for smooth mobility. (Fig. **2G**) As the cage passes through the Harrison cage glider, the bilateral tailored tip smoothly diverges to the exiting and the traversing nerve roots and safely protects the neural structures (Fig. **2C**).

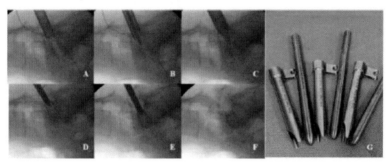

Fig. (2). Intraoperative C-arm images. A: The working cannula was carefully advanced and docked on the annulus with the open bevel pointing away from the exiting and traversing nerve root to retract the neural structures away. B: Through the working cannula, annulus release and endplate preparation were done using a mixture of the endoscopic drill. C: The working cannula was replaced with the Harrison cage glider to provide guidance for the appropriate size of the cage to be inserted with fluoroscopy. D, E, F: Under fluoroscopic guidance, we inserted the appropriately sized 3D-printed titanium cage packed with autograft into the disc space through the Harrison cage glider. After half of the cage was inserted in the intervertebral disc space, the cage glider could be removed safely to adjust the advance direction. G: The Harrison cage glider.

Reduction of the Spondylolisthesis and Correction of the Focal Scoliosis by Endo-TLIF

Advancement of the uniportal full endoscopic surgical techniques allows the reduction of the spondylolisthesis and correction of focal scoliosis by Endo-TLIF (Fig. **5**). The essential procedures increase segmental mobility by disc adhesion releasing technique and a sizeable interbody cage insertion. Kim and Wu *et al.* have described the use of Endo-TLIF in a case report in which they completely resected the ipsilateral facet joint and introduced a sizeable interbody cage to reduce the translational deformity in a grade 2 spondylolisthesis patient [16]. They described an application of Endo-TLIF in mild to moderate degenerative scoliosis and reported the excellent early clinical results and improvement in coronal Cobb's angle [2, 16].

SURGICAL STEPS

Preoperative Preparation

Patients' history, clinical examination, radiographic interpretation of lumbar anteroposterior, lateral, flexion, extension views, and MRI-stenosis analysis were recorded. Computed tomography (CT) scan is performed for preoperative evaluation of the pedicle size and to rule out any congenital malformation, disc calcifications, and vacuum disc signs. A 3D reconstruction CT scan helps give the surgeon a visual impression of the amount of bone resection is needed. The operative side is decided based on the side of the main symptoms.

Anesthesia and Skin Incision

The procedures could be performed with either epidural anesthesia with sedation or general anesthesia. The patient was prone on a Wilson Frame over a radiolucent operating table with the spine in slight flexion. The endoscopic systems use the irrigation pump and set the fluid infusion pressure at 25–40 mmHg. A surgeon stands on the symptomatic side and uses the upper pedicle screw skin incision for the uniportal endoscope insertion and docking for each corresponding level of posterolateral approach interbody fusion (Fig. **1C**). The vertical 1.6 cm skin incision is done to facilitate working cannula placement. An extended fascia incision of 3 cm is made to allow mobility of the working channel and subsequent rod placement after interbody cage insertion.

Insertion of Endoscope

A 13.7 mm diameter working cannula with a beveled tip was inserted *via* the transforaminal approach (Fig. **1C**). We performed an intraoperative anteroposterior and lateral view to confirm the correct level of decompression at this point. An endoscope of 15° viewing angle, outer diameter 10 mm, working channel diameter of 6 mm, and working length 125 mm was inserted for the surgical procedure.

Surgical Procedures

A clear endoscopic view is obtained after hemostasis with radiofrequency ablation of the cephalad lamina and the facet joint (Fig. **3A**). The inferior articular process was drilled in a curvilinear direction, starting from the spinolaminar junction to the superolateral region of the inferior articular process (Figs. **3B** & **3C**). A complete inferior articular facetectomy is performed and harvested as an autograft (Fig. **3D**). Trimming the pars interarticularis with an endoscopic drill may be required to provide more working space for interbody fusion (Fig. **3E**). The underlying superior articular process is exposed after the inferior articular facet was removed (Fig. **3F**). The superior articular process was resected from the medial to the lateral direction to its base. The local bone graft was used as an autograft for the fusion (Figs. **3G & 3H**).

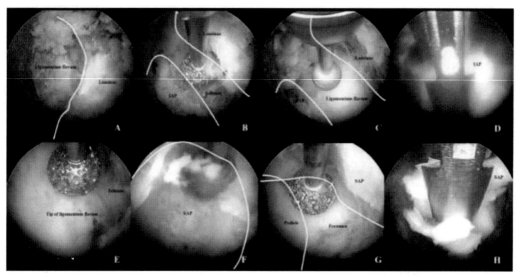

Fig. (3). Exposure of the ligamentum flavum in the interlaminar window and the laminae. Endo TLIF facet resection was done on right L5-S1. (A): Exposure of the ligamentum flavum in the interlaminar window and the laminae. (B): After exposure to the IAP, endoscopic drilling was started at the junction between cephalad lamina and IAP. (C): Endoscopic drilling was exposing the deep layer of ligamentum flavum and last thin cortical layer of IAP. (D): IAP was resected and harvested as a bone graft. (E): The isthmus was trimmed with an endoscopic drill to provide more working space, and the tip of ligamentum flavum was exposed. (F): Exposure of the SAP after IAP removal. (G) Endoscopic drilling was done at the base of SAP along caudal lamina. (H) SAP was resected and harvested for a bone graft.

The ligamentum flavum overlying the disc and neural elements are removed with endoscopic Kerrison rongeurs and forceps (Fig. **4A**). Epidural bleeding may occur during this step of the procedure. Typically, it can be controlled with radiofrequency, which is also valuable for releasing adhesions encountered during the access to the intervertebral interspace *via* annulotomy. The working cannula is rotated clockwise and advanced carefully, with the opened bevel pointing away from the exiting and traversing nerve root to retract the neural structures away gently. The working cannula can be strategically positioned to expose the intervertebral disc (Fig. **4B**). Forceps, plasma coagulators, blunt probes, and drills are employed to open the annulus up further (Fig. **4C**), after which the working cannula is advanced into the disc space's opening to keep the disc space. The endplate preparation is performed for the interbody fusion under endoscopic vision using a mixture of the endoscopic drill, forceps, a blunt bent probe, and a plasma coagulator (Fig. **4D**). The optimal fusion bed preparation would be evidenced by decortication of the endplate cartilage with punctate bleeding of subchondral bone (Fig. **4E**).

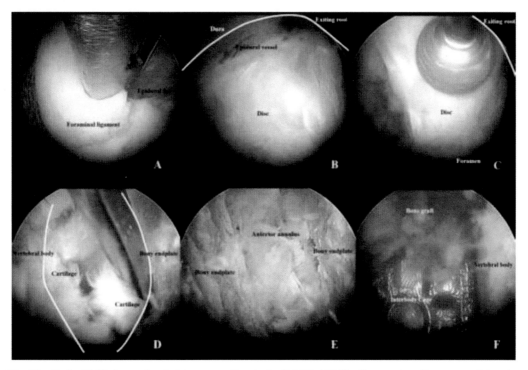

Fig. (4). Endo-TLIF disc and endplate preparation in the L5-S1. (A) The ligamentum flavum overlying the disc and neural elements was removed with endoscopic Kerrison rongeur and forceps. (B) Working cannula advanced and rotated to protect the exiting nerve root and the traversing nerve root docking on the disc. (C) Endoscopic disc drilling was performed to remove syndesmophytes, disc adhesions, and open up intervertebral disc space. (D) Disc and cartilage were denuded of the endplate using a mixture of drilling, endoscopic probe, and forceps. (E) Complete endplate preparation was done to the anterior annulus just short of the anterior longitudinal ligament under direct magnified endoscopic visualization. (F) Intervertebral cage was inserted and checked that is was in an optimal position under endoscopic visualization.

Once endplate preparation was complete, the working cannula was further advanced into the intervertebral disc space with the tip of the working cannula. The authors recommend placing the working cannula in the dorsal third of the disc space to hold the disc space open while placing the bone graft in the anterior portion of the intervertebral disc space. Serial dilators gradually widen the disc space to accommodate the best-sized trial for the cage implant. After trial removal, a mixture of autograft and allograft was placed in the ventral and contralateral disc space under fluoroscopic guidance through the endoscopic working cannula. Finally, a trial was reinserted to compact the bone graft and guide the cage's appropriate size to be inserted with fluoroscopy. Under fluoroscopic guidance, the measured 3D-printed titanium cage packed with autograft is inserted into the disc space through the Harrison cage glider (Figs. **2C - F**). Cage insertion under fluoroscopic guidance was facilitated by gentle retraction of the neural elements, endoscopically visualized (Fig. **4F**). The cage was then adjusted into an optimal position under direct endoscopic vision. The authors placed a drain routinely, which would be removed on day one postoperatively.

Pedicle Screw and Rod Insertion with Appropriate Compression and Distraction

Percutaneous pedicle screws were inserted under fluoroscopic guidance in standard fashion with or without cement augmentation in the select osteoporotic patient. Cement was injected through the percutaneous trocar before the insertion of self-tapping pedicle screws. Two bent rods of appropriate length and lordosis were prepared and inserted using the percutaneous rod holder. After the cement was sufficiently hardened, the pedicle screws were performed compression and final tightening the set screws over the rod. The intervertebral body cage, deployed in a good position, usually restored the disc height. The wound was closed in layers.

Post-Operative Care

All Endo-TLIF patients were admitted. On postoperative day one, the patients could be mobilized, and they had CT and standing XR performed as per hospital protocol. The drain is typically removed on postoperative day one or two. Patients were followed up at one week, three months, six months, and 1-year post-operation.

Potential Risks

There were several complications reported in uniportal and biportal endoscopic procedures: Incidental durotomy (3.3%) [1], transient paresthesia (1–3%), epidural hematoma, with a revision rate of 1.9%, and headache (1–2%) [2 - 4].

CLINICAL SERIES

In a severely collapsed disc space, large syndesmophytes or a calcified disc obstructing the disc space's entry and severe disc adhesion in the annulus portion of intravertebral disc space. A 3.5~4.5 mm endoscopic diamond burr is most beneficial to resect the syndesmophytes and mobilized spontaneously fused disc spaces. The index level's segmental mobility was increased by the disc adhesion releasing technique to allow the large-sized interbody cage insertion to accomplish the more significant restoration of disc height even in severe collapsed intervertebral disc space. Endplate-preserving decortication techniques are critical to prevent cage subsidence. In our series, we found no subsidence in our retrospective cohort of 30 levels of Endo-TLIF in 27 patients during the mean follow-up of 12 months. Average VAS score reductions were 2.5±1.1, 3.2±0.9, and 4.3± 1.0 at one week post-operation, three months post-operation, and final follow-up, respectively, $p < 0.05$. There was a significant increase in mid-sagittal computer tomographic anterior, middle, and posterior disc height of 6.99±2.30, 6.28±1.44, 5.12±1.79 mm, respectively, $p < 0.05$. CT mid coronal disc height showed an increase of 7.13±1.90 mm, $p < 0.05$. There was a significant improvement in the CT coronal wedge angle of 2.35±4.73 and the CT segmental focal sagittal angle of 1.98±4.69, $p < 0.05$ [1].

DISCUSSION

The results of endoscopic fusion through the uniportal transforaminal trans-Kambin route and biportal-assisted endoscopic fusion have provided positive clinical outcomes [2, 3]. Kim and Wu *et al.* reported favorable clinical and radiological results with the uniportal full endoscopic posterolateral transforaminal lumbar interbody fusion [11]. There were comparison studies between biportal endoscopic fusion and open fusion procedures, which showed significantly less blood loss and early postoperative pain control; there was a trend in lower complications rate but no difference in fusion rate. However, there is a lack of literature describing the long-term follow-up results of the fusion rate in the Endo-TLIF and the biportal-assisted endoscopic fusion. There is no comparative study of our technique Endo-TLIF with open conventional fusion. Therefore, a discussion would be focused on early clinical or radiological favorable results of the Endo-TLIF, and it's involved technical advancements rather than the comparison with microscopic MIS TLIF.

Transforaminal endoscopic interbody fusion has several advantages in preserving muscle attachment and the integrity of the facet joint. Additionally, the surgery could be done under local anesthesia and moderate sedation. It is especially crucial for patients with significant comorbidities as uniportal transforaminal endoscopic fusion operates within a small safe corridor of Kambin's triangle, requiring a narrow width cage with an expandable cage to fit through the limited access to the intervertebral disc space [17]. With a narrow width cage used in uniportal transforaminal endoscopic fusion, there would be higher stress concentration on the endplates, which may cause a higher incidence of subsidence, especially if the endplate was violated during endplate preparation under fluoroscopy with a periodic endoscopic inspection [6, 7]. Compared to the transkambin approach, the endplate preparation was performed under direct endoscopic vision throughout the entire process in Endo-TLIF. Kim and Wu *et al.*

reported the Endo-TLIF case series using the endoscopic disc drilling and endplate denudation techniques with 12 months mean follow-up period [3, 16]. No subsidence occurred compared to the 6% rate of subsidence resulting from Trans-Kambin transforaminal interbody fusion [8]. The exiting nerve root is potentially in danger of injury, most commonly *via* neuropraxia. Reported dysesthesia rates vary between 0% to 22% in the uniportal transforaminal endoscopic fusion [5, 6]. Since a cage is inserted through Kambin's triangle, there might be a high possibility of exiting nerve root injury during insertion. Direct decompression of the central spinal canal and nerve roots may also be limited in the trans-Kambin approach.

A large interbody cage can better reconstruct the anterior column of the lumbar spine and promotes interbody fusion, and minimizes the risk of implant retropulsion. The main advantage of biportal endoscopic interbody fusion is the ability to use large interbody cages to perform interbody fusion with clear vision using an endoscope. Also, during the Endo-TLIF, the complete resection of the ipsilateral facet joint created enough space for a sizeable interbody cage used in microscopic tubular transforaminal lumbar interbody fusion or the biportal endoscopic interbody fusion. Uniportal full endoscopic transforaminal interbody fusion was demonstrated in a patient with grade 2 spondylolisthesis by Kim and Wu *et al*. They used a sizeable interbody cage to reduce the translational deformity with excellent clinical results [16]. They recently used this technique to perform interbody fusion in patients with severe collapsed disc space and reported favorable clinical outcomes with CT-based radiologic positive results [4]. In collapsed disc spaced, Endo-TLIF can be challenging. Difficulties may arise from non-parallel endplates, deformity, and small size neuroforamen (Figs. **5A** - **H**) [18 - 20]. Complications are of concern, and surgeons should have a heightened level of awareness for these anatomical variations. To achieve consistently good results with the Endo-TLIF, surgeons should be versatile in unilateral laminotomy with bilateral decompression.

Kim and Wu *et al*. reported the early clinical results in Endo-TLIF application in adult degenerative scoliosis [4]. The evaluation showed a significant improvement in the CT coronal and sagittal focal angle for Endo-TLIF cases, decreasing the effect of coronal wedging and sagittal kyphosis caused by severe disc collapse affected lumbar segment. However, they did not have evidence or advocate Endo-TLIF for more than 20 degrees of severe scoliosis deformity. More soft tissue and bony releases and the addition of more fusion levels might be necessary. Traditional fusion procedures may be more appropriate for these types of patients.

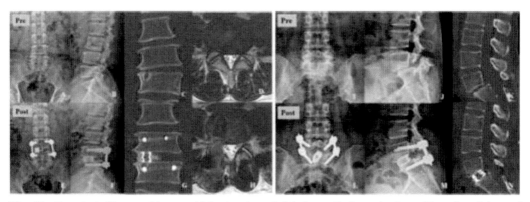

Fig. (5). Case 1: A 42-year-old man with back pain and right leg radiating pain showed lateral wedging and collapsed disk space at the L4-5 level. Endo-TLIF L4-5 with the right paraspinal approach was performed. (**A, C**) Preoperative right-sided concave lateral wedging of L4-5 and endplate bony erosion. (**B**) Preoperative loss of lumbar lordosis. (**D**) Preoperative right foraminal and lateral recess stenosis. (**E, G**) The interbody cage insertion in the wedging site jacked up the upper vertebra endplate with increased disc height and decreased concave coronal deformity. (**F**) Postoperatively, the lumbar lordosis was improved. (**H**) Postoperative relief of foraminal and lateral recess stenosis. Case 2: A 48-year-old woman with back pain and neurogenic claudication showed spondylolytic spondylolisthesis with collapsed disc space at the L5-S1 level. Endo-TLIF L5-S1 with left paraspinal approach was performed. (**J, K**) Preoperative isthmic spondylolisthesis with vacuum disc at L5-S1 level. (**L**) Postoperative good position of the interbody cage and implants. (**M, N**) Lateral X-ray image and midsagittal cut CT scan showed reduced spondylolisthesis with good placement of cage and bone graft.

CONCLUSION

Due to the increase in the elderly population, minimally invasive spine surgery, especially endoscopic spine surgery, is urgently needed. It has been found that endoscopic spine surgery has many advantages over conventional surgery through a long research period.

In addition, endoscopic lumbar interbody fusion will not end only with a minimized option, but only if it can give an advantage compared to the existing surgery. A recent study confirmed that endplate preservation through endplate denudation could reduce subsidence and increase the fusion rate. It was confirmed that the disc height could be sufficiently restored through the adhesion releasing technique.

CONSENT FOR PUBLICATION

Not applicable.

CONFLICT OF INTEREST

The authors declare no conflict of interest, financial or otherwise.

ACKNOWLEDGEMENT

Declared none.

REFERENCES

[1]   Vos T, Flaxman AD, Naghavi M, *et al.* Years lived with disability (YLDs) for 1160 sequelae of 289 diseases and injuries 1990-2010: a systematic analysis for the Global Burden of Disease Study 2010. Lancet 2012; 380(9859): 2163-96.
[http://dx.doi.org/10.1016/S0140-6736(12)61729-2] [PMID: 23245607]

[2]   Kim M, Kim HS, Oh SW, *et al.* Evolution of Spinal Endoscopic Surgery. Neurospine 2019; 16(1): 6-14.
[http://dx.doi.org/10.14245/ns.1836322.161] [PMID: 31618807]

[3]   Wu PH, Kim HS, Lee YJ, *et al.* Uniportal Full Endoscopic Posterolateral Transforaminal Lumbar Interbody Fusion with Endoscopic Disc Drilling Preparation Technique for Symptomatic Foraminal Stenosis Secondary to Severe Collapsed Disc Space: A Clinical and Computer Tomographic Study with Technical Note. Brain Sci 2020; 10(6): E373.
[http://dx.doi.org/10.3390/brainsci10060373] [PMID: 32549320]

[4]   Heo DH, Park CK. Clinical results of percutaneous biportal endoscopic lumbar interbody fusion with application of enhanced recovery after surgery. Neurosurg Focus 2019; 46(4): E18.
[http://dx.doi.org/10.3171/2019.1.FOCUS18695] [PMID: 30933919]

[5]   Ahn Y, Youn MS, Heo DH. Endoscopic transforaminal lumbar interbody fusion: a comprehensive review. Expert Rev Med Devices 2019; 16(5): 373-80.
[http://dx.doi.org/10.1080/17434440.2019.1610388] [PMID: 31044627]

[6]   Wagner R, Haefner M. Uniportal Endoscopic Lumbar Interbody Fusion. Neurospine 2020; 17 (Suppl. 1): S120-8.
[http://dx.doi.org/10.14245/ns.2040130.065] [PMID: 32746525]

[7]   Ao S, Zheng W, Wu J, *et al.* Comparison of Preliminary clinical outcomes between percutaneous endoscopic and minimally invasive transforaminal lumbar interbody fusion for lumbar degenerative diseases in a tertiary hospital: Is percutaneous endoscopic procedure superior to MIS-TLIF? A prospective cohort study. Int J Surg 2020; 76: 136-43.
[http://dx.doi.org/10.1016/j.ijsu.2020.02.043] [PMID: 32165279]

[8]   Morgenstern C, Yue JJ, Morgenstern R. Full Percutaneous Transforaminal Lumbar Interbody Fusion Using the Facet-sparing, Trans-Kambin Approach. Clin Spine Surg 2020; 33(1): 40-5.
[http://dx.doi.org/10.1097/BSD.0000000000000827] [PMID: 31162179]

[9]   Heo DH, Son SK, Eum JH, Park CK. Fully endoscopic lumbar interbody fusion using a percutaneous unilateral biportal endoscopic technique: technical note and preliminary clinical results. Neurosurg Focus 2017; 43(2): E8.
[http://dx.doi.org/10.3171/2017.5.FOCUS17146] [PMID: 28760038]

[10] Park MK, Park SA, Son SK, Park WW, Choi SH. Clinical and radiological outcomes of unilateral biportal endoscopic lumbar interbody fusion (ULIF) compared with conventional posterior lumbar interbody fusion (PLIF): 1-year follow-up. Neurosurg Rev 2019; 42(3): 753-61.
[http://dx.doi.org/10.1007/s10143-019-01114-3] [PMID: 31144195]

[11] Kim HS, Wu PH, Lee YJ, Kim DH, Jang IT. Technical Considerations of Uniportal Endoscopic Posterolateral Lumbar Interbody Fusion: A Review of Its Early Clinical Results in Application in Adult Degenerative Scoliosis. World Neurosurg 2020.
[PMID: 32531438]

[12] Holly LT, Schwender JD, Rouben DP, Foley KT. Minimally invasive transforaminal lumbar interbody fusion: indications, technique, and complications. Neurosurg Focus 2006; 20(3): E6.

[http://dx.doi.org/10.3171/foc.2006.20.3.7] [PMID: 16599422]

[13]   Kim HS, Wu PH, Jang IT. Lumbar Endoscopic Unilateral Laminotomy for Bilateral Decompression Outside-In Approach: A Proctorship Guideline With 12 Steps of Effectiveness and Safety. Neurospine 2020; 17 (Suppl. 1): S99-S109.
[http://dx.doi.org/10.14245/ns.2040078.039] [PMID: 32746523]

[14]   Lim KT, Meceda EJA, Park CK. Inside-Out Approach of Lumbar Endoscopic Unilateral Laminotomy for Bilateral Decompression: A Detailed Technical Description, Rationale and Outcomes. Neurospine 2020; 17 (Suppl. 1): S88-98.
[http://dx.doi.org/10.14245/ns.2040196.098] [PMID: 32746522]

[15]   Lim KT, Nam HGW, Kim SB, Kim HS, Park JS, Park CK. Therapeutic Feasibility of Full Endoscopic Decompression in One- to Three-Level Lumbar Canal Stenosis *via* a Single Skin Port Using a New Endoscopic System, Percutaneous Stenoscopic Lumbar Decompression. Asian Spine J 2019; 13(2): 272-82.
[http://dx.doi.org/10.31616/asj.2018.0228] [PMID: 30472819]

[16]   Kim HS, Wu PH, Jang I-T. Technical note on Uniportal full endoscopic posterolateral approach transforaminal lumbar interbody fusion with reduction for grade 2 spondylolisthesis. Interdiscip Neurosurg 2020; 21: 21.
[http://dx.doi.org/10.1016/j.inat.2020.100712]

[17]   Morgenstern R, Morgenstern C, Jané R, Lee SH. Usefulness of an expandable interbody spacer for the treatment of foraminal stenosis in extremely collapsed disks: preliminary clinical experience with endoscopic posterolateral transforaminal approach. J Spinal Disord Tech 2011; 24(8): 485-91.
[http://dx.doi.org/10.1097/BSD.0b013e3182064614] [PMID: 21336171]

[18]   Lee CW, Yoon KJ, Kim SW. Percutaneous Endoscopic Decompression in Lumbar Canal and Lateral Recess Stenosis - The Surgical Learning Curve. Neurospine 2019; 16(1): 63-71.
[http://dx.doi.org/10.14245/ns.1938048.024] [PMID: 30943708]

[19]   Kim JH, Kim HS, Kapoor A, *et al.* Feasibility of Full Endoscopic Spine Surgery in Patients Over the Age of 70 Years With Degenerative Lumbar Spine Disease. Neurospine 2018; 15(2): 131-7.
[http://dx.doi.org/10.14245/ns.1836046.023] [PMID: 29991242]

[20]   Hwa Eum J, Hwa Heo D, Son SK, Park CK. Percutaneous biportal endoscopic decompression for lumbar spinal stenosis: a technical note and preliminary clinical results. J Neurosurg Spine 2016; 24(4): 602-7.
[http://dx.doi.org/10.3171/2015.7.SPINE15304] [PMID: 26722954]

CHAPTER 17

Technical Pearls for Difficult Cases, Controversies and Complications of Lumbar Endoscopy

Ji-Yeon Kim[1], Hyeun sung Kim[1,*], Kai-Uwe Lewandrowski[2,3,4] and Tae Jang[1]

[1] *Department of Neurosurgery, Nanoori Hospital, Seoul City, South Korea*

[2] *Center for Advanced Spine Care of Southern Arizona and Surgical Institute of Tucson, Tucson AZ, USA*

[3] *Associate Professor of Orthopaedic Surgery, Universidad Colsanitas, Bogota, Colombia, USA*

[4] *Visiting Professor, Department Orthopaedic Surgery, UNIRIO, Rio de Janeiro, Brazil*

Abstract: Spinal endoscopy has the stigma of being reserved for only a few that figure out how to master the steep learning curve and develop clinical practice settings where an endoscopic spine surgery can thrive. In essence, endoscopic treatment of herniated discs specifically and nerve root compression in the lumbar spine in general amounts to replacing traditional open spine surgery protocols with spinal endoscopic surgery techniques. In doing so, the endoscopic spine surgeon must be confident that the degenerative spine's common painful problems can be handled with the endoscopic spinal surgery techniques with at least comparable clinical results and complication rates. This chapter illustrates several complex clinical examples and proposes treatment algorithms with pertinent pearls and tips for revision and complication cases.

Keywords: Complications, Controversies, Endoscopic techniques, Herniated disc.

INTRODUCTION

The increasing utilization of percutaneous endoscopic lumbar discectomy has also brought to light its advantages and clinical outcomes [1 - 5]. As with any new technology, there is a surge of utilization followed by a rise in less favorable results and complications highlighting the procedure's limitations. Percutaneous endoscopic lumbar discectomy (PELD) – whether in its transforaminal [1, 6 - 15] or interlaminar form [1, 16 - 21] – has procedure-specific shortcomings and additional limitations dictated by the underlying degenerative disc disease that is

---

[*] **Corresponding author Hyeun-Sung Kim:** Department of Neurosurgery, Nanoori Hospital, Gangnam, Seoul, South Korea; Tel: +82-10-2440-2631; E-mail: neurospinekim@gmail.com

Kai-Uwe Lewandrowski, Jorge Felipe Ramírez León, Anthony Yeung, Hyeun-Sung Kim, Xifeng Zhang, Gun Choi, Stefan Hellinger and Álvaro Dowling (Eds.)

worth discussing. In this chapter, the authors list the common problems responsible for inferior clinical outcomes, complications, controversies, and technical tips and pearls on how to resolve them.

1. Early Recurrence

To achieve successful long-term outcomes with the PELD, avoiding complications is essential. Early relapse after PELD is one of the problems though that may occur after PELD (Fig. **1**). While there may be patient-related factors, procedural details include incomplete decompression that may be responsible for an early recurrence.

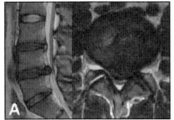 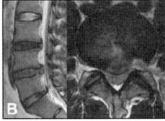 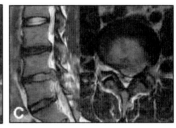

Fig. (1). Recurrence after PELD. Recurrence after PELD may be related to the early segmental loading to the operation segment after percutaneous endoscopic lumbar discectomy. (A) Preoperative MRI, (B) Immediate postoperative MRI, (C) Recurrence 3 months after PELD.

Giving patients clear postoperative instructions, including short-term bed rest, lifting limitations, choreographed walking schedules, is crucially important in avoiding problems induced by poor patient compliance during the early postoperative recovery. Physical therapy should be cautiously started 6 - 12 weeks after surgery, if at all, as many patients recover without such active exercise programs. The most controversial aspect of the endoscopic discectomy operation is to decide when to end it. In other words, when having sufficient amounts of disc tissue been removed to complete the procedure. The answer to this seemingly trivial question is not apparent. This team of authors recommends removing all unstable, delaminated, fissured, and devitalized tissue from the intervertebral disc spaces. It is during this portion where the intradiscal "inside-out" technique is most advantageous. While this subject is complex and no straightforward answer exists to the question of whether there are any prognosticators that the endoscopic spine surgeon could discern during the operation to help decide the extent of the discectomy, it is just as reasonable to assume that the underlying disease and the ability of the operated diseased remaining intervertebral disc is capable of withstanding the repetitive compressive loads of daily activities and of preventing vertical collapse is as much responsible for early recurrence. The latter question is clearly out of the surgeons' hands. Therefore, each patient should be monitored closely during the early recovery period for signs and symptoms of recurrent disc herniation.

2. VASCULAR INJURY

One of the dreaded complications of PELD is an injury to the vascular structures anterior and lateral to the spine. Especially, injuries to the segmental artery and major vessels are of concern. Segmental artery injury mainly occurs during transforaminal work, especially when using the exiting nerve root approach, because the segmental artery passes under the exiting nerve root (Fig. **2**). This segmental artery injury may induce serious retroperitoneal hematoma after PELD. The authors recommend that the endoscopic spine surgeon control bleeding from the segmental artery with radiofrequency coagulation. In the authors' experience, conversion to open surgery has not been necessary. If a symptomatic retroperitoneal hematoma should form, it can be treated with open or interventional radiology hematoma evacuation. Observation and supportive care measures are usually sufficient to manage such a retroperitoneal hematoma [22 - 24]. The authors are unaware of any publication detailing the application of embolization procedures to manage this unpleasant problem.

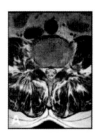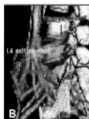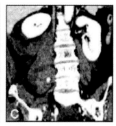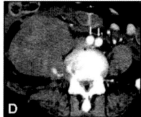

Fig. (2). Retroperitoneal hematoma (C,D) after percutaneous endoscopic lumbar discectomy for far lateral disc (A) due to segmental artery injury (B) [22].

3. NEURAL INJURY

Neural injury after PELD, although uncommon, will likely occur at one point or another during the carrier of an endoscopic spine surgeon. These are characterized by motor weakness and sensory loss. These injuries are commonly related to retraction-related neuropraxia. True surgical transection of traversing or exiting nerve root during routine lumbar endoscopy is very uncommon, and this team of authors is unaware of any such reports. Therefore, neuropraxia related problems will likely resolve spontaneously with supportive care measures, and patients should be reassured. Neuropraxia should be distinguished from dysesthesia, which frequently occurs after PELD [3, 18]. The burning sensation with decreased sensation and proprioception – although irritating to the patient – typically resolves with transforaminal epidural steroid injections and medical management with gabapentin or pregabalin within a few weeks. In rare cases, neural injury can induce a permanent neurologic deficit commonly of the exiting root injury, a cauda equina syndrome, motor weakness, and sympathetic injury. Therefore, the importance of adequate and thorough training of the aspiring endoscopic spine surgeon in formalized postgraduate fellowship training programs emphasizing careful nerve root retraction and judicious use of thermal radiofrequency ablation avoiding thermal damage [22] is of utmost importance. Avoiding these devastating complications is simply at the heart of maintaining a high-quality endoscopic spine surgery program. However, one should be prepared for managing them, and patients should be thoroughly informed preoperatively about the pros and cons of endoscopic spine surgery in general.

4. INFECTION

Another serious complication is an infection of the intradiscal area. First-line treatment should be with a minimum six weeks course of intravenous antibiotics. The antibiotics should only be started after a culture biopsy has been obtained to tailor the regimen to the patient's bacterial culture results. Patients started on empiric antibiotic programs with first- or second-generation cephalosporins may develop antibiotic resistance and a chronic or indolent infection refractory to antibiotic treatment. In some cases, formal surgical debridement is needed to control the infection [59]. An endoscopic lavage of the interior of the infected intervertebral disc is reasonable and can be attempted. However, open irrigation and debridement may be preferred, particularly if the patient does not improve clinically. Spinal fusion may ultimately be necessary as infection typically produce a rapid progression of the degenerative process at the involved surgical level or may prompt such extensive debridement that it cannot be avoided. Therefore, patients should be thoroughly educated about this devastating complication.

CASES EXAMPLES

In the following, the authors will briefly introduce common case scenarios that may prove difficult for the endoscopic spine surgeon who is attempting to treat common and complex disc herniation problems of the lumbar spine. While there may be many ways to manage these complex situations, the authors present their preferred method of handling these situations without claiming a dogmatic management style. Therefore, the cases presented herein will be concisely described with emphasis on video illustration rather than treatment. Therefore, the authors respectfully request the prospective readers view the provided procedural videos to learn more about the authors' preferred management style in the clinical case scenarios listed below.

1. Paracentral Lumbar HNP

For patients with a paracentral disc herniation a targeted fragmentectomy is recommended (Fig. **3**).

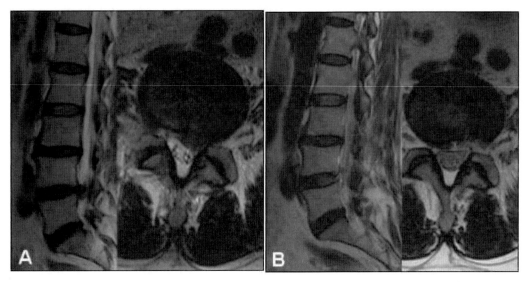

Fig. (3). Percutaneous transforaminal endoscopic lumbar discectomy for paracentral lumbar HNP. A. Preoperative MRI, B. Postoperative MRI.

The relevant steps of the targeted fragmentectomy are detailed in the following video showcasing the endoscopic revision surgery:

Video-MIS Text 22-PELD case 01-Paracentral Lumbar HNP-01

2. Upward Migrated Lumbar HNP

For patients with an upward migrated the following procedural steps are recommended.

- Exiting nerve root approach.
- Round working channel to protect the exiting root.
- It is important to approach close to the axilla area and identify the remnant disc (Fig. **4**).

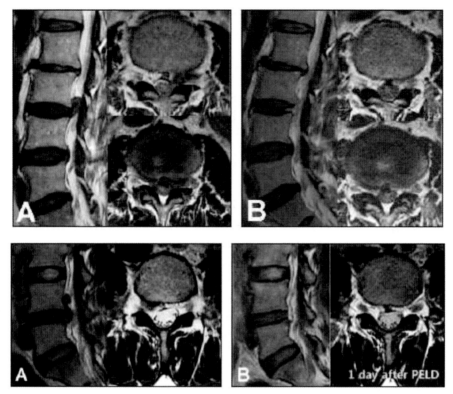

Fig. (4). Percutaneous endoscopic lumbar discectomy for upward migrated HNP. Case 1. L3-4: A. Preoperative MRI, B. postoperative MRI, Case 2. L4-5: A. Preoperative MRI, B. postoperative MRI.

The relevant pearls and tips of the PELD for upward migrated are detailed in the following video showcasing the endoscopic surgery details:

Video-MIS Text 23-PELD case 02-Upward migrated lumbar HNP-01

3. Foraminal Lumbar HNP

For patients with an foraminal herniated disc the following procedural steps are recommended [25, 26]:

- Exiting nerve root approach.
- Round working channel: exiting root protection.
- It is important to identify the remnant disc (Fig. **5**).

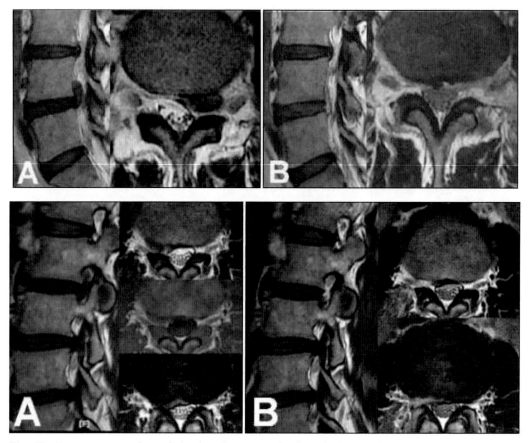

Fig. (5). Percutaneous endoscopic lumbar discectomy for foraminal HNP. Case 1. L4-5: A. Preoperative MRI, B. postoperative MRI, Case 2. L2-3: A. Preoperative MRI, B. postoperative MRI.

An example case of PELD for a foraminal HNP is shown in the following video:

Video-MIS Text 24-PELD case 03-Foraminal lumbar HNP-01

4. Far Lateral Lumbar HNP

For patients with an far lateral herniated disc the following procedural steps are recommended [25 - 27]:

- Exiting nerve root approach.
- Round working channel to protect the exiting root.
- The L5-S1 far lateral disc is not an easy to approach using the rigid endoscope when there is a high iliac crest (Fig. **6**).

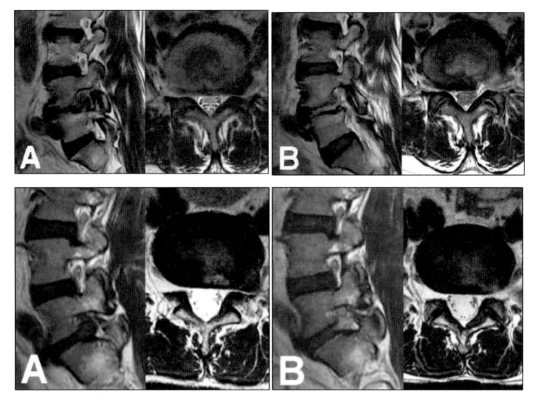

Fig. (6). Percutaneous endoscopic lumbar discectomy for far lateral HNP. Case 1. L4-5: A. Preoperative MRI, B. postoperative MRI, Case 2. L5-S1: A. Preoperative MRI, B. postoperative MRI.

An example case of PELD for a far lateral HNP is shown in the following video:

Video-MIS Text 25-PELD case 04-Far lateral Lumbar HNP-01

5. Severe Canal Compromise Type Lumbar HNP

For patients with a herniated disc and severe canal compromise the following procedural steps are recommended [28]:

- Outside-in approach for epidural exposure.
- Dural exposure.
- Identify any remnant disc because central stenosis is frequently combined with a multi-fragmented disc (Fig. **7**).

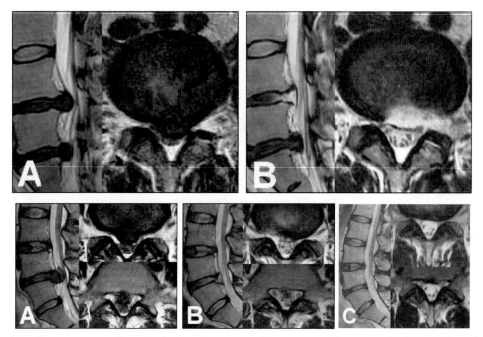

Fig. (7). Percutaneous endoscopic lumbar discectomy for severe canal compromised HNP. Case 1. A. Preoperative MRI, B. postoperative MRI, Case 2. A. Preoperative MRI, B. postoperative MRI, C. 1 year follow up.

An example case of PELD for a HNP in a patient with severe central canal compromise is shown in the following video:

Video-MIS Text 26-PELD case 05-Severe Canal Compromise Type Lumbar HNP-01

6. Severe Canal Compromised, Epidural Migrated Lumbar HNP

For patients with a herniated disc and severe canal compromise the following procedural steps are recommended [28]:

- Outside-in approach is useful for epidural exposure.
- Dural exposure.
- Sometimes, a large fragment can be located dorsal to the posterior longitudinal ligament (PLL). Therefore, the area dorsal to the PLL that is ventral to the dura must be checked for additional disc fragments.
- At the end of the case, make sure the epidural space is free without obstructions (Fig. **8**).

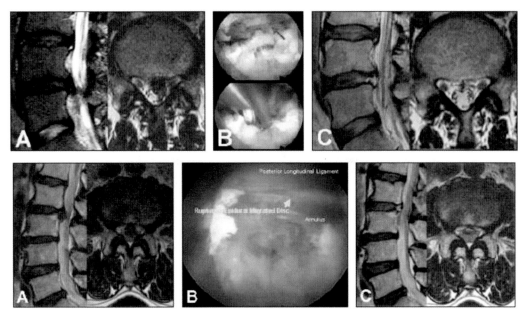

Fig. (8). Epidural migration of a ruptured disc. In cases of a ruptured disc that is separated completely from the disc space pass over the posterior longitudinal ligament, successful removal of the migrated disc sometimes failed. Therefore, the free epidural space should be checked. Case 1. A. Preoperative MRI, B. Intraoperative image, C. Postoperative MRI. Case 2. A. Preoperative MRI, B. Intraoperative image, C. Postoperative.

An example case of Severe Canal Compromised, Epidural Migrated Lumbar HNP is shown in the following video:

Video-MIS Text 27-PELD case 06-Severe Canal Compromised, Epidural Migrated Lumbar HNP-01

7. Downward Migrated Lumbar HNP

For patients with a downward herniated disc and severe canal compromise the following procedural steps are recommended [9, 27]:

- Perform a targeted fragmentectomy for moderate to high grade inferior migrated herniated discs.
- Epidural exposure.
- Foraminoplasty / Suprapedicular approach.
- The free traversing root should be identified.
- If the incomplete extraction of the disc material is suspected, the authors recommend an immediate postop MRI scan (Fig. **9**).

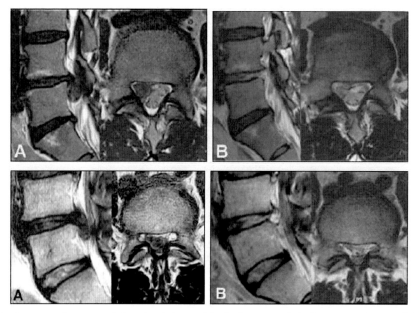

Fig. (9). In the cases of a ruptured disc that is located in the low part of the lower vertebral pedicle, removal of the pathologic disc is not easy. Case 1. A. Preoperative MRI, B. Postoperative MRI, Case 2. A. Preoperative MRI, B. Postoperative MRI.

An example case of downward migrated herniated disc is shown in the following video:

Video-MIS Text 28-PELD case 07-Down Migrated Lumbar HNP-01

8. Recurred HNP After Open Lumbar Discectomy

For patients with a recurred HNP after open lumbar discectomy the following procedural steps are recommended [3, 29]:

- Careful dissection of epidural adhesion
- Expect incidental durotomies and avoid nerve root injury at all cost (Fig. **10**).

An example case of recurred HNP after open lumbar discectomy is shown in the following video:

Video-MIS Text 29-PELD case 08- Recurred HNP after open lumbar discectomy-01

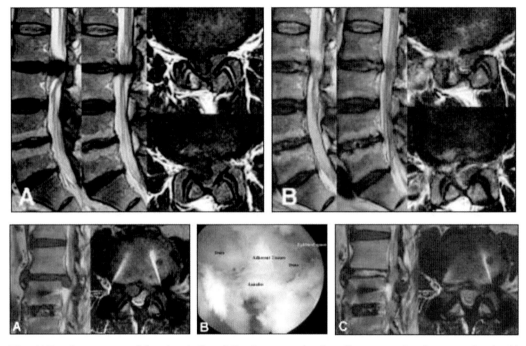

Fig. (10). Recurrence of herniated disc following open lumbar discectomy is often associated with inseparable adhesions, and so disc extraction must be performed meticulously and sufficient dissection of the herniated disc from the dura is necessary for root decompression. Case 1. A. Preoperative MRI, B. Postoperative MRI, Case 2. A. Preoperative MRI, B. Intraoperative, C. Postoperative MRI.

9. Recurrent HNP After Transforaminal PELD

For patients with a recurrent HNP after transforaminal PELD the following procedural steps are recommended [3, 29]:

- Perform dareful dissection of an adhesion
- Adhesion of both the exiting and traversing nerve roots are often be seen during revision of transforaminal PELD.
- Be prepared for repair of dural tearing.
- Be vigilant and carefully retract nerve roots to avoid injury (Fig. **11**).

An example case of recurrent HNP after previous transforaminal PELD is shown in the following video:

Video-MIS Text 30-PELD case 09- Recurred HNP after PELD-01

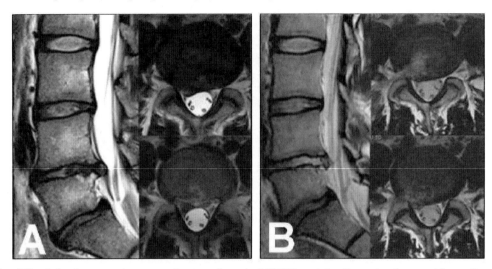

Fig. (11). Adhesions can also occur after transforaminal PELD, and the disc extraction must be performed meticulously, with sufficient dissection of the herniated discs from the dura, which is necessary for root decompression. A. Preoperative MRI, B. Postoperative MRI.

10. Recurrent HNP after Intradiscal Therapy

For patients with a recurrent HNP after intradiscal therapy the following procedural steps are recommended [3, 29]:

- Careful dissection of adhesions.
- Adhesions can often be seen in the revision of intradiscal therapy at the prior entry point through the annulus.
- There is a higher risk of dural tears and nerve root injury. Be prepared to manage them (Fig. **12**).

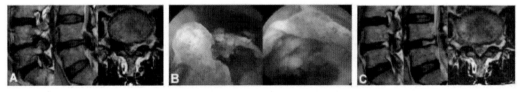

Fig. (12). Adhesions can also occur after a minimally invasive procedure, and the disc extraction must be performed meticulously and sufficient dissection of the herniated discs from the dura is necessary for root decompression. A. Preoperative MRI, B. Intraoperative, C. Postoperative MRI.

An example case of recurrent HNP after intradiscal therapy is shown in the following video:

Video-MIS Text 31-PELD case 10- Recurred HNP after intradiscal therapy-01

11. Focal Calcification within Lumbar HNP

For patients with a focal calcification within a lumbar HNP the following procedural steps are recommended:

- In the cases of focal calcification within a mixed HNP, calcification and disc protrusion can be removed using the punch and rongeur.
- But in the cases of huge calcification or severe calcification of the HNP, a drill or shaver will be needed for removal of the calcification (Fig. **13**).

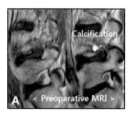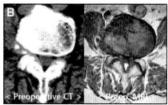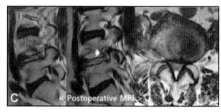

Fig. (13). If the focal calcification is mixed with soft disc protrusion, it will induce symptomatic radicular pain. If the point of calcification is not huge, it can be broken down and the calcified discs removed effectively using a punch or rongeur. A,B. Preoperative CT/MRI, C. Postoperative MRI.

An example case of focal calcification within a lumbar HNP is shown in the following video:

Video-MIS Text 32-PELD case 11-Focal calcification mixed Lumbar HNP-01

12. Combined Foraminal Stenosis and HNP

For patients with a combined foraminal stenosis and HNP the following procedural steps are recommended [30 - 32]:

- Removal of hard bony structures.
- There is a probability of an exiting nerve root injury (Fig. **14**).

An example case of combined foraminal stenosis and HNP is shown in the following video:

Video-MIS Text 33-PELD case 12-Stenosis Combined Foraminal HNP

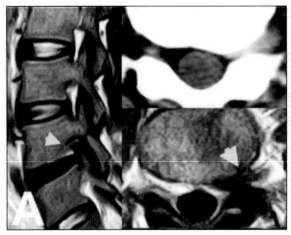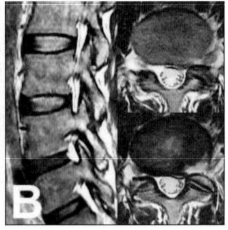

Fig. (14). In cases of foraminal stenosis, the foraminal stenosis is commonly combined with bony overgrowth. To achieve sufficient foraminal decompression, removal of the overgrowth of bony structures will be needed. A. Preoperative CT/MRI, B. Postoperative MRI.

13. Discal Cyst

For patients with a discal cyst the following procedural steps are recommended [33]:

- Fluid may gush out sometimes when a cyst ruptures.
- It is important to identify the stalk of a cyst.
- It is important to clear the cyst wall and identify the free dura and the nerve root (Fig. **15**).

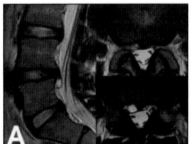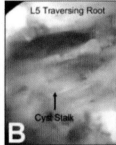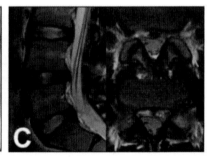

Fig. (15). Percutaneous endoscopic discal cystectomy. It is important to identify the stalk of a cyst and the free traversing root. A. Preoperative MRI, B. Intraoperative, C. Postoperative MRI.

An example case of a discal cyst is shown in the following video:

Video-MIS Text 34-PELD case 13-Cyst mixed lumbar HNP-01

14. Two-level Lumbar HNP

For patients with two-level lumbar HNP the following procedural steps are recommended:

- Two adjacent HNP that require PELD can be approached through a single skin incision.
- The remainder of the procedure standard for each level (Fig. **16**).

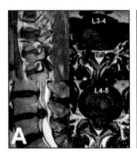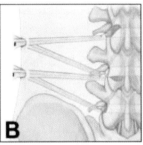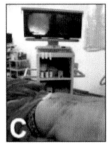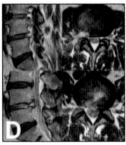

Fig. (16). Adjacent 2 level symptomatic disc can be operated with the 1 skin incision using the percutaneous rigid endoscope. A. Preoperative MRI, B,C. Intraoperative images, D. Postoperative MRI.

An example case of a two-level lumbar HNP is shown in the following video:

Video-MIS Text 35- PELD case 14-Adjacent 2 Level Lumbar HNP-01

DISCUSSION

The peer-reviewed published literature has established that complications with the lumbar endoscopy procedure are rare. The purpose of this chapter was not to relitigate this point but to provide the reader of Contemporary Endoscopic Spinal Surgery with several illustrative examples of difficult cases and some technical pearls and tips on how to handle problems that the endoscopic spine surgeon may encounter. When attempting more complex scenarios or patients with prior surgery – regardless of whether it was done open or endoscopically – the endoscopic spine surgeon should be aware of a high risk of durotomy, nerve root injuries, and complications. Epidural fibrosis, granulation tissue in a previously operated terrain should be expected and could tether the traversing and exiting nerve roots. Thus, the risk of nerve root injury is higher. Patients should be educated about the higher risk of postoperative dysesthesia. Although typically self-limiting, this unavoidable sequela from an otherwise expertly executed endoscopic spine surgery can be quite annoying to patients. Preoperative education is therefore critical to avoid unnecessary postoperative emergency room visits, readmissions, or imaging studies that ultimately do not change management but raise the cost of care. True nerve root injuries are thankfully uncommon. Patients with neuropraxia-related motor weakness, sensory and proprioception loss should be reassured. Additional treatments besides supportive care measures are often not necessary. Patients should be worked up again if other pain generators emerge as the failure to cure or an unfavorable postoperative course is not always related to the previous endoscopic surgery. Other problems may exist in the same patient.

The authors hope that the authors' illustrative video case examples will aid the aspiring endoscopic spine surgeon to better position him- or herself when trying to establish their own endoscopic spinal surgery program at their local health care facility. The individual skill level and the equipment infrastructure may vary quite a bit from one surgeon or clinical setting to another. Spine surgeons should seek out master surgeons who offer formalized postgraduate training programs to learn the more advanced skills required to handle the complex problems presented in this chapter. The learning curve is steep. Mastering it often hinges on good mentorship.

CONCLUSION

Endoscopic spine surgery requires a skill set distinctly different from what is taught in traditional postgraduate spinal surgery programs. Surgeons that have received training in endoscopes in the treatment of other body parts and organ systems may have an easier transition to learning spinal endoscopy. As shown in this chapter, more complex clinical cases can be treated with the procedure increasingly obviating the need for open spine surgery. While there are other translaminar minimally invasive spinal surgery techniques, the endoscopic access and treatment methods offer by far the most direct and least disruptive therapies to treat common painful conditions of the degenerative lumbar spine disease.

CONSENT FOR PUBLICATION

Not applicable.

CONFLICT OF INTEREST

The authors declare no conflict of interest, financial or otherwise.

ACKNOWLEDGEMENTS

Declared none.

REFERENCES

[1]   Kim DH, Choi G, Lee SH. Endoscopic Spine Procedures. Thieme Medical Publishers 2011; p. 11.

[2]   Abdullah AF, Wolber PG, Warfield JR, Gunadi IK. Surgical management of extreme lateral lumbar disc herniations: review of 138 cases. Neurosurgery 1988; 22(4): 648-53.
[http://dx.doi.org/10.1227/00006123-198804000-00005] [PMID: 3374776]

[3]   Ahn Y, Lee SH, Park WM, Lee HY, Shin SW, Kang HY. Percutaneous endoscopic lumbar discectomy for recurrent disc herniation: surgical technique, outcome, and prognostic factors of 43 consecutive cases. Spine 2004; 29(16): E326-32.
[http://dx.doi.org/10.1097/01.BRS.0000134591.32462.98] [PMID: 15303041]

[4]   McCulloch JA. Principles of Microsurgery for Lumbar Disc Diseases. New York: Raven Press 1989.

[5]   Mekhail N, Kapural L. Intradiscal thermal annuloplasty for discogenic pain: an outcome study. Pain Pract 2004; 4(2): 84-90.
[http://dx.doi.org/10.1111/j.1533-2500.2004.04203.x] [PMID: 17166191]

[6]   Ditsworth DA. Endoscopic transforaminal lumbar discectomy and reconfiguration: a postero-lateral approach into the spinal canal. Surg Neurol 1998; 49(6): 588-97.
[http://dx.doi.org/10.1016/S0090-3019(98)00004-4] [PMID: 9637618]

[7]   Tsou PM, Yeung AT. Transforaminal endoscopic decompression for radiculopathy secondary to intracanal noncontained lumbar disc herniations: outcome and technique. Spine J 2002; 2(1): 41-8.
[http://dx.doi.org/10.1016/S1529-9430(01)00153-X] [PMID: 14588287]

[8]   Tsou PM, Alan Yeung C, Yeung AT. Posterolateral transforaminal selective endoscopic discectomy and thermal annuloplasty for chronic lumbar discogenic pain: a minimal access visualized intradiscal surgical procedure. Spine J 2004; 4(5): 564-73.
[http://dx.doi.org/10.1016/j.spinee.2004.01.014] [PMID: 15363430]

[9]   Ruetten S, Komp M, Godolias G. An extreme lateral access for the surgery of lumbar disc herniations inside the spinal canal using the full-endoscopic uniportal transforaminal approach-technique and prospective results of 463 patients. Spine 2005; 30(22): 2570-8.
[http://dx.doi.org/10.1097/01.brs.0000186327.21435.cc] [PMID: 16284597]

[10]   Jasper GP, Francisco GM, Telfeian AE. Endoscopic transforaminal discectomy for an extruded lumbar disc herniation. Pain Physician 2013; 16(1): E31-5.
[PMID: 23340542]

[11]   Eustacchio S, Flaschka G, Trummer M, Fuchs I, Unger F. Endoscopic percutaneous transforaminal treatment for herniated lumbar discs. Acta Neurochir (Wien) 2002; 144(10): 997-1004.
[http://dx.doi.org/10.1007/s00701-002-1003-9] [PMID: 12382128]

[12]   Gibson JN, Cowie JG, Iprenburg M. Transforaminal endoscopic spinal surgery: the future 'gold standard' for discectomy? - A review. Surgeon 2012; 10(5): 290-6.
[http://dx.doi.org/10.1016/j.surge.2012.05.001] [PMID: 22705355]

[13]   Yeung AT, Tsou PM. Posterolateral endoscopic excision for lumbar disc herniation: Surgical technique, outcome, and complications in 307 consecutive cases. Spine 2002; 27(7): 722-31.
[http://dx.doi.org/10.1097/00007632-200204010-00009] [PMID: 11923665]

[14]   Yeung AT, Yeung CA. Advances in endoscopic disc and spine surgery: foraminal approach. Surg Technol Int 2003; 11: 255-63.
[PMID: 12931309]

[15]   Yeung AT. The evolution of percutaneous spinal endoscopy and discectomy: state of the art. Mt Sinai J Med 2000; 67(4): 327-32.
[PMID: 11021785]

[16]   Maroon JC. Current concepts in minimally invasive discectomy. Neurosurgery 2002; 51(5) (Suppl.): S137-45.

[PMID: 12234441]

[17]   Kim HS, Park JY. Comparative assessment of different percutaneous endoscopic interlaminar lumbar discectomy (PEID) techniques. Pain Physician 2013; 16(4): 359-67.
[PMID: 23877452]

[18]   Choi G, Lee SH, Raiturker PP, Lee S, Chae YS. Percutaneous endoscopic interlaminar discectomy for intracanalicular disc herniations at L5-S1 using a rigid working channel endoscope. Neurosurgery 2006; 58(1) (Suppl.): ONS59-68.
[http://dx.doi.org/10.1227/01.NEU.0000362000.35742.3D] [PMID: 16479630]

[19]   Ruetten S, Komp M, Godolias G. A New full-endoscopic technique for the interlaminar operation of lumbar disc herniations using 6-mm endoscopes: prospective 2-year results of 331 patients. Minim Invasive Neurosurg 2006; 49(2): 80-7.
[http://dx.doi.org/10.1055/s-2006-932172] [PMID: 16708336]

[20]   Ruetten S, Komp M, Merk H, Godolias G. Use of newly developed instruments and endoscopes: full-endoscopic resection of lumbar disc herniations *via* the interlaminar and lateral transforaminal approach. J Neurosurg Spine 2007; 6(6): 521-30.
[http://dx.doi.org/10.3171/spi.2007.6.6.2] [PMID: 17561740]

[21]   Ruetten S, Komp M, Merk H, Godolias G. Full-endoscopic interlaminar and transforaminal lumbar discectomy *versus* conventional microsurgical technique: a prospective, randomized, controlled study. Spine 2008; 33(9): 931-9.
[http://dx.doi.org/10.1097/BRS.0b013e31816c8af7] [PMID: 18427312]

[22]   Kim HS, Ju CI, Kim SW, Kim JG. Huge Psoas Muscle Hematoma due to Lumbar Segmental Vessel Injury Following Percutaneous Endoscopic Lumbar Discectomy. J Korean Neurosurg Soc 2009; 45(3): 192-5.
[http://dx.doi.org/10.3340/jkns.2009.45.3.192] [PMID: 19352485]

[23]   Ahn Y, Kim JU, Lee BH, Lee SH, Park JD, Hong DH. Massive Retroperitoneal Hematoma after Transforaminal Percutaneous Endoscopic Lumbar Discectomy: Reoprt of Two Cases. Rachis 2008; (4): 10-1.

[24]   Ahn Y, Kim JU, Lee BH, *et al.* Postoperative retroperitoneal hematoma following transforaminal percutaneous endoscopic lumbar discectomy. J Neurosurg Spine 2009; 10(6): 595-602.
[http://dx.doi.org/10.3171/2009.2.SPINE08227] [PMID: 19558294]

[25]   Choi G, Lee SH, Bhanot A, Raiturker PP, Chae YS. Percutaneous endoscopic discectomy for extraforaminal lumbar disc herniations: extraforaminal targeted fragmentectomy technique using working channel endoscope. Spine 2007; 32(2): E93-9.
[http://dx.doi.org/10.1097/01.brs.0000252093.31632.54] [PMID: 17224806]

[26]   Lübbers T, Abuamona R, Elsharkawy AE. Percutaneous endoscopic treatment of foraminal and extraforaminal disc herniation at the L5-S1 level. Acta Neurochir (Wien) 2012; 154(10): 1789-95.
[http://dx.doi.org/10.1007/s00701-012-1432-z] [PMID: 22782651]

[27]   Sasani M, Ozer AF, Oktenoglu T, Canbulat N, Sarioglu AC. Percutaneous endoscopic discectomy for far lateral lumbar disc herniations: prospective study and outcome of 66 patients. Minim Invasive Neurosurg 2007; 50(2): 91-7.
[http://dx.doi.org/10.1055/s-2007-984383] [PMID: 17674295]

[28]   Lee SH, Kang BU, Ahn Y, *et al.* Operative failure of percutaneous endoscopic lumbar discectomy: a radiologic analysis of 55 cases. Spine 2006; 31(10): E285-90.
[http://dx.doi.org/10.1097/01. brs.0000216446.13205.7a] [PMID: 16648734]

[29]   Lee DY, Shim CS, Ahn Y, Choi YG, Kim HJ, Lee SH. Comparison of percutaneous endoscopic lumbar discectomy and open lumbar microdiscectomy for recurrent disc herniation. J Korean Neurosurg Soc 2009; 46(6): 515-21.
[http://dx.doi.org/10.3340/jkns.2009.46.6.515] [PMID: 20062565]

[30] Knight MT, Vajda A, Jakab GV, Awan S. Endoscopic laser foraminoplasty on the lumbar spine--early experience. Minim Invasive Neurosurg 1998; 41(1): 5-9.
[http://dx.doi.org/10.1055/s-2008-1052006] [PMID: 9565957]

[31] Knight MT, Goswami A, Patko JT, Buxton N. Endoscopic foraminoplasty: a prospective study on 250 consecutive patients with independent evaluation. J Clin Laser Med Surg 2001; 19(2): 73-81.
[http://dx.doi.org/10.1089/104454701750285395] [PMID: 11443793]

[32] Nellensteijn J, Ostelo R, Bartels R, Peul W, van Royen B, van Tulder M. Transforaminal endoscopic surgery for lumbar stenosis: a systematic review. Eur Spine J 2010; 19(6): 879-86.
[http://dx.doi.org/10.1007/s00586-009-1272-6] [PMID: 20087610]

[33] Ha SW, Ju CI, Kim SW, Lee S, Kim YH, Kim HS. Clinical outcomes of percutaneous endoscopic surgery for lumbar discal cyst. J Korean Neurosurg Soc 2012; 51(4): 208-14.
[http://dx.doi.org/10.3340/jkns.2012.51.4.208] [PMID: 22737300]

CHAPTER 18

Treatment of Degenerative Lumbar Spondylolisthesis with Endoscopic Decompression of the Lumbar Spinal Canal

Zhang Xifeng[1,2,*], Yan Yuqiu[2], Yuan Huafeng[3], Cong Qiang[3] and Wu Shang[4]

[1] *Department of Orthopedics, First Medical Center, PLA General Hospital, Beijing, 100853, China*

[2] *Department of Orthopedics, Beijing Yuho Rehabilitation Hospital, Beijing 100853, China*

[3] *Department of Orthopedics, Shenyang 242 Hospital, Shenyang, Liao Ning 110031, China*

[4] *Department of Orthopedics, Affiliated Hospital of Yangzhou University, Yangzhou, 225001, China*

Abstract: Degenerative spondylolisthesis is a common problem in the elderly. The associated spinal stenosis in the central canal and the foramina may cause sciatica-type claudication symptoms affecting the lower back and extremities. Walking endurance is typically reduced. Eventually, patients may decide on surgical decompression if conservative care measures, including spinal injections, physical therapy, activity modifications, and pain medication, no longer provide relief. In the elderly, extensive spine surgery is always of concern regarding operation length, blood loss, postoperative pain management, and medical comorbidities whose management may easily spin out of control following major spine surgery. In a small subset of spondylolisthesis patients, decompression alone may suffice, particularly in those where the spinal motion segment has become rigid due to endstage degenerative disc disease, vertical collapse, and auto fusion. On the other hand, stenosis is often severe in these types of patients, for which reason extensive decompression may be necessary, and postoperative iatrogenic instability may ensue. In this article, the authors present the technique of endoscopic canal and foraminal decompression in patients with such advanced spondylolisthesis. They discuss the technical caveats and limitations of the procedure.

Keywords: Degenerative spondylolisthesis, Endoscopic decompression, Spinal stenosis.

* **Corresponding author Zhang Xifeng:** Department of Orthopedics, First Medical Center, PLA General Hospital, Beijing, 100853, China and Department of Orthopedics, Beijing Yuho Rehabilitation Hospital, Beijing 100853, China; Tel: +86 (10) 8821 9862; E-mail: xifengzhang301@outlook.com

Kai-Uwe Lewandrowski, Jorge Felipe Ramírez León, Anthony Yeung, Hyeun-Sung Kim, Xifeng Zhang, Gun Choi, Stefan Hellinger and Álvaro Dowling (Eds.)

INTRODUCTION

Spondylolisthesis may cause severe stenosis in the central spinal canal, the bilateral lateral recesses, and neuroforamina [1, 2]. Decompression without instrumentation may be tried but may fail if the patient develops postoperative instability [3]. This topic has been subject to extensive clinical investigation in the Spine Patient Outcome Research Trials (SPORT) and other studies [4 - 9]. Limited decompression with laminotomy or laminoforaminotomy has been tried [10]. With the recent advent of minimally invasive spinal surgeries, including endoscopic decompression techniques, this somewhat controversial subject has been revisited as the collateral exposure-related damage may not be as extensive. Endoscopic decompression strategies may be useful in patients with rigid end-stage degenerative disc disease and the complete vertical collapse of the intervertebral disc space. In those cases, a spontaneous fusion of the anterior column may be present *via* bridging sentinel osteophytes or even through the interbody space itself. In these types of patients, endoscopic decompression for claudication-related spinal stenosis symptoms may be an alternative to traditional open decompression without the associated blood loss, postoperative pain, and recovery associated with laminectomy with and without fusion. In this chapter, the authors present two illustrative cases and review the technical steps involved where this strategy was used successfully to the patients' advantage.

CASE PRESENTATIONS

Case 1

The first patient was a 77-year-old female whose chief complaint was difficulty walking and standing erect, typical of lumbar spinal stenosis. Symptoms recently had worsened over the past 2 months when walking endurance was reduced to 20 meters. The patient's motor strength on spot testing did not show obvious deficits. However, there was tenderness in the lower back, hyporeflexia in the lower extremities, a negative straight leg raise test bilaterally, and normal vascular examination suggesting that the patient's symptoms were predominately related to neurogenic claudication. Advanced CT and MRI imaging studies of the lumbar spine showed severe central, lateral recess and foraminal stenosis with associated grade 1 spondylolisthesis at the L4/5 level (Fig. **1**).

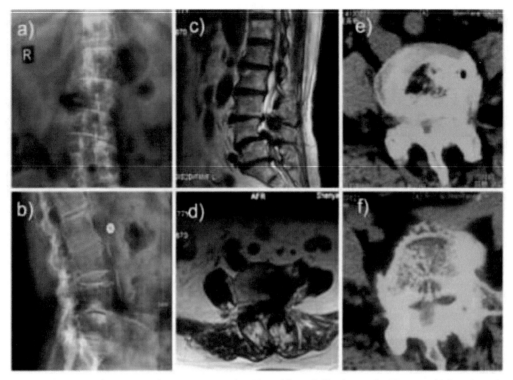

Fig. (1). Shown are the preoperative anteroposterior (a) and lateral (b) views of a 77-year-old female patient with claudication symptoms. Sagittal (c) and axial (d) MRI scans and axial CT scan sections (e-f) through the L4/5 level showed severe central, lateral recess, and foraminal stenosis preoperatively associated with rigid grade 1 spondylolisthesis. Dynamic extension-flexion views did not demonstrate any radiographic evidence of translational instability.

The indication for decompression surgery was established given the patient's severe disability with corresponding findings on the imaging studies and failed non-operative care. The patient has clear symptoms of degenerative lumbar spondylolisthesis leading to lumbar spinal stenosis, and imaging confirmed lumbar spondylolisthesis and lumbar spinal stenosis. The surgical decompression was planned with use of the endoscopic spinal surgery techniques and transforaminal approach in prone position under local anesthesia with 1% lidocaine and fluoroscopic image-guidance was adopted. Employing standard transforaminal endoscopic surgery protocol, the symptomatic right-sided neuroforamen was accessed with an 18-G spinal needle through which a guidewire was placed. A serial dilation over the guidewire, an endoscopic working channel was placed posterolaterally onto the hypertrophic facet joins. The authors preferred decompression tool is a motorized endoscopic drill which fits right through the central working channel of the endoscope. Thus, resection of the superior articular process to the base of the pedicle inferiorly, and to the medial edge of the lateral recess was performed allowing access to the ligamentum flavum which was also resected with endoscopic rongeurs. The decompression was considered complete when the lateral aspect of the cural sac was decompressed as evidenced by loosely pulsating epidural fat. Radiofrequency was used to stop bleeding before removing the endoscopic working cannula.

Postoperatively, the patient suffered from dysesthesia related to surgical irritation of the dorsal root ganglion. The patient's condition recovered well after the operation, and the symptoms were significantly relieved compared to the preoperative functional status. Re-examination of three-dimensional CT 2 days after operation showed that a significant portion of the right superior articular process and facet joint structures causing central stenosis were sufficiently removed. Another postoperative MRI scan done two months postoperatively, showed that the lumbar spinal canal was enlarged compared to the preoperative MRI study (Fig. **2**).

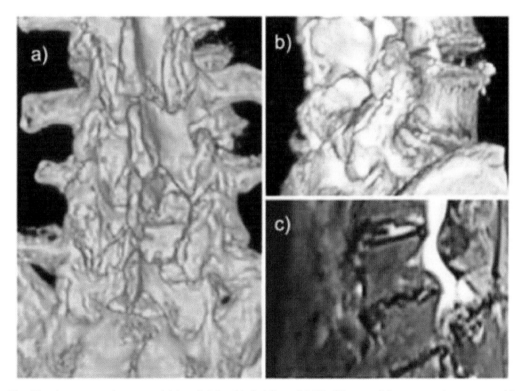

Fig. (2). A postoperative coronal (a) and right-sided oblique (b) 3D-CT scan of the same patient presented in figure 1 is shown. The CT scan was done two days after surgery and showed near-complete removal of the superior articular process. A postoperative sagittal MRI (c) scan taken two months after the endoscopic decompression surgery confirms central canal decompression from the right-sided transforaminal approach.

Case 2

This patient is a 66-years-old female with a chief complaint of low back and right lower extremity pain for the last one year. Her symptoms had been worsening over the previous month, for which reason she presented for surgical consultation. Her symptoms were activity-related and classic for neurogenic claudication. They were alleviated by rest in the supine position and aggravated by standing or sitting up straight for a long time. Her walking distance to the pain limit was 200 meters. Physical examination also revealed antalgic gait, apparent lumbosacral tenderness provoked by percussion. Her sensory examination was intact and symmetrical for pinprick and temperature sensation in both lower limbs was normal. Overall, the motor strength examination revealed 5/5 normal muscle strength in the lower extremities, including the right, in all major motor groups. Nerve tension signs such as femoral nerve stretch test or the straight leg raise test were negative on both sides. Radiographic studies of the patient's lumbar spine showed grade 1 L4/5 spondylolisthesis on plain film x-rays. The preoperative CT and MRI scans of the lumbar spine confirmed L4/5 grade 1 spondylolisthesis with associated lumbar spinal stenosis (Fig. **3**).

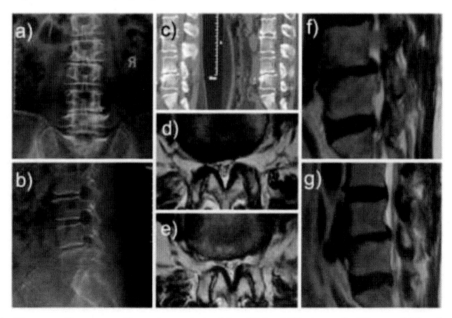

Fig. (3). Shown are the preoperative anteroposterior (a) and lateral (b) views of a 66-year-old female patient with claudication symptoms. Sagittal (c) CT, and axial (d-e), and sagittal MRI scans (f-g) confirmed predominantly right-sided foraminal and lateral recess stenosis with some thickening of the ligamentum flavum consistent with grade 1 spondylolisthesis. Dynamic extension-flexion views did not demonstrate any radiographic evidence of translational instability.

The patient had failed conservative care and presented for surgical consultation. The surgeon team indicated right-sided interlaminar endoscopic decompression despite the degenerative lumbar spondylolisthesis at the L4/5 level. The patient's spondylolisthesis was considered rigid, for which reason a fusion surgery was not deemed necessary. During the preoperative discussion with the patient, the possibility that postoperative instability may ensue, was raised. The patient was aware that a fusion procedure with interbody fusion with posterior supplemental pedicle screw fixation may be necessary as a salvage operation.

With the patient in the prone position and sterilely prepped and draped in standard surgical fashion, local anesthesia with 1% lidocaine was instituted by infiltrating the L4/5 paraspinal tissues and the facet joint complex. A small amount of local anesthetic was injected into the neuroforamen. Under C-arm fluoroscopy, the L4/5 intervertebral window was cannulated with an 18-G spinal needle. Serial dilation over a guidewire similar to the technique employed in the patient of case 1. The endoscopic working cannular was placed laterally to the facet joint complex. The decompression was performed similarly as in case 1 with an endoscopic power drill until a subtotal resection of the superior articular process is accomplished. Again, the decompression was taken medially and superiorly until the dural sac's lateral aspect was fully decompressed. Postoperatively, the patient's VAS score decreased by 6 points. The JOA score increased from 10 points to 28 points. Ultimately, this patient did very well with the transforaminal endoscopic decompression, and no further surgery was required for the L4/5 spondylolisthesis. Postoperative imaging studies are shown in Fig. (**4**).

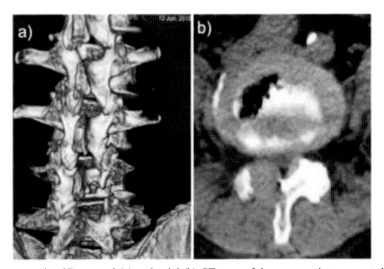

Fig. (4). A postoperative 3D coronal (a) and axial (b) CT scan of the same patient presented in Fig. (3) is shown. The endoscopic interlaminar decompression surgery accomplished adequate central and lateral recess decompression on the right side.

DISCUSSION

Degenerative spondylolisthesis is one of the common diseases of the lumbar spine frequently requiring surgery [11 - 13]. The associated lumbar spinal stenosis often causes symptoms. Degenerative lumbar spondylolisthesis was defined by Newman et al. as a displacement of the lower vertebral body forward, with or without neurological symptoms [14 - 21]. The symptoms of low back pain caused by this disease are mainly caused by lumbar spinal stenosis and lumbar instability. The populations in many developed countries are increasingly aging, creating the need for simplified surgical treatments. Minimally invasive surgeries are of particular relevance and have been the center of ongoing clinical research and investigation.

The mainstay of surgical treatment of degenerative lumbar spondylolisthesis with spinal stenosis is spinal canal decompression. Concurrent fusion is advocated by most surgeons who perform open decompression involving removing portions or the entire lumbar facet joints since the decompression renders the motion segment unstable. However, this topic is controversial. The evidence-based literature suggests little or no added benefit or improvement in clinical outcomes from adding interbody and instrumented posterolateral fusion to lumbar decompression surgery. However, there is consensus that it does raise the complication- and reoperation rates mostly because of hardware-related problems.

The randomized and controlled SPORT studies published by Weinstein et al. found that surgical treatment of lumbar spinal stenosis improves patient's functioning and clinical outcomes compared to conservative care [4 - 9]. Research by Sun et al. found that fusion, in addition to laminectomy, does not improve the quality of life and clinical satisfaction of patients after surgery but increases the surgical risk and postoperative complication rate [22]. However, Liang et al. believe that decompression combined with intervertebral body fusion and internal pedicle screw fixation delivers more reliable clinical outcomes with higher patient satisfaction because of more complete decompression and better leg pain resolution [23]. One Chinese retrospective study compared the short-term effects of spinal decompression and spinal decompression with internal fixation and fusion in treating degenerative lumbar spondylolisthesis [24]. This study found that spinal canal decompression and spinal canal decompression with internal fixation and fusion are safe and effective surgical methods for treating degenerative lumbar spondylolisthesis. However, spinal canal decompression alone has less surgical trauma, less bleeding, and fewer postoperative complications and is associated with lower cost.

Our two patients with degenerative with grade 1 lumbar spondylolisthesis with spinal stenosis were both elderly women. Because of the degenerative lumbar spondylolisthesis, the typical symptoms of lumbar spinal stenosis, intermittent claudication, and the lack of mechanical symptoms, we opted for spinal canal decompression. Both patients improved promptly, and long-term postoperative follow-up results were favorable, with significant improvements in the VAS and JOA score. There is no question that the endoscopic lumbar decompression – regardless of whether done through the transforaminal or interlaminar approach - reduces approach trauma, blood loss, and postoperative pain while achieving results similar to or even better than spinal canal decompression, internal fixation, and fusion. However, future clinical investigations will have to confirm this notion.

CONCLUSION

Simplified endoscopic decompression in elderly patients with rigid degenerative lumbar spondylolisthesis and symptomatic spinal stenosis should be considered in patients with unilateral claudication symptoms and without any radiographic evidence of translational motion on dynamic extension flexion views. Endoscopic decompression without fusion may be a viable alternative to open lumbar laminectomy and lowers perioperative burden to the patient and lowers societal cost.

CONSENT FOR PUBLICATION

Not applicable.

CONFLICT OF INTEREST

The authors declare no conflict of interest, financial or otherwise.

ACKNOWLEDGEMENTS

Declared none.

REFERENCES

[1]   Guigui P, Ferrero E. Surgical treatment of degenerative spondylolisthesis. Orthop Traumatol Surg Res 2017; 103(1S): S11-20.
[http://dx.doi.org/10.1016/j.otsr.2016.06.022] [PMID: 28043848]

[2]   Matz PG, Meagher RJ, Lamer T, *et al.* Guideline summary review: An evidence-based clinical guideline for the diagnosis and treatment of degenerative lumbar spondylolisthesis. Spine J 2016; 16(3): 439-48.
[http://dx.doi.org/10.1016/j.spinee.2015.11.055] [PMID: 26681351]

[3]   Bydon M, Alvi MA, Goyal A. Degenerative Lumbar Spondylolisthesis: Definition, Natural History, Conservative Management, and Surgical Treatment. Neurosurg Clin N Am 2019; 30(3): 299-304.

[http://dx.doi.org/10.1016/j.nec.2019.02.003] [PMID: 31078230]

[4] Abdu WA, Sacks OA, Tosteson ANA, *et al.* Long-Term Results of Surgery Compared With Nonoperative Treatment for Lumbar Degenerative Spondylolisthesis in the Spine Patient Outcomes Research Trial (SPORT). Spine 2018; 43(23): 1619-30.
[http://dx.doi.org/10.1097/BRS.0000000000002682] [PMID: 29652786]

[5] Pearson AM, Lurie JD, Tosteson TD, Zhao W, Abdu WA, Weinstein JN. Who should undergo surgery for degenerative spondylolisthesis? Treatment effect predictors in SPORT. Spine 2013; 38(21): 1799-811.
[http://dx.doi.org/10.1097/BRS.0b013e3182a314d0] [PMID: 23846502]

[6] Rihn JA, Hilibrand AS, Zhao W, *et al.* Effectiveness of surgery for lumbar stenosis and degenerative spondylolisthesis in the octogenarian population: analysis of the Spine Patient Outcomes Research Trial (SPORT) data. J Bone Joint Surg Am 2015; 97(3): 177-85.
[http://dx.doi.org/10.2106/JBJS.N.00313] [PMID: 25653317]

[7] Tosteson AN, Lurie JD, Tosteson TD, *et al.* Surgical treatment of spinal stenosis with and without degenerative spondylolisthesis: cost-effectiveness after 2 years. Ann Intern Med 2008; 149(12): 845-53.
[http://dx.doi.org/10.7326/0003-4819-149-12-200812160-00003] [PMID: 19075203]

[8] Weinstein JN, Lurie JD, Tosteson TD, *et al.* Surgical *versus* nonsurgical treatment for lumbar degenerative spondylolisthesis. N Engl J Med 2007; 356(22): 2257-70.
[http://dx.doi.org/10.1056/NEJMoa070302] [PMID: 17538085]

[9] Weinstein JN, Lurie JD, Tosteson TD, *et al.* Surgical compared with nonoperative treatment for lumbar degenerative spondylolisthesis. four-year results in the Spine Patient Outcomes Research Trial (SPORT) randomized and observational cohorts. J Bone Joint Surg Am 2009; 91(6): 1295-304.
[http://dx.doi.org/10.2106/JBJS.H.00913] [PMID: 19487505]

[10] Koreckij TD, Fischgrund JS. Degenerative Spondylolisthesis. J Spinal Disord Tech 2015; 28(7): 236-41.
[http://dx.doi.org/10.1097/BSD.0000000000000298] [PMID: 26172828]

[11] Chan AK, Sharma V, Robinson LC, Mummaneni PV. Summary of Guidelines for the Treatment of Lumbar Spondylolisthesis. Neurosurg Clin N Am 2019; 30(3): 353-64.
[http://dx.doi.org/10.1016/j.nec.2019.02.009] [PMID: 31078236]

[12] Schroeder GD, Kepler CK, Kurd MF, *et al.* Rationale for the Surgical Treatment of Lumbar Degenerative Spondylolisthesis. Spine 2015; 40(21): E1161-6.
[http://dx.doi.org/10.1097/BRS.0000000000001116] [PMID: 26274525]

[13] Shao K, Ji LX. [Progress on surgical treatment of isthmic spondylolisthesis]. Zhongguo Gu Shang 2019; 32(3): 283-7. [Progress on surgical treatment of isthmic spondylolisthesis].
[http://dx.doi.org/10.3969/j.issn.1003-0034.2019.03.017] [PMID: 30922014]

[14] Fitzgerald JA, Newman PH. Degenerative spondylolisthesis. J Bone Joint Surg Br 1976; 58(2): 184-92.
[http://dx.doi.org/10.1302/0301-620X.58B2.932080] [PMID: 932080]

[15] Newman PH. Spondylolisthesis, its cause and effect. Ann R Coll Surg Engl 1955; 16(5): 305-23.
[PMID: 14377314]

[16] Newman PH. Spondylolisthesis. Physiotherapy 1974; 60(1): 14-6.
[PMID: 4445291]

[17] Newman PH. Degenerative spondylolisthesis. Orthop Clin North Am 1975; 6(1): 197-8.
[http://dx.doi.org/10.1016/S0030-5898(20)31211-6] [PMID: 1089933]

[18] Newman PH. Stenosis of the lumbar spine in spondylolisthesis. Clin Orthop Relat Res 1976; &NA;(115): 116-21.
[http://dx.doi.org/10.1097/00003086-197603000-00020] [PMID: 1253474]

[19]   Newman PH. Surgical treatment for spondylolisthesis in the adult. Clin Orthop Relat Res 1976; &NA;(117): 106-11.
[http://dx.doi.org/10.1097/00003086-197606000-00014] [PMID: 1277660]

[20]   Newman PH. Spondylolisthesis. Acta Orthop Belg 1981; 47(4-5): 437-40.
[PMID: 7336897]

[21]   Wiltse LL, Newman PH, Macnab I. Classification of spondylolisis and spondylolisthesis. Clin Orthop Relat Res 1976; (117): 23-9.
[PMID: 1277669]

[22]   Sun W, Xue C, Tang XY, *et al.* Selective versus multi-segmental decompression and fusion for multi-segment lumbar spinal stenosis with single-segment degenerative spondylolisthesis. J Orthop Surg Res 2019.
[http://dx.doi.org/10.1186/s13018-019-1092-2]

[23]   Liang HF, Liu SH, Chen ZX, Fei QM. Decompression plus fusion *versus* decompression alone for degenerative lumbar spondylolisthesis: a systematic review and meta-analysis. Eur Spine J 2017; 26(12): 3084-95.
[http://dx.doi.org/10.1007/s00586-017-5200-x] [PMID: 28647763]

[24]   Yukun Z. Analysis of the efficacy of 62 cases of pure spinal canal decompression in the treatment of first-degree degenerative spondylolisthesis in the elderly. Chongqing Medicine 2014; 43: 276-80.

SUBJECT INDEX